ANTIGLOBULINS, CRYOGLOBULINS AND GLOMERULONEPHRITIS

DEVELOPMENTS IN NEPHROLOGY

Cheigh JS, Stenzel KH, Rubin AL: Manual of clinical nephrology of the Rogosin Kidney Center. 1981. ISBN 90-247-2397-3.

Nolph KD ed.: Peritoneal dialysis. 1981. ISBN 90-247-2477-5.

Gruskin AB, Norman ME eds: Pediatric nephrology. 1981.
ISBN 90-247-2514-3.

Schück O ed: Examination of the kidney function. 1981. ISBN 0-89838-565-2.

Strauss J ed: Hypertension, fluid-electrolytes and tubulopathies in pediatric nephrology. 1982. ISBN 90-247-2633-6.

Strauss J ed: Neonatal kidney and fluid-electrolytes. 1983.
ISBN 0-89838-575-X.

Strauss J ed: Acute renal disorders and renal emergencies. 1984.
ISBN 0-89838-663-2.

Didio LJA, Motta PM eds: Basic, clinical, and surgical nephrology. 1985.
ISBN 0-89838-698-5.

Friedman EA, Peterson CM eds: Diabetic nephropathy: Strategy for therapy.
1985. ISBN 0-89838-735-3.

Dzúrik R, Lichardus B, Guder W eds: Kidney metabolism and function. 1985.
ISBN 0-89838-749-3.

DiDio LJA, Motta PM eds: Basic, clinical, and surgical nephrology. 1985.
ISBN 0-89838-698-5.

Oreopoulos DG ed: Geriatric nephrology. 1986. ISBN 0-89838-781-7.

Pajamin EP ed: Acute Continuous Renal Replacement Therapy. 1986.
ISBN 0-89838-793-0.

Cheigh JS, Stenzel KH, Rubin AL eds: Hypertension in Kidney Disease. 1986.
ISBN 0-89838-797-3.

Deane N, Wiheman RJ, Benis GA eds: Guide to Reprocessing of Hemodialyzers.
1986. ISBN 0-89838-798-1.

Ponticelli C, Minetti L, D'Amico G eds: Antiglobulins, Cryoglobulins and Glomerulonephritis. 1986. ISBN 0-89838-810-4.

Antiglobulins, cryoglobulins and glomerulonephritis

Second International Milano Meeting of Nephrology
30 September − 1 October 1985

edited by

CLAUDIO PONTICELLI
Maggiore Hospital, Milan

LUIGI MINETTI
Ca' Grande Hospital, Milan

GIUSEPPO D'AMICO
San Carlo Hospital, Milan

1986 **MARTINUS NIJHOFF PUBLISHERS**
a member of the KLUWER ACADEMIC PUBLISHERS GROUP
DORDRECHT / BOSTON / LANCASTER
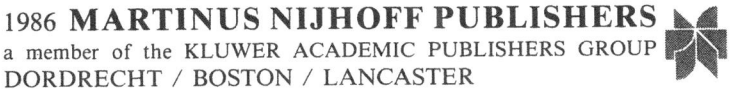

Distributors

for the United States and Canada: Kluwer Academic Publishers, 101 Philip Drive, Assinippi Park, Norwell, MA 02061, USA
for the UK and Ireland: Kluwer Academic Publishers, MTP Press Limited, Falcon House, Queen Square, Lancaster LA1 1RN, UK
for all other countries: Kluwer Academic Publishers Group, Distribution Center, P.O. Box 322, 3300 AH Dordrecht, The Netherlands

Book information

ISBN-13:978-94-010-8406-2   e-ISBN-13:978-94-009-4289-9
DOI: 10.1007/978-94-009-4289-9

Library of Congress Cataloging in Publication Data

International Milano Meeting of Nephrology (2nd :
    1985)
    Antiglobulins, cryoglobulins, and glomerulonephritis.

    (Developments in nephrology)
    Includes index.
    1. Glomerulonephritis--Immunological aspects--
Congresses. 2. Autoantibodies--Congresses. 3. Cryo-
globulins--Congresses. 4. Cryoglobulinemia--Congresses.
I. Ponticelli, Claudio. II. Minetti, Luigi.
III. D'Amico, G. (Guiseppe) IV. Title. V. Series.
RC918.G55I58 1985   616.6'12   86-8549

Copyright

Contents

List of First Authors

George N. ABRAHAM, The University of Rochester, Medical Center, Department of Medicine, Clinical Immunology. Rheumatology Unit, 601 Elmwood Avenue, BOX 695, Rochester, New York 14642 (USA).

Vincent AGNELLO, Lahey Clinic Medical Center, Immunology Laboratory, 41 Mall Road, Burlington, Massachussetts 01805 (USA).

Giovanni BARBIANO DI BELGIOJOSO, Divisione di Nefrologia e Dialisi, Ospedale Ca Granda, Piazza Ospedale Maggiore 3, 20162 Milano (Italy).

Constantin A. BONA, The Mount Sinai Medical Center, One Gustave L. Levy Place, New York, N.Y. 10029 (USA).

Dennis A. CARSON, Department of Basic and Clinical Research, Scripps Clinic and Research Foundation, 10666 North Torrey Pines Road, La Jolla, California 92037 (USA).

Stewart J. CAMERON, Clinical Science Laboratories, Guy's Tower (17th & 18th Floors), Guy's Hospital, London Bridge SE1 9RT (UK).

Daniel CORDONNIER, Centre Hospitalier Regional et Universitaire de Grenoble, Department of Nephrology, B.P. 217 X, 38043 Grenoble Cedex (France).

Franco DAMMACCO, Institute of Medical Pathology, University of Bari, Medical School, 7012 Bari (Italy).

Franco FERRARIO, Ospedale Provinciale 'S. Carlo Borromeo', Divisione di Nefrologia e Dialisi, Via S. Pio II, 3, 20153 Milano (Italy).

Peter M. FORD, Queen's University, Rheumatic Diseases Unit, 26 Barrie Street, Kingston, Ontario, K7L 316 (Canada).

David GELTNER, Kaplan Hospital, Department Internal Medicine, P.O.B. 1, Rehovot (Israel).

Irma GIGLI, UCSD Medical Center, Division of Dermatology, 225 Dickinson Street, San Diego, California 92103 (USA).

Richard J. GLASSOCK, Department of Medicine, Lac Harbor — UCLA Medical Center, 1000 Carson Stret, Torrance, California 90509 (USA).

X

Peter D. GOREVIC, Division of Allergy, Rheumatology, and Clinical Immunology, Health Sciences Center, State University of New York at Stony Brook, Stony Brook, New York 11794 (USA).

Franco INVERNIZZI, Clinica Medica II, Ospedale Maggiore — Università di Milano, Via Francesco Sforza 35, 20122 Milano (Italy).

Paul H. LAMBERT, WHO Immunology Research and Training Centre, Department of Pathology, Centre Medical Universitaire, 1 Rue Michel Servet, 1211 Geneva 4 (CH).

Quirino MAGGIORE, Divisione di Nefrologia 'G. Monasterio', Ospedale Regionale, Via Sbarre Inferiori 39, 89100 Reggio Calabria (Italy).

Michael J. MIHATSCH, Institut Fur Pathologie der Universitat, Schonbeistrasse 40, 4056 Basel (CH).

Patrick NAISH, North Staffordshire Royal Infirmary, Princes Road, Hartshill, Stoke-on Trent ST4 7LN (UK).

Claudio PONTICELLI, Divisione di Nefrologia e Dialisi, Ospedale Maggiore, Via Commenda 15, 20122 Milano (Italy).

Jean Charles RENVERSEZ, Centre Hospitalier Regional et Universitaire, Biochimie Medicale — A, Proteins et Lipides, B.P. 217 X, Grenoble Cedex 38043 (France).

Patrick J.G. SISSONS, Royal Postgraduate Medical School, Hammersmith Hospital, Ducane Road, London W12 0HS (UK).

Antonio TARANTINO, Divisione di Nefrologia e Dialisi, Ospedale Maggiore, Via Commenda 15, 20122 Milano (Italy).

An-Chuan WANG, Medical University of South Carolina, Department of Basic and Clinical Immunology and Microbiology, 171 Ashley Avenue, Charleston, South Carolina 29425 (USA).

Curtis B. WILSON, Department of Immunology, Research Institute of Scripps Clinic, 10666 North Torrey Pines Road, La Jolla, California 92037 (USA).

Introduction

RICHARD J. GLASSOCK

Introducing a scientific symposium is an uncertain and difficult task. The remarks must not be too specific lest the participant's later contributions be intruded upon, yet an overview of the goals and objectives of the conference should be presented in an inquisitive and stimulating fashion. Perhaps a compromise position would be to make a few general statements and pose a limited number of questions which hopefully would then be addressed during the formal or informal portions of the meeting. A conclusion incorporating some perspectives of the relevance of the specific topic to the more global issues of disease and its consequences might be appropriate.

The goals and objectives of this conference, as set forth by its organizers, Professors Ponticelli, D'Amico and Minetti, are rather simple and straightforward; namely, to review and elucidate the immunopathophysiology of cryoimmunoglobulins and auto-antibodies to immunoglobulins (Ig) and, secondarily, to explore the possible participation of these disordered states in glomerular injury. As such, this conference is principally devoted to an analysis of two properties of certain species of the globulin fraction of serum proteins, specifically the ability to self associate on the basis of immune interactions and to form insoluble aggregates when exposed to reduced ambient temperature. As we shall see, these two properties are often distinctly related.

Session I will appropriately deal with fundamental aspects of the first property, focusing on the auto-antibodies formed to C-terminal half of the $C\gamma2$ domain of Ig (Rheumatoid Factors) [1] and autoantibodies to the variable, antigen combining, sites of Ig (anti-idiotypic antibodies) [2]. That autoantibodies to specific topographic sites on normal or altered Ig molecules occur in health and disease has been recognized since the first description of rheumatoid factors by Waaler in 1940 [3]. Since virtually the entire topographic surface of a protein molecule is potentially capable of eliciting a specific antibody response [4], it is perhaps surprising that only certain domains of the Ig molecule have a propensity to evoke an antibody response. Indeed, it is likely that this phenomenon is governed by immune response genes at the major histocompatibility complex. The role by Rheumatoid Factor in pathogenesis of disease has been poorly understood [1]. It seems unlikely that such auto-antibodies play a direct role in tissue injury and conceivably could even have a protective influence. Hopefully, contributions will help to sort out this confusing area.

The production of anti-idiotypic antibody following antigen exposure and an immune response is well recognized [2]. The regulatory influence of these antiglobulins may have great potential for exploitation in prevention and therapy of disease [2]. In this context, three phenomena relate to the idiotype/anti-idiotype network need to be considered; namely, 1) the conservation of idiotypes in certain types of autoantibodies, 2) the existence of regulatory (stimulating and suppressive) idiotype/anti-idiotype combination, and, 3) the stereochemical mimicking of self-antigens by anti-idiotypic antibody [2]. These issues and their relevance to human and experimental immunopathology of glomerular disease will be an important aspect of this conference. In addition to the role of these autoantibodies in regulation of the immune response it is becoming clear that they may also play a role in the pathogenesis of glomerular injury [2] and in the formation of cryoimmunoglobulins [5]. This data will be reviewed in Session II and III of the conference. A caveat is in order here. While globulin-antiglobulin interactions most certainly occur in the course of pathologic events responsible for glomerulonephritis, a major question remains as to whether these interactions truly participate in the genesis of injury or whether they occur pari-passu and play no vital or necessary role in tissue injury. In my view, this is the central question facing investigators in this field.

Cryoimmunoglobulinemia, the subject of Sessions IV, V, and VI, has now been recognized for over 50 years [6–8]. The biophysical and biochemical basis of cryoprecipitation is not fully understood but undoubtedly involves some change in tertiary or quaternary structure which in turn alters the interaction of the molecule in solution with the solvent [8, 9]. Plasma proteins, other than immunoglobulins also precipitate in the cold and some of these, most notably fibronectin, may play a part in the cold insolubility of immunoglobulins [10]. An immune interaction, even among monoclonal Ig may serve as the trigger for the conformational changes responsible for cryoprecipitation [5]. The association between the largely *in vitro* phenomenon of cryoprecipitation and the *in vivo* phenomenon of glomerular and vascular injury has long been recognized. In some instances, e.g., distal cutaneous necrosis at reduced ambient temperature inducing *in vivo* precipitation and occlusion of vascular beds seems directly responsible for tissue injury. In other situations, e.g., glomerulonephritis, where temperature related phenomena are *unlikely* to occur, the physical properties of cryoprecipitates seems more of an epiphenomenon and the glomerular injury is consequent to a more fundamental aspect of the process, namely, self-association of Ig molecules forming aggregates which may be physically trapped in glomeruli. Here the role of glomerular filtration in producing a localized increase in plasma protein concentration, regional alteration in ionic environment, receptors for discrete sites on conformationally altered Ig molecules are likely to play important roles in determining the susceptibility of the glomerulus.

Exploration of autoantibodies to immunoglobulins and the phenomenon of cryoprecipitation offers many important avenues of research in the field of glomerulonephritis. As the discussion evolves in this timely conference, this will become more evident. On behalf of the participants, let me extend sincere thanks to the organizers for the choice of the topic and the excellent melding of basic and clinical investigation which should lead to a stimulating exchange of ideas.

References

1. Roitt IM, Hay FC, Nineham LJ and Male DK: Rheumatoid Arthritis. In: Clinical Aspects of Immunology. 4th Ed. Ed. by PJ Lachmann and DK Peters. Blackwell Scientific Publications. Oxford 1982, pp 1165–1172.
2. Zanetti M and Wilson CB: A role for anti-idiotypic antibodies in immunologically mediated nephritis. Am J Kidney Disease 1985 (In Press).
3. Waaler F: On the occurrence of a factor in human serum activating the specific agglutination of sheep blood corpuscles. Acta Pathol Microbiol Scana 17:172–179, 1940.
4. Berzofsky JA: Intrinsic and extrinsic factors in protein antigenic structure. Science 229: 932–940, 1985.
5. Weber RG, Clem LW and Voss EW: The molecular mechanism of cryoimmunoglobulin precipitation. II. Thermodynamic basis for self-association as determined by fluorescence polarization. Molec Immunol 21:61–67, 1984.
6. Wintroloe MM and Buell MV: Hyperproteinemia associated with multiple myeloma. Bull. Johns Hopkins Hosp 52:156, 1933.
7. Laurence J and Nachman R: Cryoglobulinemia. Disease-a-Month 27:6, 1981.
8. Grey HM and Kohler PF: Cryoimmunoglobulins. Semin. Hematol. 10:87, 1973.
9. Lalezari P, Kumar M, Kumar K and Lawrence C: Inhibition of cold insolubility of an IgA cryoglobulin by decane dicarboxylic and related compounds. Am J Hematol 15:279–288, 1983.
10. Strevey J, Beaulieu A, Menard C, Valet J, LaTuleppe L and Hebert J: The role of fibronectin in the cryoprecipitation of monoclonal cryoglobulins. Clin Exp Immunol 55:340–346, 1984.
11. Brouet JC, Clauvel JP, Danon F, Klein M and Seligmann M: Biologic and clinical significance of cryoglobulins. A report of 86 cases. Am J Med 53:775–788, 1974.
12. Gamble CN and Ruggles SW: The immunopathogenesis of glomerulonephritis associated with mixed cryoglobulinemia. N Engl J Med 299:81–86, 1978.
13. Meltzer M, Franklin EC, Elias K, McCluskey RJ and Cooper N: Cryoglobulinemia – a clinical and laboratory study. Am J Med 40:837–842, 1966.

Part I. Physiology and pathology of antiglobulins

1. Subsets of rheumatoid factors determined by cross idiotypes

VINCENT AGNELLO, M.D.

The first studies of cross idiotypes among rheumatoid factors involved monoclonal IgM anti globulins (mRF) obtained mainly from patients with mixed cryoglobulinemia (Kunkel, 1973). Two distinct idiotype groups were described, a major group WA comprising approximately 60% of those proteins and a minor group PO comprising 20%; 20% were uncharacterized. More recently a third rheumatoid factor cross idiotype has been defined, the Bla group, that is distinct from the PO and WA groups (Agnello, 1980). The rheumatoid factors (RF) in this group are unique in that in addition to reactivity with an antigen on IgG they cross react with an antigen on DNA-nucleoprotein.

A monoclonal rheumatoid factor that cross reacts with DNA nucleoprotein

The prototype rheumatoid factor for this third group was a monoclonal IgM protein, Bla isolated from the serum of a patient with Waldenstrom's macroglobulinemia. The cross reactivity of this rheumatoid factor was first shown in the antinuclear antibody test. In contrast to the usual antinuclear antibody reaction the nuclear reactivity of Bla could be completely blocked by aggregated IgG. The cross reaction could also be demonstrated in gel diffusion as shown in Fig. 1. The nature of the DNA-nucleoprotein antigen reactive with Bla was partially characterized and appeared to be a tertiary structure on the nucleosome core which involved both DNA and some portion of the amino terminus end of the histone H2a–H2b fraction (Agnello, 1980). The reactivity of Bla with aggregated IgG and DNA nucleo-protein could be quantitatively demonstrated using a sensitive competitive inhibition radioimmunoassay that had been previously developed with Bla mRF for the detection of immune complexes (Gabriel, 1977). The binding of Bla mRF to IgG-sepharose in this assay could be maximally inhibited by both aggregated IgG and DNA nucleoprotein. The combining site of Bla

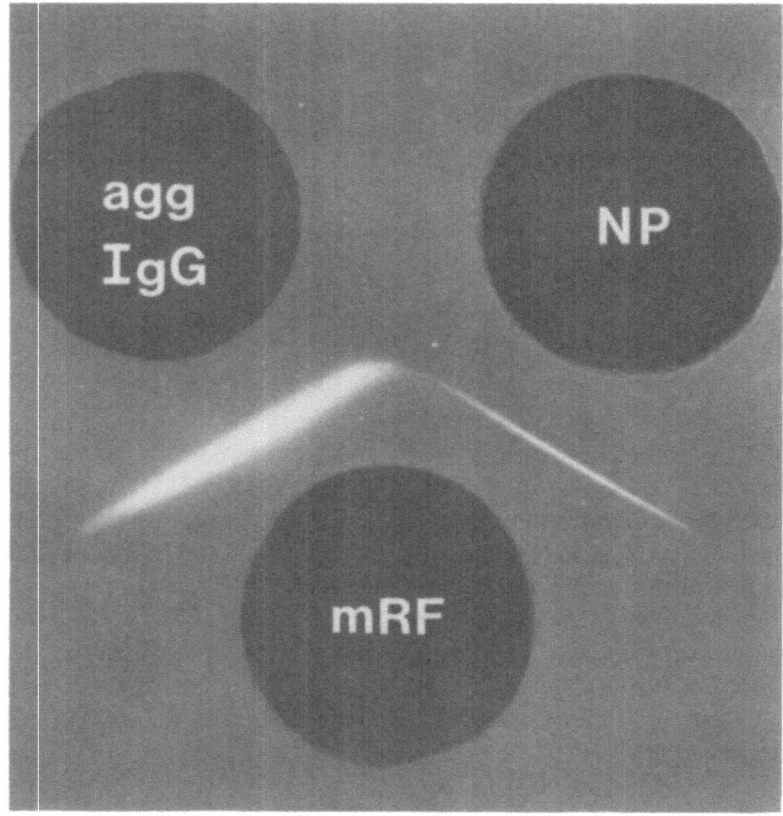

Figure 1. 0.6% agarose gel diffusion plate. Precipitation of purified Bla monoclonal rheumatoid factor (mRF) 1 mg/ml with aggregated IgG (agg IgC) 10 mg/ml and 3 mg/ml of DNA-nucleoprotein (NP) (Agnello, 1980).

could be shown to be involved in the cross reactivity using an anti-idiotype serum to Bla. The anti-idiotype serum blocked equally well the binding of Bla to aggregated IgG and DNA nucleoprotein.

Table I. Incidence of cross-reactive RF.

	Number of RF-positive patients	Number of Patients Positive
Classic RA	62	27
MCTD	7	5
Overlap syndromes	10	4
SLE	8	0
Mixed cryoglobulinemia	11	0
Miscellaneous	12	1

Polyclonal rheumatoid factors that cross-react with DNA-nucleoprotein

Polyclonal rheumatoid factors with cross reactivity similar to that of Bla were found in a variety of diseases using three different assays: gel precipitation, blocking of ANA with aggregated IgG and radioimmunoassay in which nucleosome binding by rheumatoid factors is inhibited by aggregated IgG (Table I). Approximately 40% of RF in sera of patients with classic rheumatoid arthritis are the cross reactive type. The incidence is probably higher, since in two other studies in which isolated rheumatoid factors were tested, the incidences were 66% and 93% (Johnson, 1979; Aitcheson, 1980). Only a small group of patients with mixed connective tissue disease and positive RF were studied. Of these, in 5 of 7 the RF was the cross-reactive type. In two of these the cross reactive RF was only detectable after isolation by IgG-sepharose affinity chromatography. However, this type of cross reactive rheumatoid factor does not invariably occur in all RF positive sera as shown by studies of mixed cryoglobulinemia where no cross reactive RF were found even after isolation studies. None were found in systemic lupus erythematosus but isolation studies were not done, hence their occurrence is not totally excluded.

Nine of the 11 mixed cryoglobulin cases were idiopathic mixed cryoglobulinemia (Table II). All of the rheumatoid factors which could be typed belonged to the WA group. Two sera had positive antinuclear reactions, Tal and Dri. Neither had the Bla type rheumatoid factor.

The reactivity of one polyclonal rheumatoid factor with DNA-nucleoprotein is shown in Fig. 2. The antigen on the DNA-nucleoprotein which reacted with ORL, the polyclonal RF, could be shown to involve the same DNA-histone H2a-H2b structure which reacted with Bla, the monoclonal RF.

Table II. Patients with idiopathic cryoglobulinemia.

Patient	Cross-idiotype	Major clinical findings
Blo	WA	Palpable purpura; nephritis
Tal	—	Palpable purpura; mononeuritis multiplex; Sjögren's syndrome
McD	WA	Palpable purpura; nephritis
Dri	WA	Palpable purpura
Pac	WA	Nephritis; Sjögren's syndrome
Arl	WA	Palpable purpura; polyneuropathy
Cha	—	Cerebral vasculitis
Bel	NT	Palpable purpura; nephritis
Sou	WA	Palpable purpura

NT — not tested, sera protein failed to label with I^{125}.

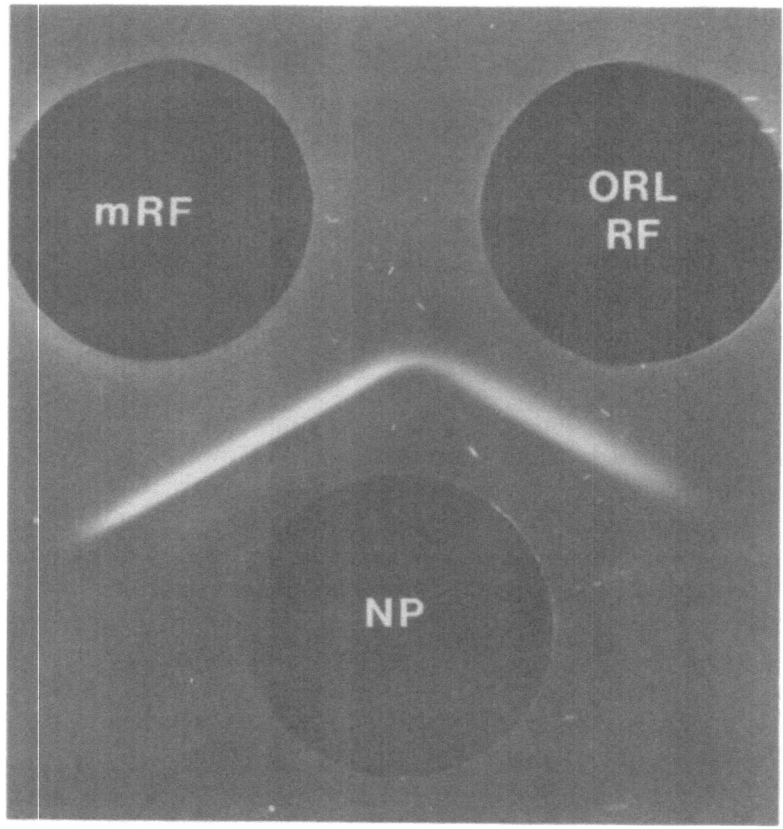

Figure 2. 0.6% agarose gel diffusion plate. Precipitation of 1 mg/ml Bla mRF and 1 mg/ml Orl polyclonal RF with NP (Agnello, 1980).

Characterization of the Bla cross idiotype

Antisera to Bla and Orl were prepared as described for the WA and PO typing reagents (Kunkel, 1973) except that solid phase immunoabsorbents were used (Agnello, 1980). The format used for characterization of the Bla cross idiotype is shown in Fig. 3. The method of antigen binding inhibition was used. The binding of the test RF to IgG sepharose was inhibited by the typing antisera. In this system a WA protein should be inhibited by anti McD, the WA reagent but not anti Lay, the PO reagent. The reverse should be the case for a PO protein.

The Bla cross idiotype was established by demonstrating that (1) Bla binding was inhibited by anti Orl but not anti McD or anti Lay, and (2) Orl binding was inhibited by anti Bla but not anti McD or anti Lay. However, only approximately 20% of the polyclonal ORL RF bore the Bla cross idio-

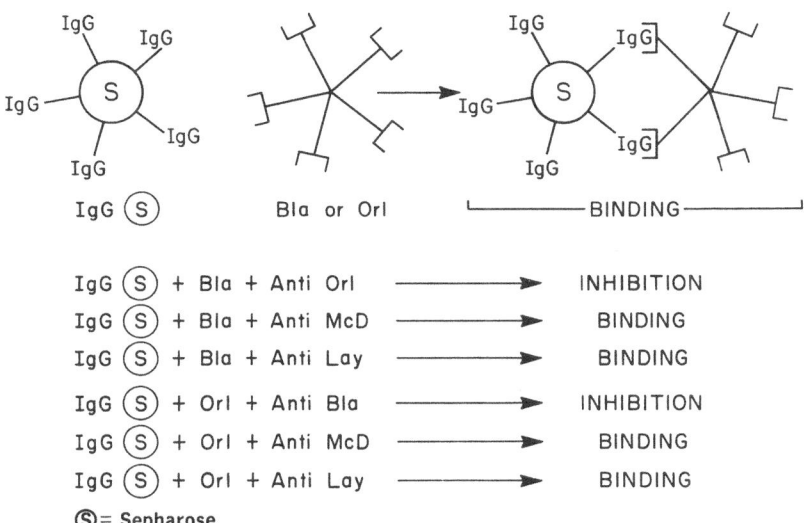

Figure 3. Format for establishing Bla cross idiotype.

type. This result was consistent with the portion of ORL RF which could bind to DNA-nucleoprotein.

Disparity in typing the PO group using antigen-binding and hemagglutination inhibition techniques

One incidental finding in investigating RF cross idiotype was that the PO cross idiotype could be demonstrated by hemagglutination inhibition, the

Table III. PO cross idiotype demonstrated in the hemagglutination system.

		Inhibition protein conc. (mg/ml)					
		.20	.10	.05	.025	.0125	.006
	Lay	0	0	0	0	1$^+$	2$^+$
	Pom	0	0	0	0	1$^+$	2$^+$
+	McD	2$^+$	2$^+$	2$^+$	2$^+$	2$^+$	2$^+$
+	Wa	2$^+$	2$^+$	2$^+$	2$^+$	2$^+$	2$^+$
*	Bla	2$^+$	2$^+$	2$^+$	2$^+$	2$^+$	2$^+$
¶	Puf	2$^+$	2$^+$	2$^+$	2$^+$	2$^+$	2$^+$

antiserum, anti Lay absorbed   0   complete inhibition
coat Pom   -   2$^+$ maximum agglutination
+ RFs of Wa group
* RF of BLA group
¶ IgM without RF activity

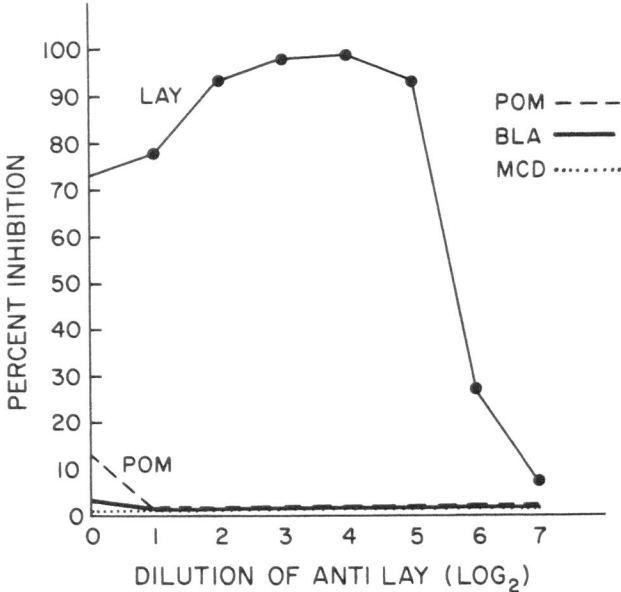

Figure 4. Inhibition of 0.2 µg of various radiolabelled monoclonal RF binding to IgG-Sepharose by anti-Lay. In contrast to the strong inhibition of Lay, Pom is only minimally inhibited.

technique originally used in its description but could not be demonstrated by the antigen-binding inhibition technique. Pom and Lay inhibited equally well the anti Lay agglutination of Pom coated cells whereas proteins of the WA and Bla groups gave no inhibition (Table III). The same anti Lay did not inhibit the binding of WA or Bla to IgG-sepharose but in contrast to the hemagglutination results gave only minimal inhibition of Pom (Fig. 4). These findings suggest that the antigen binding inhibition technique defines only those idiotypes relating to combining site, whereas the hemagglutination detects a broader range of cross idiotypes which do not necessarily involve the combining site. If this interpretation is correct, then the PO group is a non-binding site RF cross idiotype.

'Hidden' cross reactive rheumatoid factors

The finding that RF cross reactive with DNA-nucleoprotein were 'hidden' in some sera of patients with mixed connective tissue disease (Agnello, 1980; Agnello, 1980b) and rheumatoid arthritis (Johnson, 1979; Aitcheson, 1980) suggested that these RF may be bound in complexes in some sera. It had previously been noted in immune complex studies that some sera of patients with rheumatoid arthritis and mixed connective tissue disease con-

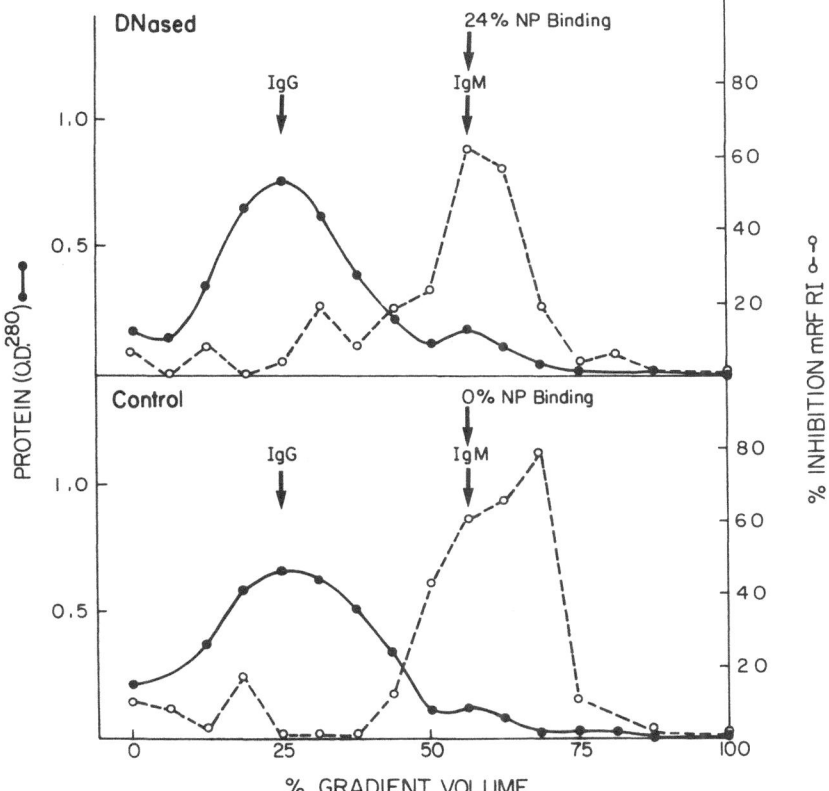

Figure 5. 10–40% sucrose density gradient of Bak serum. Protein (OD^{280}) distribution is shown
(●—●). IgG and IgM concentrations for each fraction were determined. The fractions with the
highest concentrations of each protein are shown by the arrows. Each Fraction was tested for
inhibition in the mRF assay (o—o) and for DNA-nucleoprotein (NP) binding. Only the NP
binding in the peak IgM tube is shown. The serum was compared before (control) and after
DNAse treatment.

tained complexes which preferentially reacted with Bla mRF compared to
C1q (Gabriel, 1977); Agnello, 1980). Two sera of patients with mixed connective tissue disease that had 'hidden' cross reactive RF were studied using
Bla mRF and C1q. The studies in patient Bak are shown in Fig. 5. Reactivity with Bla mRF was found in the region of IgM and beyond. The peak
inhibition was found beyond the fraction of highest IgM concentration. The
fractions were also tested for DNA-nucleoprotein binding. No binding was
found. After DNAse treatment of the serum, inhibition in mRF decreased
in the fractions beyond the peak IgM and nucleosome binding which could
be inhibited by aggregated IgG was detectable. The binding of the peak IgM
tube was now 24%. The finding suggests the presence of complexes consisting of cross reactive RF and an antigen containing DNA.

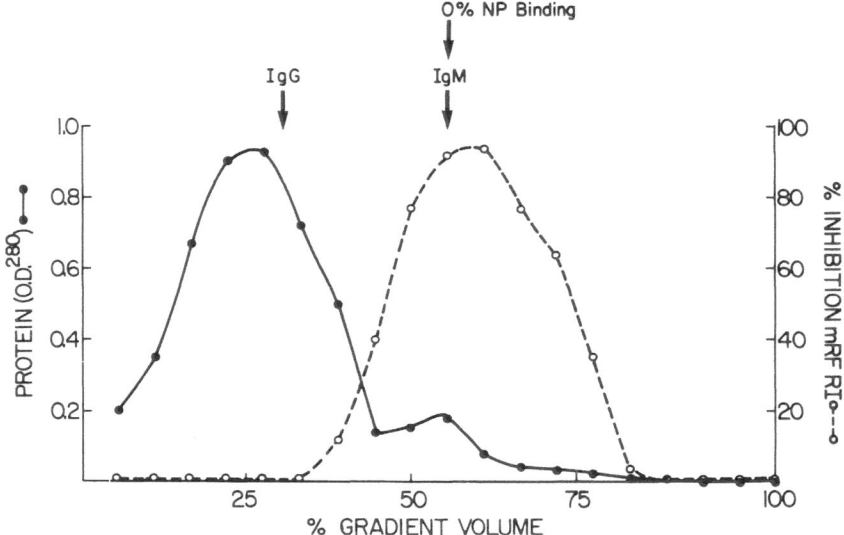

Figure 6. 10–40% sucrose density gradient fractionation of Orl serum. Protein (OD[280]) distribution is shown (•—•). IgG and IgM concentrations for each fraction were determined. The fractions with highest concentrations of each protein are shown by the arrows. Each fraction was tested for inhibition in the mRF assay (o—o) and for DNA nucleo-protein (NP) binding; only the NP binding in the peak IgM tube is shown.

Similar studies were done with ORL serum (Fig. 6). Complexes were detected in the region of IgM and beyond. Cross reactive RF was not detectable. DNAse treatment had no effect. However, the reaction of the complexes with mRF could be eliminated by reduction and alkylation of the complexes or by absorption of the complexes with IgG-sepharose suggests that RF was involved in the complexes. To determine whether anti idiotype antibody was present in the RF complexes, isolation studies were performed. Complexes were first isolated on sepharose 6B and the IgG containing complexes isolated by affinity chromatography on protein A sepharose. The IgG in the protein A eluate was isolated by dissociation on a pH 2.8 glycine HCl sucrose density gradient. The IgG was labelled with I[125] pepsin treated and tested for binding to Bla and ORL. No binding could be detected. From these experiments it appears that IgG anti idiotype antibodies were not present in the complexes or at least were not a major component.

Clinical significance of RF cross idiotypes

The clinical significance of the occurrence of various RF cross idiotypes in disease is not known. There appears to be a high incidence of rheumatoid factors of the WA group in idiopathic mixed cryoglobulinemia (Kunkel, 1973; Powell, 1983). This type also occurs in rheumatoid arthritis (Forre, 1979; Carson, 1981) and in normals as suggested by immunofluorescent studies of pokeweed mitogen-stimulated normal peripheral lymphocytes (Bonagura, 1982). The exact incidence of the WA group in rheumatoid arthritis and normals is not known; however, in the immunofluorescent cellular studies all individuals studied, normal and with rheumatoid arthritis, had the WA cross idiotype (Bonagura, 1982). Bla cross idiotype occurs in high incidence in mixed connective tissue disease and rheumatoid arthritis. The incidence in normals is not known. It remains to be determined whether the occurrence of various cross idiotypes in disease states are merely a reflection of the potential pool which exists in normals or if the production of specific cross idiotypes are associated with different diseases. The cellular studies on the WA cross idiotype favor the former possibility. The occurrence of the Bla cross idiotype in 90% of patients with rheumatoid arthritis but not in idiopathic mixed cryoglobulinemia favors the latter.

References

Agnello V, Arbetter A, Ibanez de Kasep G, Powell R, Tan EM and Joslin F: J Exp Med 151:1514–1527, 1980.

Agnello V, Ibanez de Kasep G and Mitamura T: In: Y Shiokawa, T Abe and Y Yamauchi, Eds, New Horizons in Rheumatoid Arthritis, Amsterdam: Excerpta Medicus, 1980b, pp 71–75.

Aitcheson C, Peebles C, Joslin F and Tan EM: Arth Rheum 23:528–538, 1980.

Bonagura VR, Kunkel HG and Pernis B: J Clin Invest 69:1356–1365, 1982.

Carson DA, Pasquali J, Tsoukas CD, Fong S, Slovin SF, Lawrence SK, Sloughter L and Vaughan JH: Springer Semin Immunopathol 4:161–179, 1981.

Forre O, Dublong JH, Michaelsen TE and Natvig JB: Scand J Immunol 9:281–289, 1979.

Gabriel JR, A and Agnello V: J Clin Invest 59:990–1001, 1977.

Johnson PM: Scan J Immunol 9:461–466, 1979.

Kunkel HG, Agnello V, Joslin FG, Winchester J and Capra JD: J Exp Med 137:331–342, 1973.

Powell R and Agnello V: Clin Immunol Immunopath 29:146–151, 1983.

2. Structure and function of rheumatoid factor: implications for its role in the pathogenesis of mixed cryoglobulinemia

ROBERT D. GOLDFIEN, SHERMAN FONG, POJEN CHEN and
DENNIS A. CARSON

Rheumatoid factors (RF) are antibodies directed against the constant region (Fc) of IgG. Although originally described in association with rheumatoid arthritis [1, 2], they occur in a wide range of pathological and non-pathological states, and it soon became evident that RF were not specific for rheumatoid arthritis. Early studies demonstrated the regular appearance of RF during the course of chronic infections such as subacute bacterial endocarditis [3], leprosy and various chronic liver diseases [4] including infectious hepatitis. They were also found to occur frequently in patients with autoimmune diseases such as systemic lupus erythematosus and scleroderma [4–6], and with certain neoplastic conditions, mainly Waldenstrom's macroglobulinemia and chronic lymphocytic leukemia (CLL). Patinets with mixed cryoglobulinemia have provided an important source of monoclonal IgM-RF, as it regularly participates in immune complex formation in these patients.

Here we will trace the evolution of our current understanding of RF, and then describe studies performed in this laboratory and others concerning the structural characteristics and genetic aspects of RF. With these considerations in mind, we will try to draw some conclusions about the role of RF in both physiological and pathological states.

In the early 1960's the notion arose that RF were somehow elicited in response to antigenic stimulation, especially of a chronic nature. The first experimental induction of RF was described by Abruzzo and Christian [7]. They gave rabbits repeated inoculations with formalin-fixed bacteria and demonstrated that RF-like-substances appeared in the serum. Aho et al. [8]subsequently showed that RF appeared in the serum of a small percentage of normal individuals following prophylactic vaccinations. These studies were important for several reasons. First, they added considerable weight to the developing concept of RF as being a normal component of the immune system, and second, they clearly pointed out that there could be significant levels of RF without arthritis, or indeed any demonstrable pathology. It was not clear why in some cases RF was associated with severe illness, and in others, without symptoms. All of the early studies dealt only with macroglobulins, i.e., IgM-RF. The first hint that IgG-RF might exist came in a study by Kunkel et al. [9] of 11 patients. Seven of these patients had classical rheumatoid arthritis, and 4 had undefined vasculitic illnesses. By ultracentrifugal analysis of serum from these patients, a variety of γ globulin complexes were noted ranging from 9S to 17S. The complexes were dissociated by urea or acid buffers to homogeneous 7S (γ globulin) proteins. The authors postulated that the γ globulin-anti-γ globulin complex, though devoid of RF activity (assayed by sheep cell agglutination), might contain an IgG counterpart of the usual IgM-RF.

The physiology of RF has been studied in a number of *in vitro* systems. In 1979, Izui et al. [10] demonstrated the appearance of high titers of IgM-RF in normal, autoimmune, and nude mice, following injection of bacterial lipopolysaccharide (LPS). LPS was known to be a potent adjuvant, as well as a polyclonal (antigen non-specific) B cell activator, and had been shown to stimulate production of anti-DNA antibodies in mice [11, 12]. The authors reported that the rise in IgM-RF titer occurred in parallel with both anti-DNA and anti-dinitrophenol antibodies, suggesting that polyclonal B cell activation was the probable cause for RF synthesis.

RF production also appears to occur regularly during the secondary humoral immune response. Nemazee and Sato [13], using a plaque forming cell assay, found that repeated immunization of A/J mice with a number of protein antigens elicited an IgM-anti-IgG response comparable in magnitude to the response directed against the immunizing protein. No RF was found after primary immunization. The IgM-RF were consistently IgG1 specific. Taken together, the data implicated circulating immune complexes as the stimulus for RF secretion. In addition, no class switching occurred among the RF population (i.e. no IgG-RF could be detected). These results were confirmed by Coulie and Van Snick [14]. These investigators isolated hybridomas after booster immunizations in 129/SV mice. In several fusion experiments, up to 10% of clones isolated were found to be IgG specific. In follow-up studies with several mouse strains, they noted the production by spleen cell cultures of large amounts of IgM-RF between 2 and 4 days following secondary immunization with protein antigens. They also found a striking prevalence of anti-UgG1 RF, and suggested that this might be due to the predominance of the IgG1 isotype in the humoral response to the immunizing antigen.

Despite the above findings of increased RF production by spleen cells, there was little, if any, increase in serum IgM-RF levels. We have made a similar observation in humans by using Epstein-Barr virus to induce IgM-RF production *in vitro* [15]. By limiting dilution analysis, we documented a 2–3 fold increase in IgM-RF precursor B cells following tetanus toxoid immunization in the healthy ones. However, serum IgM-RF levels were often unchanged or only slightly elevated. Whether this is due to rapid consumption of RF by immune complexes, or a primarily extravascular localization of RF is unclear. Some evidence for the latter hypothesis comes from studies of a unique murine B cell subset displaying the Ly-1 marker (Ly-1 B cells). This surface antigen, originally described as a T-cell surface marker, has been detected on a small percentage of splenic B cells and a high percentage of peritoneal B cells [16]. Similarly, in humans, the cognate T cell marker, Leu 1 is found on the majority of B cells from chronic lymphocitic leukemia patients [17], and a percentage of B cells in normal lymph node [18]. Studies by Hayakawa et al. have implicated these Ly-1 B cells in autoantibody production in mice [19], and reconstitution studies suggested that they might constitute a separate lineage [20]. Of special interest is the observation that Ly-1 B cells, while detectable only at very low levels in peripheral blood, spleen and lymph nodes, constituted almost 50% of B cells recovered from the peritoneal cavity in normal mice. Whether or not these cells truly represent a distinct lineage is not settled. However, they clearly are a functionally coherent group of B cells which might act as a source for autoantibody precursors.

A subset of human B cells with similar properties to the Ly-1 B cell has been defined by the ability to form rosettes with mouse red blood cells (MRBC). Fong et al. [21] isolated MRBC+ cells from human peripheral blood and found that this subset contained an increased percentage of EBV-inducible IgM-RF precursor B cells. In another study, this B cell population was noted to be increased in patients with rheumatoid arthritis [22]. Recently, B cells carrying T1 (LY-1 like antigen) have been reported to account for up to 48% of peripheral blood B cells in rheumatoid arthritis patients, although the percentage did not correlate with disease activity [23].

Taken together, these data suggest the existence of a distinct subset of B cells which normally secrete IgM-RF and other IgM autoantibodies. Under normal circumstances these cells remain in extravascular tissues, perhaps with a predilection for the gut-associated lymphoid tissue.

Idiotypes and genetics of RF

In 1973, Kunkel et al. [24], using highly adsorbed rabbit antisera, found that the majority of monoclonal IgM-RF from patients with mixed cryoglobulinemia shared a cross reactive idiotype. The RF were all IgM kappa. Subsequent amino acid sequence analysis [25] showed that the light chain variable regions of two of these RF, designated Sie and Wol, were highly homologous, differing in only 8 of 109 residues. Indeed, a fairly large number of monoclonal IgM-RF have now been isolated and appear to arise preferentially from a serologically minor V kappa (sub)subgroup, designated VkIIIb [26–29].

Work in our laboratory has been directed towards defining more precisely the structural basis for the crossreactive idiotypes on IgM-RF cryoglobulins. Because of the difficulties of doing genetic studies in an outbred population, and poor results with hybridoma techniques in humans, we have employed a novel approach. We immunized rabbits with peptides corresponding to the hypervariable regions (complementarity determining regions [CDR]) of human IgM-RF. The resulting antisera were used as sequence probes to analyze panels of RF protein from patients with mixed cryoglobulinemia. The sequences and derivation of these peptides are shown in Table I. In a pilot study [29], we were able to define a private idiotype using the antiserum to the third heavy chain CDR of IgM-RF Sie. We then synthesized peptides corresponding to the light and heavy chain CDR of several RF. Knowing that the kappa light chains of human RF were highly homologous, we screened a series of RF cryoglobulins with the antiserum directed against the second light chain CDR sequence of RF Sie (anti-PSL2, see Table I) [30]. Table II shows the amino acid sequences of 8 RF screened and the reactivity of these RF with anti-PSL2. Six of the 8 RF have identical sequences in this region, and all reacted with the anti-PSL2 antiserum by ELISA and by immunoblotting. The RF Pom, which differs by 2 amino acids was weakly positive, and the RF Lay was non-reactive. These results together with sequence data suggest that the crossreactive idiotype on the majority of IgM-RF stems from amino acid sequence identity of the kappa IIIb second CDR. This analysis has been extended to 24 RF cryoglobulins, of which 19 or 79% were reactive [31] with anti-PSL2 (Table III). Analysis

Table I. Amino acid sequences of peptides.

Name*	Protein	Residues spanned [+]	Amino acid sequence [‡]
1) PPH1	Pom	22–35	AASGFTFSSSAMSC
2) PPH2	Pom	49–65	AWKYENGNDKHYADSVNH (GGC)
3) PPH3	Pom	95–102	DAGPYVSPTFFAH (GGC)
4) PWH2	Wol	49–65	GQIPLRFNGEVKNPSGVV (GGC)
5) PWH3	Wol	95–102	EYGFDTSDYYYYY (GGC)
6) PSH1	Sie	22–35	KTSGGTFSGYTISC
7) PSH2	Sie	49–65	GSPAKWTDPFQGVYIKWE (GGC)
8) PSH3	Sie	95–102	EWKGQVNVNPFDY (GGC)
9) PSL2	Sie	49–61	YGASSRATGIPDR (C)
10) PSL3	Sie	88–99	CQQYGSSPQTFG

* The first letter, P, denotes peptide; the second letter refers to the cognate protein, P = Pom, W = Wol, S = Sie; H or L stands for the heavy or light chain, respectively, and the number corresponds to the first, second, or third CDR.
[+] Numbering according to Kabat et al. [40].
[‡] The one letter code is used; residues in parentheses were added to allow chemical coupling to keyhole limpet hemocyanin (see 29).

Table II. Amino acid sequences of the kappa chains of human monoclonal IgM-RF paraproteins in the second CDR and adjacent framework region.

IgM-RF	Reactivity with anti-PSL2	Region* Residue* FR-2 49	CDR-2 50	51	52	53	54	55	56	FR-3 57	58	59	60	61
1. Sie	+	Tyr	Gly	Ala	Ser	Ser	Arg	Ala	Thr	Gly	Ile	Pro	Asp	Arg
2. Wol	+													
3. Pom	+/−					Thr							Ala	
4. Lay	−					Thr		Glu	Ala				Ser	
5. Got	+													
6. Neu	+													
7. Pay	+													
8. Gar	+													

* The region and the residue number were assigned by Kabat et al. [40].
Adapted from Chen et al. [30].

of this panel of RF with the anti-PSL3 antiserum showed a somewhat lower percentage of positive reactions. Recently, more monoclonal IgM-RF kappa light chains have been sequenced [32], with the striking finding that four of these light chains share identical amino acid sequences from residues 1–95 (the entire V kappa region).

Antisera directed against the heavy chain CDR of 3 IgM-RF were used to screen the same set of RF cryoglobulins, with a completely different result. No crossreactivity was seen among this sizeable panel of RF (Table III). Thus, there are probably many unrelated heavy chains used in the formation of RF cryoglobulins, compared to a restricted set of light chains.

The high degree of idiotypic crossreactivity and striking sequence homology of monoclonal IgM-RF cryoglobulins among a genetically heterogen-

Table III. Idiotype expression of 24 human monoclonal IgM-RF.

IgM-RF	PSL2	PSL3	PSH3	PWH2	PWH3	PPH1	PPH2	PPH3
Cur	+ +	+ +	−	−	−	ND	−	−
Gar	+ +	+ +	−	−	−	−	−	−
Glo	+ +	+ +	−	−	−	−	−	−
Got	+ +	+ +	−	−	−	−	−	−
Neu	+ +	+	−	−	−	−	−	−
Pal	+ +	+ +	ND*	ND	ND	ND	ND	ND
Pay	+ +	+ +	−	−	−	−	−	−
Pom	+/−	−	−	−	−	+ +	+ +	+ +
Sie	+ +	+ +	+ +	−	−	−	−	−
Wol	+ +	−	−	+ +	+ +	−	−	−
Boc	+ +	+ +	−	−	−	ND	−	−
Flo	+ +	+ +	−	−	−	ND	−	−
Gal	−	+ +	+	−	−	ND	−	−
Lew	+ +	−	−	−	−	ND	−	−
She	−	−	−	−	−	ND	−	−
Lay	−	−	−	ND	ND	ND	−	−
Teh	+ +	ND	−	ND	ND	ND	ND	ND
Bel	+ +	+ +	−	−	−	−	−	−
Dri	+ +	+ +	−	−	−	−	−	−
Mcd	+ +	+ +	−	−	−	−	−	−
Blo	+ +	−	−	−	−	−	−	−
Ark	+ +	−	−	−	−	−	−	−
Tal	−	−	−	−	−	−	−	−
Sou	+ +	−	−	−	−	−	−	−
Total positive	19	14	2	1	1	1	1	1
Total assayed	24	23	23	21	21	16	22	22
% Positive	79	60	9	5	5	6	5	5

* ND — not done.
Adapted from [31] and [39].

eous population imply that common V kappa genes are being expressed. In addition, the set of V kappa genes is expressed with relatively little somatic mutation. These V kappa genes have been well-conserved in evolution. We have still analyzed a relatively small number of IgM-RF from patients with mixed cryoglobulinemia. Considering the unique ability of the anti-peptide reagents to provide specific sequence data, it would be of interest to study a much larger number of RF cryoglobulins from patients with diverse ethnic backgrounds.

Role of RF in the normal immune response

The physiological and structural data summarized above support the concept that IgM RF have an important role in the normal immune system. Thus, the autoantibodies occur regularly during the secondary immune response, and disappear following the elimination of antigen; RF precursor cells are present in high frequency and can be induced by polyclonal B cell activation; they may be found preferentially among a restricted B cell subset defined by either lineage or maturational stage; and they are coded for by evolutionarily-conserved germline V kappa genes. However, the exact role of IgM-RF in the immune system is still highly speculative. One current concept is that they act as enhancing antibodies [13, 33, 34], facilitating antibody-antigen interactions, and hastening clearance of immune complexes from the circulation. An interesting feature of murine IgM-RF is the predominant binding to IgG1. Although IgG1 is the major isotype found in this species, it fixes complement poorly. Therefore, RF might function to allow more efficient complement activation. Finally, RF could conceivably function to crosslink low affinity IgG antibodies, increasing their apparent affinity for antigen, and thus their utility. Perhaps this could have served an important role in the evolution of the humoral immune system, as new pathogens appeared, which were poorly recognized by the available germline repertoire. In this context, it would make biological sense for RF precursors to preferentially locate in sites of continual exposure to novel antigenic stimuli, such as the gut.

Role of RF in pathogenesis

In rheumatoid arthritis, mixed cryoglobulinemia and lymphoproliferative diseases, RF have been implicated in the expression of disease manifestations *per se* rather than simply representing an epiphenomenon. One must consider why RF can cause disease on the one hand, and aid in combatting disease on the other.

One variable is where the RF is secreted. As noted above, during a physiological response involving RF production, there is relatively little RF detected in the circulation. In lymphoproliferative diseases and mixed cryoglobulinemia there is abundant circulating RF with attendant immune complex phenomena, including vasculitis and glomerulonephritis. In rheumatoid arthritis, the predominant RF secretion and immune complex formation occurs in the joint synovial membrane. Perhaps the physiological RF response occurs in close proximity to the site of antigenic stimulation, and functions to enhance local immune function. This would be analogous to the local activation of the clotting mechanism which occurs at the site of endothelial injury. The appearance of RF in the systemic circulation would then imply a loss of regulation or systemic antigenemia (as in subacute bacterial endocarditis, for example).

Another important factor is the nature of the RF itself. In this regard IgG-RF provides a special case. IgG-RF are unique antibodies. They tend to form large aggregates both with themselves and with other IgG [33]. The propensity to self-aggregate probably arises from the ability to form three bonds per IgG molecule. The addition of saturating quantities of non-RF IgG tends to dissociate these complexes [9]. It is also worth emphasizing that IgG-RF usually do not occur in high titer in normal subjects. Rather, their continued synthesis usually reflects immune regulatory abnormalities such as are found in rheumatoid arthritis, hypergammaglobulinemic purpura and other autoimmune diseases.

In mixed cryoglobulinemia, the circulating RF is always an IgM, and thus self-association does not occur. The formation of abundant and large circulating immune complexes must have a different cause. The decreased solubility of IgM-IgG complexes at low temperatures, combined with an excessive load of RF-producing lymphocytes, may be the major factor. However, this interpretation ignores the question of the etiology of the RF autoantibodies. Perhaps some cases of mixed cryoglobulinemia represent paraneoplastic syndromes, in which clones of RF precursor B cells proliferate autonomously. IgM-RF might, under certain circumstances, also form large immune complexes via binding to an antigen other than the Fc fragment of IgG [36-38]. Considering the complexity and immense number of possible antigens, it would be surprising if dual specificity never occurred. According to immune network theory, many antibodies should also act as anti-idiotypes to other antibodies. In the case of IgM-RF this situation would promote the formation of unusually large IgM-IgG complexes with resultant complement activation. This could result if either the RF or the IgG were acting as an anti-idiotype. In the case of idiotype-anti-idiotype complexes, one would predict that the IgG component might be oligoclonal rather than polyclonal. The presence and composition of such complexes should be verifiable with techniques currently available.

Acknowledgement

Funding for this research supported in part by grants AM25443, AG04100, AM07144, and RR00833 from the National Institutes of Health. SF is the recipient of a Research Career Development Award (AG00279) from the National Institutes of Health. PC is an Investigator of the Arthritis Foundation. This is publication number 4226BCR from the Research Institute of Scripps Clinic.

References

1. Waaler E: On the occurrence of a factor in human serum activating the specific agglutination of sheep blood corpuscles. Acta Path Microbiol Scand 17:172-188, 1940.
2. Rose H, Ragan C, Pearce E, Lipman M: Differential agglutination of normal and sensitized sheep erythrocytes by sera of patients with rheumatoid arthritis. Proc Soc Exp Biol Med 68:1-6, 1948.
3. Williams RC, Kunkel HG: Rheumatoid factor, complement, and conglutinin aberrations in patients with subacute bacterial endocarditis. J Clin Invest 41:666-675, 1962.
4. Dresner E, Trombly P: The latex fixation reaction in non-rheumatic diseases. New Eng J Med 261:981, 1959.
5. Rodman G: The natural history of progressive systemic sclerosis (diffuse scleroderma). Bull Rheum Dis 13:301, 1963.
6. Block K: Immunoglobulin in aspects of rheumatoid arthritis and SLE. Arthritis Rheum 6:532, 1963.
7. Abruzzo L, Christian C: The induction of rheumatoid factor-like substance in rabbits. J Exp Med 114:791–806, 1961.
8. Aho K, Konttinen A, Rajasalmi M, Wager O: Transient appearance of the rheumatoid factor in connection with prophylactic vaccinations. Acta Path Microbiol Scand 56: 478–479, 1962.
9. Kunkel HG, Muller-Eberhard HM, Fudenburg HH, Tomasi TB: Gamma globulin complexes in rheumatoid arthritis and certain other conditions. J Clin Invest 40:117, 1961.
10. Izui S, Eisenberg RA, Dixon FJ: IgM rheumatoid factors in mice injected with bacterial lipopolysaccharides. J Immunol 122:2096-2102, 1979.
11. Fournie G, Lambert P, Miescher P: Release of DNA in circulating blood and induction of anti-DNA antibodies after injection of bacterial lipopolysaccharides. J Exp Med 140: 1189, 1974.
12. Izui S, Kobayakawa T, Zyrd M, Louis J, Lambert P: Mechanism for induction of anti-DNA antibodies by bacterial lipopolysaccharides in mice. II. Correlation between anti-DNA induction and polyclonal antibody formation by various polyclonal B lymphocyte activators. J Immunol 119:2157, 1977.
13. Nemazee DA, Sato VL: Induction of rheumatoid antibodies in the mouse: regulated production of autoantibody in the secondary humoral response. J Exp Med 158:529–545, 1983.
14. Coulie P, Van Snick J: Rheumatoid factors and secondary immune responses in the mouse. II. Incidence, kinetics and induction mechanisms. Eur J Immunol 13:895–899, 1983.
15. Welch MJ, Fong S, Vaughan JH, Carson DA: Increased frequency of rheumatoid factor precursor B lymphocytes after immunization of normal adults with tetanus toxoid. Clin Exp Immunol 51:299–305, 1983.

16. Hayakawa K, Hardy RR, Parks DR, Herzenberg LA: The 'Ly-1 B' subpopulation in normal, immunodefective, and autoimmune mice. J Exp Med 157:202–218, 1983.

17. Wang CY, Good RA, Ammirati P, Dymbort G, Evans RL: Identification of a p69/70 complex expressed on human T cells showing determinants with B type chronic lymphocytic leukemia cells. J Exp Med 151:1539–1544, 1980.

18. Caligaris-Cappio F, Gobbi M, Bofill M, Janossy G: Infrequent normal B-lymphocytes express features of B-chronic lymphocytic leukemia. J Exp Med 155:623, 1982.

19. Hayakawa K, Hardy RR, Honda M, Herzenberg LA, Steinberg AD, Herzenberg LA: Ly-1 B cells: Functionally distinct lymphocytes that secrete IgM autoantibodies. Proc Natl Acad Sci USA 81:2494, 1984.

20. Hayakawa K, Hardy R, Herzenberg L, Herzenberg L: Progenitors for Ly-1 B cells are distinct from progenitors for other B cells. J Exp Med 161:1554–1568, 1985.

21. Fong S, Vaughan JH, Carson DA: Two different rheumatoid-factor producing cell populations distinguished by the mouse erythrocyte receptor and responsiveness to polyclonal B cell activators. J Immunol 130:162–164, 1983.

22. Room GRW, Plater-Zyberk C, Clarke MF, Maini RN: B-lymphocyte subpopulation which forms rosettes with mouse erythrocytes increase in rheumatoid arthritis. Rheumatol Int 2:175–178, 1982.

23. Plater-Zyberk C, Maini R, Lam K, Kennedy T, Janossy G: A rheumatoid arthritis B cell subset expresses a phenotype similar to that in chronic lymphocytic leukemia. Arthritis Rheum 28:971–976, 1985.

24. Kunkel HG, Agnello V, Joslin FG, Winchester RJ, Capra JD: Cross-idiotypic specificity among monoclonal IgM proteins with anti-gammaglobulin activity. J Exp Med 137:331–342, 1973.

25. Andrews DW, Capra JD: Complete amino acid sequence of variable domains from two monoclonal human anti-gamma globulins of the Wa cross-idiotypic group: suggestion that the J segments are involved in the structural correlate of the idiotype. Proc Natl Acad Sci USA 78:3799–3803, 1981.

26. Kunkel HG, Winchester RJ, Joslin FG, Capra JD: Similarities in the light chains of anti-gamma-globulins sharing cross-idiotypic specificities. J Exp Med 139:128–136, 1974.

27. Ledford DK, Goni F, Pizzolato M, Franklin EC, Solomon A, Frangione B: Preferential association of kappa-IIIb light chains with monoclonal human IgM-kappa autoantibodies. J Immunol 131:1322–1325, 1983.

28. Pons-Estel B, Goni F, Solomon A, Frangione B: Sequence similarities among kIIIb chains of monoclonal human IgMk autoantibodies. J Exp Med 160:893–904, 1984.

29. Chen PP, Houghten RA, Fong S, Rhodes GH, Gilbertson TA, Vaughan JH, Lerner RA, Carson DA: Anti-Hypervariable region antibody induced by a defined peptide. A new approach for studying the structural correlates of idiotypes. Proc Natl Acad Sci USA 81:1784–1788, 1984.

30. Chen PP, Fong S, Normansell D, Houghten RA, Karras JG, Vaughan JH, Carson DA: Delineation of a cross-reactive idiotype on human autoantibodies with antibody against a synthetic peptide. J Exp Med 159:1502–1511, 1984.

31. Chen PP, Goni F, Houghten RA, Fong S, Goldfien RD, Vaughan JH, Frangione B, Carson DA3 Characterization of human rheumatoid factors with seven antiidiotypes induced by synthetic hypervariable-region peptides. J Exp Med 162:3281–3285, 1985.

32. Goni F, Chen PP, Pons-Estel B, Carson DA, Frangione B: Sequence similarities and cross-idiotypic specificity of L chains among human monoclonal IgM-K with anti-gammaglobulin activity. J Immunol 135:4073–4079, 1985.

33. Nemazee DA, Sato VL: Enhancing antibody: A novel component of the immune response. Proc Natl Acad Sci USA 79:3838, 1982.

34. Hobbs MV, Morgan EL, Baker NL, Weigle W: Regulation of antibody responses by rheumatoid factor 1. Polyclonal activation of human B cells by rheumatoid factor-containing preparations from seropositive plasma. J Immunol 134:223, 1985.
35. Pope RM, Teller DC, Mannik M: The molecular basis of self-association of IgG rheumatoid factors. J Immunol 115:365–373, 1975.
36. Agnello V, Arbetter A, de Kasep GI, Powell R, Tan EM, Joslin F: Evidence for a subset of rheumatoid factors that cross-react with DNA-histone and have a distinct cross-reactive idiotype. J Exp Med 151:1514, 1980.
37. Bona CA, Finley S, Waters S, Kunkel HG: Anti-immunoglobulin antibodies. III. Properties of sequential anti-idiotypic antibodies to heterologous anti-gamma globulins. Detection of reactivity of anti-idiotype antibodies with epitopes of Fc fragments. J Exp Med 156: 986–999, 1982.
38. Rubin RL, Balderas R, Tan EM, Dixon FJ, Theofilopoulos A: Multiple autoantigen binding capabilities of mouse monoclonal antibodies selected for rheumatoid factor activity. J Exp Med 159:1429, 1984.
39. Goldfien RD, Chen PP, Fong S, Carson DA: Synthetic peptides corresponding to the third hypervariable region of human monoclonal IgM rheumatoid factor heavy chains define an immunodominant idiotype. J Exp Med 162:765–761, 1985.
40. Kabat E, Wu T, Bilofsky H, Reid-Miller M, Perry H: Sequences of proteins of immunologic interest. U.S. Dept. of Health and Human Services, Washington, DC, 1983.

3. Regulatory Idiotopes and Diseases

CONSTANTIN A. BONA

Idiotypes are phenotypic markers of V region genes encoding the specificity of two polypeptide chains which constitute the antigen receptor of T or B lymphocytes. Two categories of idiotopes are expressed on the immune receptor of lymphocytes. Individual idiotypes are clonotypic antigenic determinants expressed only by a single clone. These idiotypes results from somatic recombination or somatic mutational events. Generally, they are not inherited. A second category is represented by cross-reactive idiotypes, shared by clones exhibiting the same antigen specificity as well as by some with different antigen specificities. These idiotypes are antigenic markers of V germline genes since they are expressed by the majority or all individuals of an inbred strain or of a species. The idiotypes, as antigenic markers, can elicit a humoral or cellular immune response not only in xenogeneic or allogeneic animals, but also in syngeneic or even autologous systems.

This property led Jerne [1] to formulate the idiotype network theory of the immune system which considers that the idiotopes play a role in clonal communication as well as in the regulation of proliferation of lymphocytic clones. However, working in an autologous system, we defined a category of idiotopes which play a physiological role in idiotype-driven events that we called regulatory idiotopes [2, 3]. Subsequently, we have shown that regulatory idiotopes can be defined by four criteria:

a) they are autoimmunogens; b) are markers of V-germline genes; c) are shared by antibodies with various specificities; d) their potential to become dominantly expressed due to their recognition by regulatory T cells.

These properties were delineated by studying the idiotype of A48 myeloma protein, an IgAK exhibiting β2-6 fructosan binding activity, secreted by the ABPC48 myeloma line of BALB/c origin.

1 Properties of regulatory idiotypes

A. Autoimmunogenicity

In previous studies we have shown that the injection of A48 myeloma protein into BALB/c mice led to the synthesis of syngeneic autoanti-A48Id antibodies. Indeed, a few days after the completion of the immunization schedule consisting of several immunizations, high titers of anti-A48Id antibodies can be detected in the sera of the majority of BALB/c mice. In addition, several monoclonal antibodies specific for A48Id have been obtained from immunized BALB/c mice, by Goldberg et al. [4] and Legrain et al. [5]. These data clearly demonstrated that A48 Idiotypes are autoimmunogens, and that through a self recognition process, they stimulate the expansion and differentiation of complementary clones producing anti-Id antibodies.

B. A48 regulatory idiotopes are markers of V germ line genes

Several monoclonal antibodies have been obtained from BALB/c mice immunized with A48 or anti-A48Id antibodies, with and without levan. Monoclonal antibodies expressing A48 idiotopes were selected for their ability to inhibit the binding of labeled A48 to anti-A48Id antibodies [4]. These antibodies were used to study the expression of A48Id with monoclonal anti-A48 antibodies as well as to carry out molecular studies. Previously, it was shown by Ollo et al. [6] that A48 and UPC10, another β2-6 fructosan binding monoclonal protein, derive their V_H genes from the V_H441-4 family. This is a V_H family located at the 5' and of a murine V_H locus containing only two members: V_H441-4 and V_H X24.

The monoclonal antibodies expressing A48-UPC10 regulatory idiotopes identified by two monoclonal anti-Id antibodies (i.e. IDA10 and 10-1) were used for molecular studies. It should be mentioned that these two anti-Id antibodies recognize idiotopes on the V_H region since their expression is independent of the utilization of the V_K chain, namely V_K10, borne by UPC10 and A48 monoclonal proteins [7].

Two molecular approaches were taken to determine if A48 regulatory idiotopes are markers of V_H genes. Poly A-enriched RNA, extracted from hybridomas expressing A48-UPC10 idiotopes, was probed with the V_H441-4 germ-line gene. The results presented in Table I show that the majority of monoclonal antibodies expressing A48 regulatory idiotopes bear members of the V_H441-4 family. Northern results were confirmed by Southern blotting which demonstrated that the EcoRI-digested DNA of these hybridomas included a fragment containing a rearranged V_H gene which hybridized with V_H441-4 germline gene probe [7].

Table I. Summary results of hybridization of RNA extracted from various hybridomas with V_H 441-4 germline gene probe.

Origin of hybridomas	Designation	V_H 441-4
BALB/c myeloma proteins	A48	+
	UPC10	+
	MOPC173	+
BALB/c immunized at birth with 10 µg A48 and one month later with bacterial levan	1-5-1	+
BALB/c immunized at birth with 10 ng anti-A48Id antibodies and one month later with bacterial levan	2-1-3	+
	2-8-2	−
	2-11-1	+
	2-11-3	−
	2-12-10	+
	2-12-19	−
	2-9-17	−
	2-28-9	+
	2-1-10	+
BALB/c immunized with anti-A48Id-KLH conjugate and challenged with levan	3-76-4	?
	3-76-42	?
	3-14-19	+
	3-27-6	+
	3-9-9	+
	3-101-14	+

These results showed that the hybridomas obtained from mice immunized with A48 or anti-A48Id antibodies, which secrete antibodies expressing A48-UPV10 Idiotopes also bear V_H genes derived from V_H441-4 germline genes. These results strongly suggested that A48-UPC10 regulatory idiotopes are markers of V_H441-4 germline gene. This view is supported by the data indicating that these monoclonal antibodies have different J segments.

C. *A48-UPC10 regulatory idiotopes are shared by antibodies with various specificities*

One of the most important characteristics of regulatory idiotopes which distinguishes them from conventional idiotopes, is that they are shared by antibodies with various specificities. Indeed, we predicted [8] that the major outcome of immunization with anti-Id antibodies is not the synthesis of anti(anti-Id) antibodies, but of clones sharing regulatory idiotopes and producing antibodies with various specificities. Victor-Kobrin et al. [7] have studied the antigen specificity of monoclonal antibodies obtained from

BALB/c mice immunized with anti-A48-Id antibodies. A48 and UPC10 bind to grass levan (β2-6 fructosan) and bacterial levan (β2-6 fructosan with β2-1 branch points) but not to inulin (β2-1 fructosan). The data depicted in Table II show that 3 of 13 monoclonal antibodies bind to grass and bacterial levan, like A48 and UPC10, indicating that they are specific for only β2-6 fructosan. Two of 13 bind to only grass levan and two of 13 bind to only bacterial levan. This last group probably recognizes conformational determinants found only in bacterial levan. Two of 13 bind to both β2-6 and β2-1 and one displays weak binding to only inulin. Three of 13 bound to galactan and only one was devoid of antigen binding activity. These results showed that, indeed, clones with a variety of antigen binding specificities were activated subsequent to the immunization of mice with anti-A48Id antibodies.

D. Recognition of regulatory idiotopes by T cells

Another prediction of the regulatory idiotopes concept was that the regulabory idiotopes are recognized by T cells and that these T cells are responsible for idiotypic dominance. Rubinstein et al. [9, 10] have shown that the immunization after birth of animals with A48, or the exposure of mothers during pregnancy to UPC10 proteins, led to the dominance of A48 and

Table II. Summary data of binding specificity of monoclonal antibodies obtained from animals immunized with anti-A48Id antibodies.

Monoclonal antibodies	Grass levan β2–6 fructosan	Binding to Bacterial levan β2–1, 2–6 fructosan	Inulin β2–1 fructosan	Galactan β1–6 fructosan
A48	+	+	−	−
IPC10	+	+	−	−
MOPC173	−	−	−	+
X24	−	−	−	+
J606	−	+	+	
2-1-3	+	+	+	−
2-8-2	±	+	−	−
2-11-1	+	+	−	−
2-12-10	+	+	−	−
2-28-9	−	+	−	−
3-76-4	+	−	−	−
3-14-9	+	+	+	−
3-27-6	+	−	−	−
3-9-9	−	−	−	−
3-101-14	−	−	+	−

UPC10Id in the nati-levan response. These are idiotypes which otherwise represent a minor component of a conventional immune response elicited by immunization with bacterial levan. In this study it was shown that A48 or UPC10Id-specific helper T cells were probably responsible for A48-UPC10Id dominance. Recently, S. Waters (unpublished results) obtained A48Id specific T cell lines which proliferate in the presence of soluble A48 and irradiated splenic cells as well as in the presence of A48 myeloma cells. This proliferation was inhibited by both anti-I-A and anti-A48Id antibodies. Thus, regulatory idiotopes are recognized by helper T cells which probably play a role in the dominance of idiotypes. Our concept of regulatory idiotopes predicts that this privileged category of idiotopes plays a role in idiotype-driven events, idiotype dominance, cross-reactive regulation, and in the generation of immune memory.

2. Role of regulatory idiotypes in diseases

The concept of regulatory idiotopes regards the immune system as a collection of clones selectively interacting as a multitude of connected mininetworks characterized by an idiotypic hierarchy. The idiotypic hierarchy is based on the ability of regulatory idiotopes to break self tolerance since they most likely behave as altered self. Because they behave as altered self, they can be more easily recognized by specific regulatory T cells.

Numerous autoantibodies express interspecies or interstrain cross-reactive idiotypes. This is the case of anti-AcR, anti-DNA, anti-thyroglobulin autoantibodies as well as of rheumatoid factors.

The pathological significance of the role of regulatory idiotopes is best shown in several autoimmune disorders. In some of these diseases, it is possible that the primary immunological lesion is an aberrant regulatory idiotype: anti-idiotype regulation of clones specific for self antigens.

In patients with SLE as well as in murine lupus models antibodies to DNA are responsible for glomerulonephritis and perhaps skin lesions. A wide cross-idiotype reactivity was found on both human and murine anti-DNA antibodies. Abdou et al. [11] have shown that the remission of the disease could be correlated to the generation of autoanti-Id antibodies. Hahn and Ebling [12] showed that only a fraction of anti-DNA antibodies purified from (NZB X NZW)F1 mice are nephritogenic. These antibodies which probably express regulatory idiotopes, elicit the production of autoanti-Id antibodies when they are injected into F_1 mice. The production of anti-Id antibodies causes the suppression of anti-DNA antibodies bearing the corresponding idiotype, resulting in a transient improvement in SLE symptomatology. Lefvert [13] and Dwyer et al. [14] showed that in myastenia gravis, the remission period is related to the occurrence of autoanti-Id antibodies directed against anti-AcR antibodies bearing regulatory idiotopes.

Zanetti et al. [15] have immortalized in BALB/c an autoantibody specific for thyroglobulin. This autoantibody called Id62 bears a regulatory idiotype, according to various criteria used to define this category of idiotopes. The immunization of BALB/c with this autoantibody elicites the production of high titers of autoanti-Id antibodies. Injection of animals with anti-Id 62 antibodies elicited the production of autoantibodies specific for thyroglobulin.

These results clearly indicated that antibodies specific for regulatory idiotopes of anti-TG are recognized as self and therefore can contribute to the activation of 'dormant' clones specific for other self antigens. Therefore, the regulatory idiotopes can be involved in two different pathways in autoimmunity. They can activate autoimmune clones and contribute to the break of self tolerance, and secondly, they can elicit the production of autoanti-Id antibodies during the cause of the disease and contribute to the remission periods.

Summary

This is a revies of the concept of regulatory idiotopes including data on the immunochemical and molecular characteristics of A48 regulatory idiotopes. The role of regulatory idiotopes in autoimmune diseases is discussed.

References

1. Jerne NK: Towards a network theory of the immune response. Ann Immunol (Paris) 125C, 373, 1974.
2. Bona CA, Heber-Katz E and Paul WG: Idiotype-antiidiotype regulation I. Immunization with a levan-binding myeloma protein leads to the appearance of autoanti(anti-idiotype) antibodies and to the activation of silent clones. J Exp Med 153:951–967, 1981.
3. Paul WE and Bona C: Regulatory idiotopes and immune networks: a hypothesis. Immunology Today 3:239–234, 1982.
4. Goldberg B, Paul WE and Bona CA: Idiotype-antiidiotype regulation IV. Expression of common regulatory idiotopes on fructosan binding and non-fructosan binding monoclonal immunoglobulin. J Exp Med 158:514–528, 1983.
5. Legrain P, Voegtle D, Buttin G and Cazenave PA: Idiotype-antiidiotype interactions and the control of the anti-β-6 polyfructosan response in the mouse: specificity and idiotypy of anti-ABPC48 antiidiotypic monoclonal antibodies. Eur J Immunol 11:678–685, 1981.
6. Ollo R, Auffray C, Sikorav JL and Rougeou F: Mouse heavy chain variable regions: nucleotide sequence of germline V_H gene segment. Nucleic Acid Res 9:4099–4109, 1981.
7. Victor-Kobrin C, Bonilla FA, Bellon B and Bona CA: Immunochemical and molecular characterization of regulatory idiotopes expressed by monoclonal antibodies exhibiting or lacking β2–6 fructosan binding activity. J Exp Med 162:647–662, 1985.

8. Bona C: Regulatory idiotopes in Idiotype in Biology and Medicine (eds. H Kohler, PA Cazenave and J Urbain).

9. Rubinstein LJ, Victor-Kobrin CB and Bona CA: The function of idiotypes and anti-idiotypes on the development of the immune repertoire. Developmental and Comparative Immunol. Suppl 3:109–116, 1984.

10. Rubinstein LJ, Goldberg B, Hiernaux J, Stein KE and Bona C: Idiotype-antiidiotype regulation V. The requirement for immunization with antigen or monoclonal antiidiotypic antibodies for the activation of β2–6 and β2–1 polyfructosan-reactive clones in BALB/c mice treated at birth with minute amounts of anti-A48Id antibodies. J Exp Med 155:1123–1144, 1983.

11. Abdou NI, Wall H, Lindsley HB, Halsey JF and Suzuki T: Network theory in autoimmunity: In vitro suppression of serum anti-DNA antibody binding to DNA by anti-idiotypic antibody in systemic lupus erythematosus. J Clin Invest 67:1297–1306, 1981.

12. Hahn BH and Ebling FM: Suppression of NZB × NZW murine nephritis by administration of a syngeneic monoclonal antibody to DNA. J Clin Invest 71:1728–1736, 1983.

13. Lefvert AK, James RW, Alliod C and Fulpins BW: A monoclonal antiidiotypic antibody against anti-receptor antibodies from myasthenic sera. Eur J Immunol 12:790–792, 1982.

14. Dwyer DS, Bradley RJ, Urquhart CK and Kearney JF: Naturally occurring anti-idiotypic antibodies in myasthenia gravis patients. Nature 301:611–614, 1983.

15. Zanetti M, Liu FT, Rogers J and Katz DH: Heavy and light chains of a mouse monoclonal autoantibody express the same idiotype. J Immunol 135:1245–1251, 1985.

Discussion Part I

LAMBERT: Dr. Agnello, in your study did you consider possible cross-reactivity of IgG RF with nucleoproteins?

AGNELLO: We haven't found it, but we looked at the IgG antiglobulin, which was the first described to have cross-reactivity with DNA-nucleoproteins, the JOS protein of Hammstead and found that it bears the BLA cross idiotype.

LAMBERT: Is there an effect of charge on the binding of RF to nucleoproteins?

AGNELLO: No, there is no effect of charge.

BONA: Dr Agnello, do you think that this multi-specificity of auto-antibodies is characteristic of RF? I am sure that what you described is a feature of all auto-antibodies and that in the same molecule you have generally a low affinity binding for one antigen and a higher affinity binding for another antigen.

AGNELLO: This has been described in a number of systems and it is not clear yet whether it is a general phenomenon. We tried to determine which antigen, IgG or DNA nucleoprotein reacted better with BLA. We couldn't get a specific association constant for the DNA nucleoprotein because it was not possible to produce a monovalent antigen. By doing relative studies, the reactivity with IgG was greater than with DNA nucleoprotein. Both of them were in the range of about 10. It's possible that neither are immunogen.

GELTNER: I would like to ask dr Agnello and dr Carson whether they think that cross reactivity of the IgM RF activity is directed against the Fc or the Fab region of the IgG. By definition a RF should be an anti-Fc antibody.

CARSON: We have one monoclonal protein that reacts with Fc and Fab fragments. We looked for other examples but never found another case. However, an antibody that could react, even with low affinity, with both Fc and Fab would have a particular tendency to cryoprecipitate. This is because the interaction of RF with divalent or multivalent antigens is enhanced many fold.

GELTNER: We have studied 11 patients with mixed cryoglobulinemia, separating the IgM from the IgG and were able to show that 9 of the IfM's reacted against all the IgG F(ab)2 regions. All the IgM's showed autologous anti-F(ab)2 activity. This activity did not decrease after absorption of the anti-Fc activity. We therefore concluded that although supposed to be monoclonal, IgM RF in EMC patients have an anti-Fc and anti-F(ab)2 activity on the same molecule.

AGNELLO: Do you have evidence that the reactivity is on the same antibody molecule?

GELTNER: Yes. That work was done in dr Franklin's laboratory: we took the 'monoclonal' IgM and found that it had both activities.

LAMBERT: Dr Carson, when you did your stimulation with EB virus and reached the peak of frequence, did you look for the possible occurrence of auto-antiidiotypic antibodies reacting with the cross-reacting idiotypes in your studies?

CARSON: No, I didn't. I think this experiment is difficult to do in the human system.

AGNELLO: Dr Carson, does the monoclonal 17.109 anti-idiotype react with isolated light and heavy chains?

CARSON: The monoclonal 17.109 reacts better with the intact protein than with the isolated light chain. However, the antibody was made against the intact protein. When we tried to isolate a cross-reactive monoclonal anti-idiotype we obtained a reagent that saw light chain sequences.

LAMBERT: Did you look for a possible binding of your synthetic peptides to nucleoproteins?

CARSON: No, but a lot of RF bind to nucleoproteins. I think this is a very real phenomenon, which is also seen in monoclonal RF. The antibodies against synthetic peptides are not anti-idiotypes in the conventional sense. However, they are convenient serologic probes for primary structures in that they enable us to gain information regarding the antibody when you cannot sequence the proteins.

PETERS: Dr Carson, you spoke of the loss of the cross-reactive idiotypes in patients with rheumatoid arthritis. Have you got any other clinical state where you might expect polyclonal activation?

CARSON: The rheumatoid patients don't lose the idiotype. It is just not expressed preferentially in the serum. As regards other diseases, we have looked into sporadic RF appearing with aging and found that some express the cross-reactive idiotype and some do not. We haven't studied other disorders associated with RF synthesis.

PETERS: It's hard to understand how you can have somatic mutation without actually loosing the thing you are mutating from.

CARSON: The precursors in the germ line that give rise to new B cells are still there.

WINEARLS (London): Dr Carson, you described a patient with Sjogren's syndrome. Did this patient have polyclonal RF before developing the monoclonal IgM paraprotein?

CARSON: Some of the RF in Sjogren's syndrome are oligoclonal. They have many different heavy chains, but may use the common light chain. With a conventional reagent you might call an antibody 'polyclonal', but with an anti-peptide reagent you would consider the response to be restricted.

MONTAGNINO (Milano): Dr Bona, you have recently described some RF which are both reactive against the Fc and the Fab fragment of IgG, which you called 'epibodies'. Do you think that this may also apply to cryoglobulinemia?

BONA: We found the epibodies by working in a protein system that actually has been mentioned before; this means that with Glow protein we found antibodies to the idiotype of this protein and also to Fc–Gamma, which I called epibody, and which I think to represent a particular case of mimicry of self-antigens in the network. In my mind these antibodies present the image of idiotype network within a 'paratope'. Dr Chen, in dr Carson's laboratory, showed that the molecular basis of this specificity is related to a shared sequence (VAL-SER-SER in CDR-1 of VKIII B subgroup and SER-SER-SER sequence found on Fc fragment in some Gamma sequences). This means that epibodies recognize the same aminoacid sequence on CDR-1 of light chain and on Fc-gamma, the antigen of the RF. I was very happy that dr Geltner found the same phenomenon in spontaneous and polyclonal RF. Initially I thought that epibody was restricted to anti-Id antibodies specific for RF but now it seems, that actually epibodies are seen in other systems, particularly in myastenia gravis.

AGNELLO: I have a question for dr Bona: in the human RF there doesn't appear to be V_H restriction, whereas in the mouse it appears to be highly restricted. Why the difference?

BONA: When there are species differences we can invent very easily cheap arguments, like the selection during philogeny or selection during ontogeny. The single point that I can tell you, is that the anti-idiotypes bind to both heavy and light chains of 80% of RF. And these particularities seem to be true in mice because there is an antibody specific for thyroglobulin which has the same sequence in the 60 N-terminal aminoacids in both heavy and light chains. We don't know of other systems in which V_H and V_L have so high degree of homology.

AGNELLO: Does your anti-idiotype reagent to V_H antigens inhibit antigen binding of the whole protein?

BONA: The idiotype-antiidiotype reaction is not inhibited by purified Fc from gamma 3, gamma 1, gamma 2 and gamma 2b. It is inhibited only by high amounts of heat aggregated IgG.

LAMBERT: You have implicated Ly 1. B cells as auto-antibody forming cells. To my knowledge, no switch to IgG synthesis has been yet obtained with these cells. On the other hand the major auto-antibodies appearing in autoimmune strains of mice are IgG. Could you comment about that?

BONA: I agree that this is a very important question with a respect to Ly 1.B cells, which have been proposed to be the major B sub-line involved in autoimmune response. The equivalent of this population in human is Leu-1, which is also present only in bone marrow and in some leukemias. These cells predominantly produce IgM and we do not know their diversification during the switching. We selected hybridomas from NZB LPS-stimulated lymphocytes which secrete IgG and in a few months we will have their sequences: this will provide us informations on the diversification process in Ly 1.B cells.

Part II. Role of antiglobulins in experimental glomerulonephritis

4. Pathogenetic mechanisms of infective endocarditis glomerulonephritis in the rabbit

PATRICK NAISH

Introduction

A relatively large number of animal models of inflammatory glomerular disease exist, and much information on pathogenetic mechanisms has been derived from them. Despite the fact, however, that some of them appear to be mediated by immune complex reactions, there is a paucity of models which have a close counterpart in human disease. (This is due partly to our lack of knowledge of the aetiology of the majority of human types of glomerulonephritis).

It seemed attractive, therefore, to study the model of infective endocarditis glomerulonephritis (IEGN) developed by Arnold et al. (1975). It had the advantage of closely resembling a type of human glomerular inflammation, with a known initiating antigen leading to an antibody response, circulating immune complexes, and granular deposition of immune reactants within the glomerulus.

Material and methods

IEGN's was induced in male New Zealand white rabbits by the methods of Arnold et al. (1975) with some modifications. Animals were preimmunized by three intravenous injections of c. 10^8 heat killed streptococcus salivarius at weekly intervals. A catheter was then passed through the aortic valve via the right carotid artery and the resultant aortic valve vegetations were infected by an intravenous injection of c. 10^8 live streptococci.

Studies were carried out as detailed in Sindrey et al. (1981). Briefly, blood samples were taken at regular intervals for culture, measurement of circulating immune complexes, C3, antistreptococcal antibody, and antiglobulin antibody. Proteinuria was detected by a precipitation reaction between urine obtained by bladder catheterization and 20% trichloracetic acid. Kidney tissue, taken either at postmortem (usually c. 4 weeks after infection) or by serial renal biopsy, was examined by light microscopy and immunofluorescence staining. Frozen sections were stained for rabbit IgG, IgM, C3 and for streptococcal antigen, before and after elution of immunoglobulins by citrate buffer pH 3.2. Antiglobulins were stained for by the use of fluoresceinated soluble aggregated human IgG.

A further set of experiments were performed in which immune reactants were eluted from renal tissue with citrate buffer pH 3.2. The eluates were concentrated and tested for the presence of rabbit IgG, IgM, C3, antistreptococcal antibody and streptococcal antigen. In addition, six rabbits were studied serially as above during the course of treatment with intramuscular penicillin.

Results

Development of disease

Proteinuria developed in the majority of preimmunized animals 6–11 days after infection and persisted in most of them for the rest of the course of the disease (15–25 days). Proteinuria did not develop in those rabbits which were not preimmunized. The aortic outflow tracts of infected rabbits were almost obstructed by infected vegetations, the left ventricle was dilated, the spleen enlarged and the kidneys showed some focal areas of infarction.

Circulating immune complexes (CIC) became detectable within 10 days of valve infection and proteinuria developed shortly after. Proteinuria did not persist in those animals in which CIC became undetectable again before the end of the study. Gel filtration studies (Fig. 2) showed the CIC to be of two molecular size ranges, c. 2.10^6 daltons and c. 3.10^5–9.10^5 daltons. Antistreptococcal antibody was detectable in these fractions (Fig. 3), but streptococcal antigen and antiglobulin were not.

There was a fall of serum C3 following infection, but only in a minority of animals did it reach a level of less than 2 standard deviations below the mean for normal rabbits.

Antistreptococcal antibody titres rose in $1:640$–$1:2560$ during immunization and to $1:5120$–$1:20,480$ after infection. Only three rabbits showed any rise in circulating antiglobulin titre during the course of IEGN.

Light microscopic examination of renal tissue showed some degree of focal septic infarction. In those preimmunized animals which developed

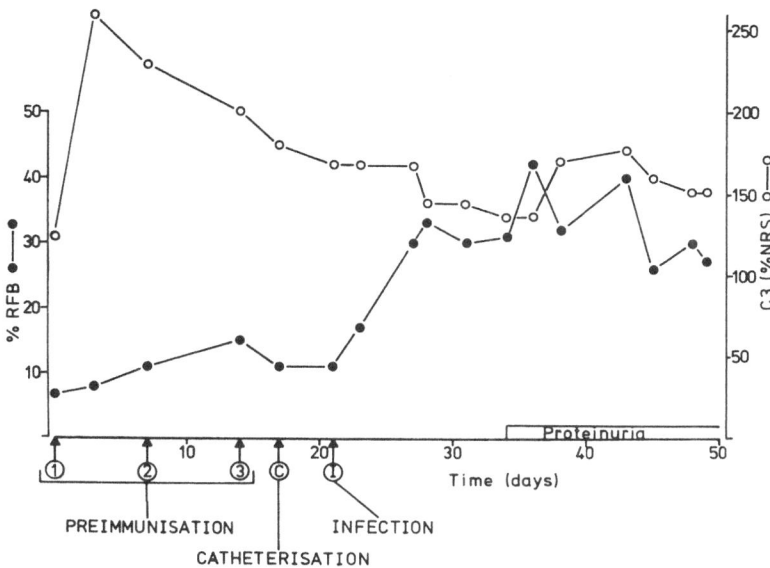

Figure 1. Course of events during induction and development of infective endocarditis glome-rulonephritis. (●—●) Rheumatoid factor binding (% RFB, i.e. circulating immune complexes). (○—○) Serum C3, expressed as percentage of value of pooled normal rabbit serum (% NRS).

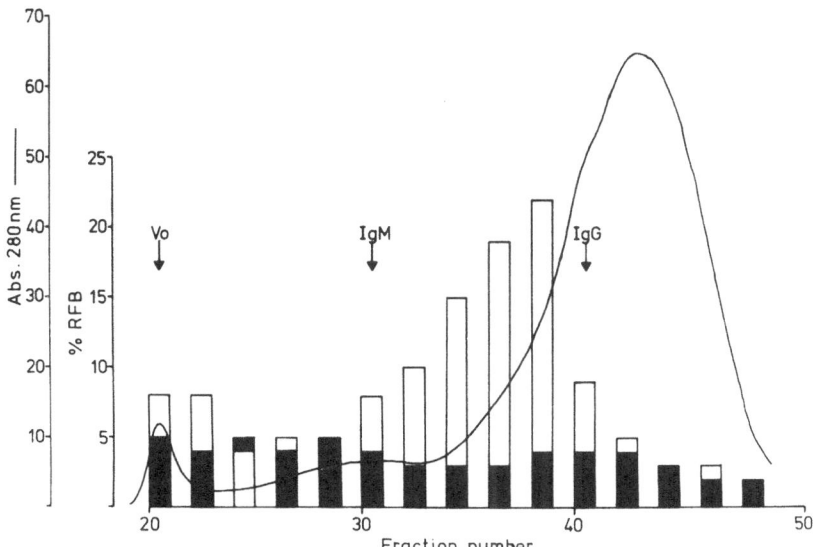

Figure 2. Sepharose 6B-CL gel filtration and RFB of fractions for normal rabbit serum (■) and serum from a rabbit with infective endocarditis glomerulonephritis (□). (——) Protein elution measured in arbitrary optical density units at 280 nm. Elution positions of IgM and IgG are shown.

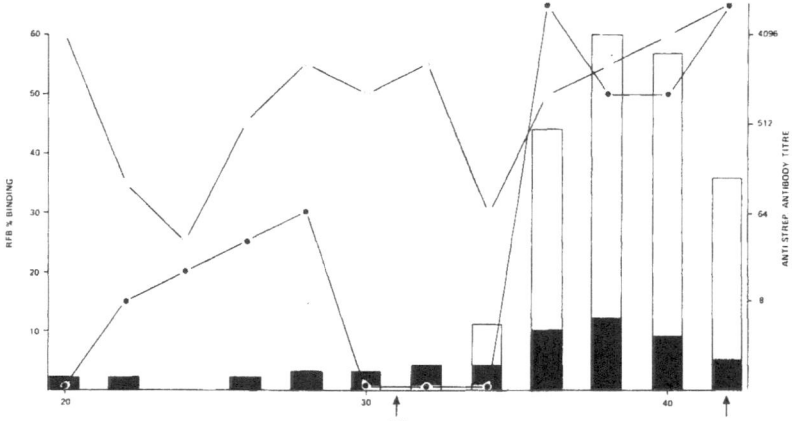

Figure 3. Sepharose 6B-CL gel filtration of sera from two rabbits showing RFB (■, □) and antistreptococcal antibody titre (●, ○) respectively.

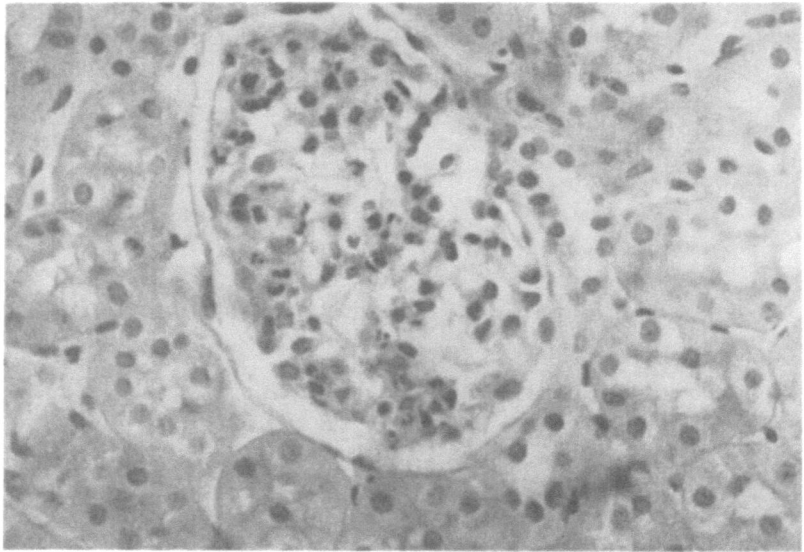

Figure 4. Light microscopy of glomerulus from rabbit with IEGN. (H & E, original × 500).

proteinuria following infection, a mild degree of endothelial and mesangial cell proliferation and neutrophil insudation was seen (Fig. 4). No glomerulonephritic changes were detected in unpreimmunized rabbits.

Granular deposition of rabbit IgG, IgM and C3 was seen on the glomerular basement membrane and in the mesangium in all but one of the proteinuric animals (Fig. 5), but only in 50 % of preimmunized animals which did not develop proteinuria. Antiglobulins within glomeruli were detectable

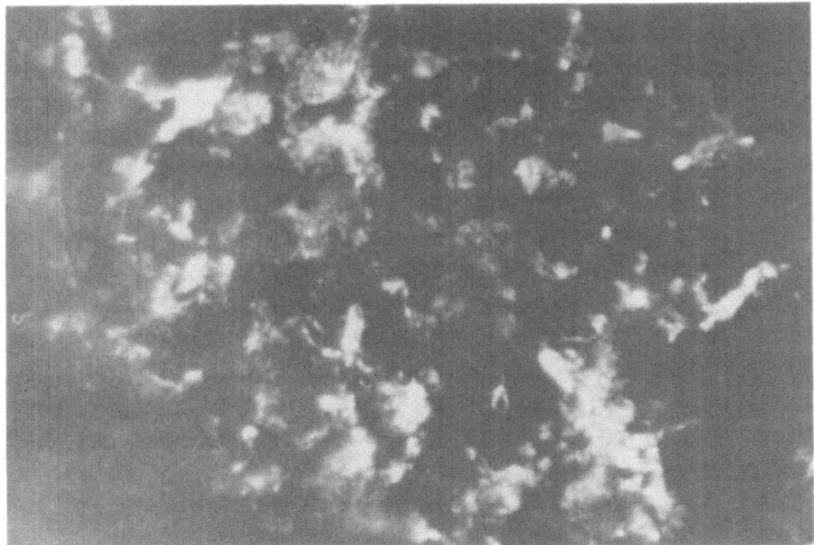

Figure 5. Immunofluorescent staining of glomerulus for rabbit IgM (original × 500).

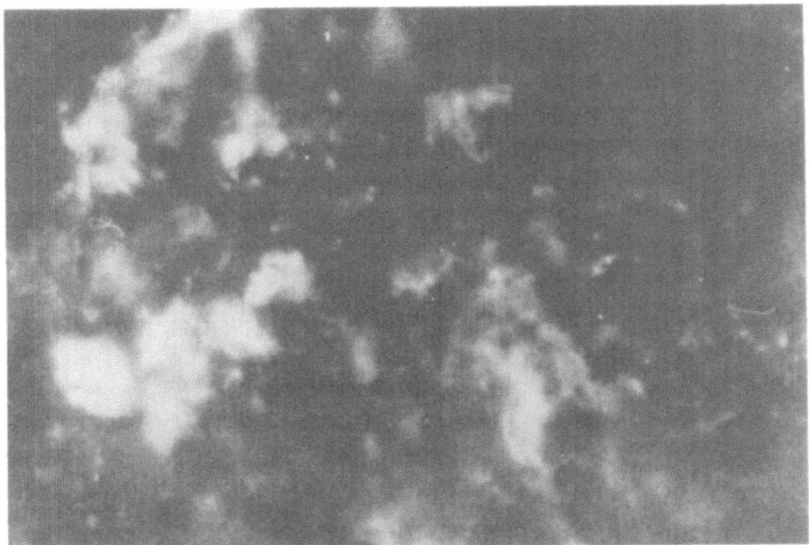

Figure 6. Immunofluorescent staining of glomerulus for antiglobulins (original × 500).

also in the majority of proteinuric, but not at all in the non-proteinuric animals (Fig. 6). A striking feature of the serial renal biopsy studies was that IgM and C3 were detectable in glomeruli some days before IgG in 3 of 5 animals so studied. Antiglobulin activity in glomeruli was associated with the presence of IgM in all but one animal (Table I). Streptococcal antigen was not detectable before or after acid elution of sections.

Table I. Immunoglobulins deposited in glomeruli and incidence of intraglomerular antiglobulins (figures in parenthesis) in rabbits grouped according to the presence or absence of circulating immune complexes and proteinuria.

	Total number of rabbits	Immunoglobulins in glomeruli			
		IgG + IgM	IgG	IgM	Negative
Circulating immune complexes and proteinuria	13 (9/13)	8 (7/8)	2 (1/2)	2 (1/2)	1 (0/1)
Proteinuria only	5 (3/5)	4 (2/4)	0 (0/0)	1 (1/1)	0 (0/0)
No circulating immune complexes or proteinuria	6 (0/6)	2 (0/2)	1 (0/1)	0 (0/0)	3 (0/3)

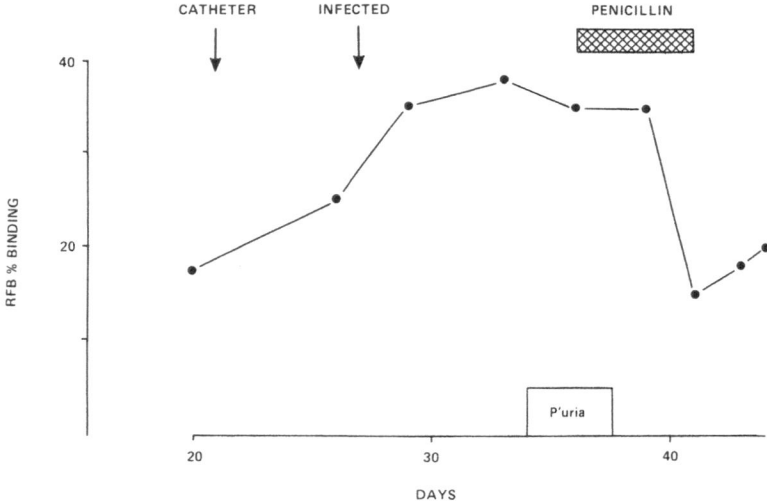

Figure 7. RFB (●—●) and proteinuria following induction of IEGN and following treatment with penicillin.

Treatment with intramuscular injections of penicillin resulted in the disappearance of CIC and proteinuria (Fig. 7). Immunoglobulins were not detectable in sections of kidney taken from animals so treated.

Elution studies of renal cortex showed the presence of IgG, IgM (by double diffusion immunoprecipitation) and antistreptococcal antibody (by agglutination of killed, trypsin treated streptococci). Streptococcal antigen could not be detected by counterimmunoelectrophoresis. Antiglobulin likewise could not be detected in eluates, as return to neutral pH resulted in precipitation in the eluate. Antistreptococcal antibody could not be detected in eluates from renal cortex of immunized, but uninfected rabbits, despite high titres of circulating antibody.

Discussion

The study of IEGN in rabbits has led to a number of interesting and important findings. The disease produced is remarkably similar to the human counterpart. CIC and proteinuria developed in the majority of animals and blood culture often became negative despite continuing evidence of glomerular inflammation and postmortem findings of a grossly infected aortic valve. Hypocomplementaemia was rare, although a fall within the normal range was common. Longterm study was unfortunately precluded by the development of left ventricular failure, due no doubt to the virtual obstruction of the aortic outflow tract.

Although some septic infarction did take place, this was very unlikely to have been the cause of proteinuria, as such lesions were seen to some extent in all infected animals regardless of the presence of proteinuria. Thorig et al. (1980) using a similar model concluded that septic infarcts were the most prominent feature of renal pathology and did not find convincing evidence of an immune complex nephritis, despite the presence of circulating immune complexes. Our preliminary experiments showed how important the timing and dosage of preimmunization was to the subsequent disease. Thorig et al. used a regime different to ours and this may explain the variation in findings.

The appearance in the blood of IgG containing macromolecules, reactive with the radiolabelled rheumatoid factor reagent, with a very similar molecular size to that found in human IEGN (4), which was followed by proteinuria, glomerular inflammation and glomerular deposition of immunoglobulin and complement, are all highly suggestive evidence of an immune complex aetiology of the initial phase of the disease. We were unable to demonstrate streptococcal antigen in either macromolecular fractions of serum or renal cortical eluates, probably because of the excess of streptococcal antibody. Similarly, the technical problem of precipitation in the eluate during the test to detect antiglobulin activity does not allow a confirmation of the findings obtained by immunofluorescence staining. However, the detection of streptococcal antibody in IgG containing fractions from gel filtration of serum of molecule size greater than 3.10^5 make it extremely likely that the CIC consisted of streptococcal-antistreptococcal proteins. The finding that the majority of such fractions were in the molecular size range above monomeric IgG, but below that of IgM, almost certainly rules out the possibility that CIC consisted of IgG and anti-IgG of IgM class. In addition, the administration of penicillin, which resulted in resolution of infected

50

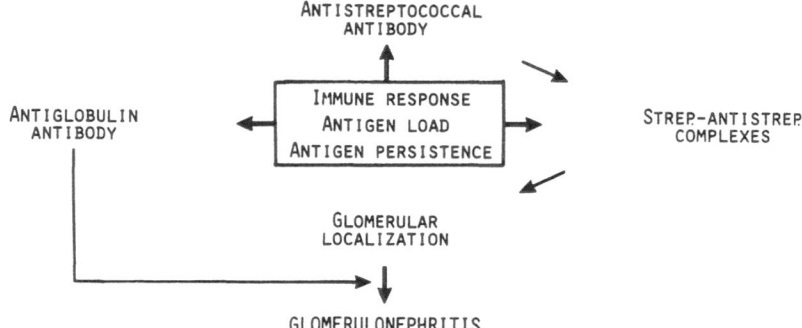

Figure 8. Representation of factors which are probably involved in the pathogenesis of glomerulonephritis of IEGN in rabbit model.

aortic lesions, also caused disappearance of CIC, proteinuria and intraglomerular immunoglobulins, further supporting the proposal that an infected aortic valve and the persistence of circulating streptococcal-antistreptococcal complexes were necessary for continuing glomerular inflammation.

Having said this, however, the striking association of the presence of intraglomerular antiglobulin activity, IgM and proteinuria and the finding of IgM in glomeruli very early in the course of proteinuria is compelling evidence to suggest that an in situ globulin-antiglobulin reaction caused the major part of the glomerular inflammation. It is very unlikely that the IgM was antistreptococcal antibody, as the animals had been repeatedly immunized over a 3 week period prior to infection, and circulating IgM antibody was not detected in the serum of preimmunized, but uninfected animals (as shown by absence of detectable antibody titres in IgM containing fractions of gel filtered serum).

A likely sequence of events may be proposed from these findings in this model of IEGN (Fig. 8). Infection of the damaged aortic valve occurring in a situation of circulating antibody excess leads to the formation of circulating streptococcal-antistreptococcal complexes, some of which deposit within glomeruli, but do not cause detectable inflammation. Subsequently, an in situ reaction between antistreptococcal IgG within the glomerulus and IgM anti-IgG leads to local complement activation, neutrophil insudation, glomerular cell proliferation and proteinuria.

IgM is frequently found in glomerular deposits of IEGN in humans and also in poststreptococcal glomerulonephritis. Rossen et al. (1975) and McIntosh et al. (1978) have provided some information that an in situ antiglobulin reaction may play a role in some forms of human glomerulonephritis. In situ recruitment of free antibody or antigen, which may be of exogenous or endogenous origin, may of course play as important, or a more important, role. Technical problems surround an investigation of the role of glomerular antiglobulins in human glomerulonephritis. However, direct staining may be possible using a more stable reagent than heat soluble IgG, or electrophoretic elutions from biopsy material, transfer of proteins to nitrocellulose paper and subsequent application of currently available and extremely sensitive detection and staining techniques may offer significant advantages over those used in the experiments described in this paper.

Summary

A reproducible model of streptococcal infective endocarditis glomerulonephritis was developed in the rabbit, in order to study the pathogenetic mechanisms of the disease. Circulating immune complexes became detectable shortly after infection of the aortic valve, followed by proteinuria. A mild proliferative glomerulonephritis developed with granular deposition of rabbit IgG, IgM and C3 within glomeruli. The presence of intraglomerular IgM and proteinuria were closely associated with the presence of antiglobulin activity within glomeruli. Despite the fact that penicillin treatment resulted in rapid resolution of most of the above features of the disease, streptococcal antigen could not be demonstrated in circulating immune complexes, or glomeruli, and could not be eluated from renal cortex.

References

1. Arnold SB, Valone JA, Askenase PW, Kashgarian M and Freedman LR: Diffuse glomerulonephritis in rabbits with Streptococcus viridans endocarditis. Lab Invest 32:681, 1975.
2. Sindrey M, Barratt J, Hewitt J, Naish P: Infective endocarditis-associated glomerulonephritis in rabbits: evidence of a pathogenetic role for antiglobulins. Clin Exp Immunol 45, 253–260, 1981.
3. Thorig L, Daha MR, Eulderink F, Kooybauer WC and Thompson J: Experimental Streptococcus sanguis endocarditis: Immune complexes and renal involvement. Clin Exp Immuno Immunol 40:496, 1980.
4. Naish P, Barratt J and Sindrey M: Assay of soluble immune complexes using radiolabelled rheumatoid factor. Meth Enzymol Vol 74:Chap 41, 1981.
5. Rossen RD, Reisberg MA, Sharp JT, Suki WN, Schloeder FX, Hill LL and Eknoyan G: Antiglobulins and glomerulonephritis. Classification of patients by the reactivity of their sera and renal tissue with aggregated and native human IgG. J Clin Invest 56:427, 1975.
6. McIntosh RM, Garcia R, Rutio L, Rabidean D, Allen JP, Carr RI and Rodriguez-Iturbe B: Evidence for an autologous immune complex pathogenetic mechanism in acute glomerulonephritis. Kidney Int 14:501, 1978.

5. Interaction of Human IgM Rheumatoid Factors with Immune Complexes in Experimental Murine Glomerulonephritis

PETER M. FORD

The occurrence of circulating IgM antiglobulin (rheumatoid factor) has been noted in a number of human diseases other than rheumatoid arthritis, in which immune complexes (IC's) are felt to have a pathogenetic role. These diseases include bacterial endocarditis, several forms of glomerulonephritis, systemic lupus, vasculitis and cryoglobulinemia. In all these diseases rheumatoid factor (RF) occurs not only in the circulation, but has been identified at the site of the damaged tissue. Furthermore RF has been identified as a component of cryoprecipitable IC's in cryoglobulinemia [1]. It has been known for many years that RF is capable of reacting with IC's *in vitro* [2] and this capacity forms the basis of one group of methods for the laboratory measurement of IC levels in body fluids [3]. More recently there has been interest in the role of RF's in human glomerulonephritis. Rossen et al. [4] noted the presence of RF in the glomeruli of patients with chronic glomerulonephritis associated with IC's and observed that RF was more likely to be found in severe than in mild disease. McIntosh et al. [5] identified RF in the blood of patients with poststreptococcal infection as soon as 7 or 8 days after the initial streptococcal infection and at the time of the onset of the renal damage and also demonstrated RF in the glomeruli of a patient with acute glomerulonephritis [6]. In patients with essential mixed cryoglobulinemia and renal involvement the RF component of the cryo has also been identified in the glomerulus [7]. In experimental animal glomerulonephritis interest in RF dates back to the work of McCormick et al. who in 1969 showed that injection of human IgM RF into rats, previously given anti-glomerular basement membrane antibody, resulted in localisation of human IgM along the basement membrane and enhancement of glomerular damage [8]. A similar mechanism occurs in the autologous phase of nephrotoxic serum nephritis with production of an antiglobulin directed against the heterologous antibody attached to the basement membrane. Zanetti and Druet [9] showed that in passive Heymann's nephritis produced in rats with a single injection of heterologous (rabbit) antibody to brush border antigen, prior induction of tolerance to rabbit immunoglobulin resulted in a diminished glomerular deposition of host IgG and prevented the onset of proteinuria as compared to non tolerant controls. Sindrey et al. [10] using a model of experimental infective endocarditis in rats found an association between glomerulonephritis and the presence of serum RF and were also able to demonstrate antiglobulin activity in the glomeruli of nephritic animals. More direct evidence for a pathogenetic role for RF was produced by Floyd and Tessar [11] who showed that in experimental vasculitis in rats, caused by a reverse passive Arthus reaction, the addition of RF to the system increased complement consumption and enhanced tissue damage.

The information presented above both from clinical observation and animal experiments would suggest a pathogenetic role for RF, however, there have been suggestions that RF in the circulation may have a protective role against the pathogenetic effects of IC's [12] although evidence to support this suggestion is sparse. Van Snick et al. [13] were able to show enhancement by IgM RF of *in vivo* clearance of IC in mice, however the IC were incubated with RF prior to injection and thus the relevance of the results is not clear. We were able to show that injection of IC's into mice given a prior IV injection of human IgM RF did not produce a significant difference in glomerular IC deposition as compared to mice given normal IV IgM, although human IgM was detected in the glomeruli of the RF group [14].

The purpose of this paper is to present information relating to the in situ glomerular reactivity of RF with IC's in different experimental systems in the mouse and to demonstrate how such reactions may play a part not only in enhancing the lesion, but also how they may contribute to the perpetuation of the process.

Passive serum sickness

Our initial studies were done using a passive serum sickness model [14]; mice were injected IV with preformed BSA-rabbit antiBSA immune complexes (prepared in 5 times antigen XS and containing 28 mg of antibody/100 g body wt. of mouse). At six hours mesangiocapillary staining for rabbit immunoglobulin and BSA could be demonstrated in mouse glomeruli (Fig. 1) and IV administration of purified human IgM with rheumatoid factor activity (14 mg/100 g body wt. – prepared by acid elution on a Sephadex G200 column) resulted in deposition of human IgM in a distribution similar to that of the immune complexes (Fig. 2) when the animals were killed 12 hrs after RF injection. Controls given IC's and normal RF negative-IgM showed no glomerular localisation of human IgM. IV administration of RF prior to given IC's did not diminish glomerular deposition of IC's as compared to controls given normal RF negative IgM, but mice given

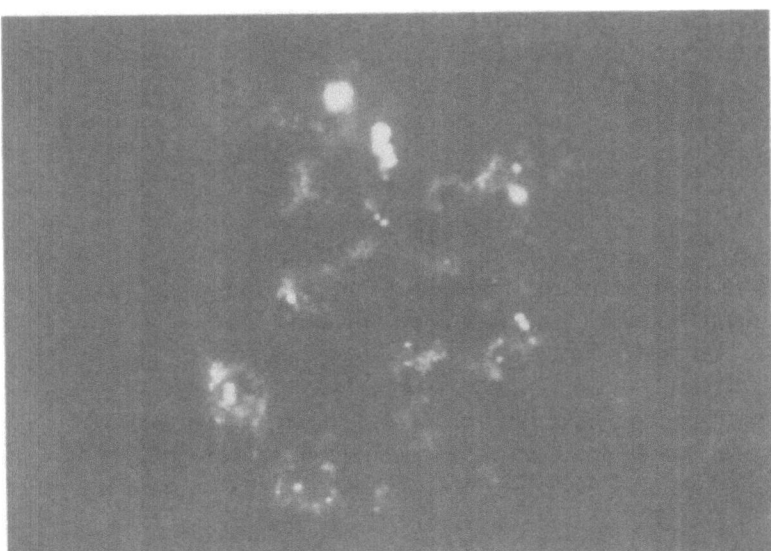

Figure 1. Passive serum sickness: mouse glomerulus stained with FITC goatantirabbit immunoglobulin (original magnification × 500) from mouse killed 6 hours after I.V. BSA-rabbit antiBSA immune complexes.

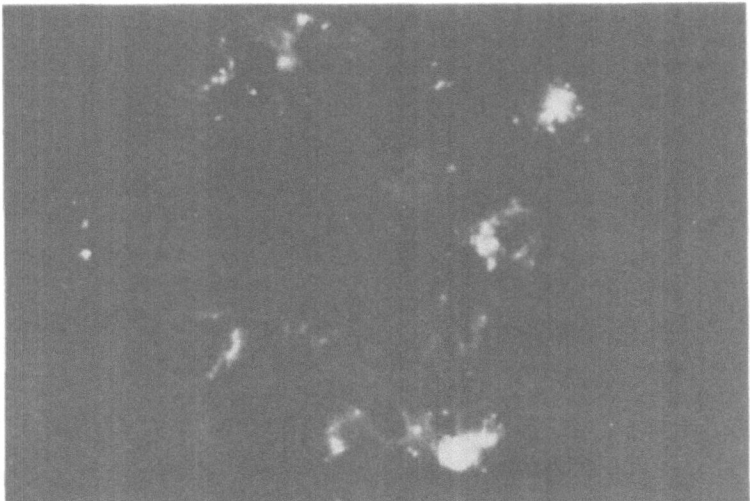

Figure 2. Passive serum sickness: mouse glomerulus stained with FAB FITC goat antihuman IgM antibody. Animal given I.V. BSA-rabbit antiBSA immune complexes followed 6 hours later by I.V. human IgM rheumatoid factor (14 mg/100 g body wt.) and killed 12 hours after the second injection. Note that staining for human IgM is in the same distribution as for the rabbit immunoglobulin in Fig. 1 (original magnification × 500).

the RF positive preparation showed glomerular localisation of human IgM six hours after IC administration. These experiments demonstrated that RF could bind *in vivo* to IC's localised in the glomerulus and that prior administration of RF did not enhance clearance of IC's to an extent that affected glomerular deposition. It was of interest to see whether the RF bound to the IC's in the glomerulus had any effect on subsequent IC deposition. To examine this further, mice which had been given IC's followed by RF as in the original experiment were given a further injection of IC's 12 hrs after the RF injection. Control animals received the same sequence of injections except that they received RF negative IgM. Examination of the kidneys 6 hrs after the final injection showed a marked enhancement of staining for rabbit immunoglobulin and BSA in the mice given RF as opposed to mice given normal IgM (FITC-Fab anti-rabbit and anti-BSA antisera were used to avoid non specific pick up by the RF). These results (Table I) suggested that the RF in the glomerulus still had free binding sites capable of combining with and fixing circulating IC's. Similar results were obtained when the final IC injection comprised rabbit antiferritin-ferritin IC's or heat aggregated human IgG. To exclude the possibility that the enhanced pickup of IC's in the RF group was due to non specific trapping as a result of

Table I. Showing staining intensity for mouse immunoglobulin and human IgM in two groups of 5 mice (20 glomeruli scored on $0-4+$ scale from a kidney section from each mouse. Each column represents the mean score). Group A received I.V. immune complexes followed 6 hours later by I.V. human IgM rheumatoid factor and 12 hours later by a further I.V. injection of immune complexes. Group B received the same sequence of injections except that the IgM was negative for rheumatoid factor activity. All animals killed 6 hours after the final injection. Note the much enhanced score for rabbit immunoglobulin staining in the group receiving rheumatoid factor positive IgM.

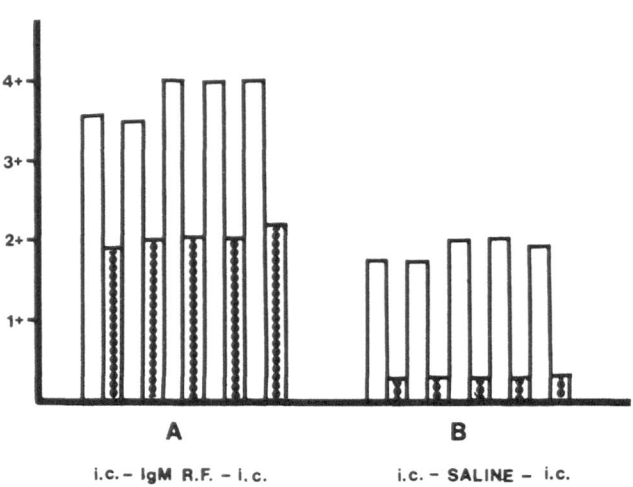

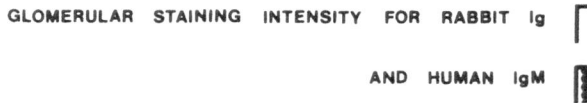

Table II. Incubation experiments: frozen sections from two groups of 5 mice, one injected with BSA-rabbit anti-BSA immune complexes I.V. followed by rheumatoid factor positive human IgM (A) and the other injected with I.V. immune complexes followed by rheumatoid factor negative human IgM (B), were incubated with either a preparation of BSA-rabbit anti-BSA immune complexes (dotted columns) or saline (black columns) washed and then stained for rabbit immunoglobulin. Note the increased staining for rabbit immunoglobulin in group A.

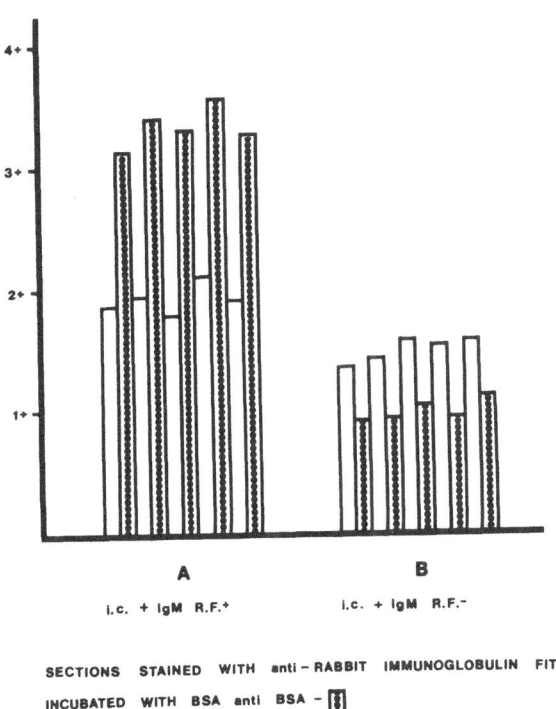

damage secondary to in situ reactivity between RF and IC's, a small IV dose of heat aggregated BSA was substituted for the final dose of IC's and no difference was seen between RF positive and negative groups. Frozen sections of kidney from two groups of mice the one given IC's followed by RF before death and the other IC's followed by RF negative IgM were washed in phosphate buffered saline and incubated with a preparation of BSA-rabbit-antiBSA IC's. Staining for rabbit immunoglobulin revealed a marked increase in staining in the RF positive group as opposed to the RF negative group (Table II). These results would appear to show that IgM RF can bind in situ to IC's in the glomerulus and that once bound, RF, presumably by virtue of unsaturated binding sites, can fix further IC's regardless of the antigen.

Chronic serum sickness

Chronic serum sickness was induced in mice by subcutaneous injection of BSA in Freund's complete adjuvant followed by daily injections intraperitoneally of 0.5 mg of BSA [15]. By 40 days, granular deposits of mouse immunoglobulin and complement may be detected by fluorescence along the basement membrane and in the mesangium, together with an increase in mesangial cellularity. IV injection of human IgM RF at this time results in localisation of human IgM in the same distribution as the mouse immunoglobulin and a minor increase in cellularity of the glomerulus at 4 days as opposed to mice given RF negative IgM who show no glomerular deposition of human IgM. We were unable to demonstrate any significant changes in renal function (Cr57 EDTA clearance or proteinuria) in RF injected animals vs normal IgM injected controls; this lack of functional effect of RF may in part be due to the impairment of complement activation noted in RF prepared by acid elution [16].

In situ immune complex formation

In addition to the more general view that immune complex glomerulonephritis is secondary to the deposition of circulation IC's there has been recent interest in the possibility that under some circumstances glomerular immune complexes may be formed by an in situ reaction between antigen and antibody [17–19]. Because in the passive serum sickness experiments we could not entirely exclude the possibility that the RF was combining with the IC's prior to deposition in the glomerulus, even though the absorption of subsequent IC's was plainly an in situ phenomenon, we chose to use our previously described model of in situ IC formation [18], where circulating IC's do not occur, to examine further the effect of RF. Essentially the in situ model used consists of giving a small dose of heat aggregated BSA and at a time when no free BSA can be demonstrated in the circulation (6 hrs), but deposits are present in the glomerulus, rabbit antiBSA is injected IV. The antibody binds to the BSA in the glomerulus with the in situ formation of immune complexes and fixation of complement. IV administration of IgM RF either before or after the injections of aggregated BSA and the rabbit antiBSA did not affect in situ IC formation, but in both cases human IgM deposited in the glomeruli in the same distribution as the in situ IC's. RF negative IgM in control mice did not deposit in the glomerulus. Furthermore by repeating the same manoevres performed in the passive serum sickness experiments we were able to show that human IgM RF bound to IC's formed in situ was able to further bind circulating BSA-rabbit antiBSA complexes as well as unrelated IC's (aggregated human IgG and ferritin-rabbit antiferritin IC's), in a pattern corresponding to that of the bound IgM [20].

It is of relevance to note that in neither the passive serum sickness nor the in situ experiments were we able to demonstrate by fluorescence the fixation of any additional complement in the glomerulus after the binding of RF, this probably relates to the effect, already referred to, of acid elution.

Cationised rheumatoid factor as the initiating event in immune complex deposition

The demonstration that positively charged (cationic) proteins could attach to endogenous glomerular polyanion in glomerular capillaries purely by virtue of the charge difference suggested that this might be one of the mechanisms involved in the attachment of circulating IC's when they carry a net positive charge or alternatively in the attachment of positively charged antigen as the initiating event in in situ IC formation. A number of investigators have now shown that when either the antigen or the antibody component of an IC carries a sufficient positive charge to render the whole complex cationic, such complexes will deposit along the basement membrane of the glomerulus to a greater degree than uncharged IC's of the same size and constitution [21, 22]. Attachment of cationised antigen to basement membrane by virtue of its charge will allow later reaction with the appropriate circulating antibody to form immune complexes in situ [23]. Less attention however has been paid to the possibility of deposition of antibody along the basement membrane by virtue of charge or other non specific mechanism, as the initiating event in in situ IC formation. Cationic antibodies can occur naturally and isoelectric focusing of antibodies from normal subjects will demonstrate a wide range of electrical charge [24]. Furthermore the net charge on an antigen initiating an immune response will induce an opposite charge on the resulting antibody, thus a negatively charged antigen will result in a positively charged antibody [25]. Ebling and Hahn [26] showed that anti DNA antibodies eluted from the kidneys of NZB/W mice were more cationic than antiDNA antibodies from the circulation. Such cationic antibodies might either enhance deposits of immune complexes from the circulation as suggested by Gauthier et al. [22] or might attach alone to the basement membrane and be the initiating event in the in situ formation of IC's. Mechanisms other than charge difference might also allow antibody alone to become attached to basement membrane and Brownlee et al. [27] demonstrated that soluble proteins including immunoglobulin could become covalently attached to non-enzymatically glycosylated collagen and furthermore such antibodies were able to react with their

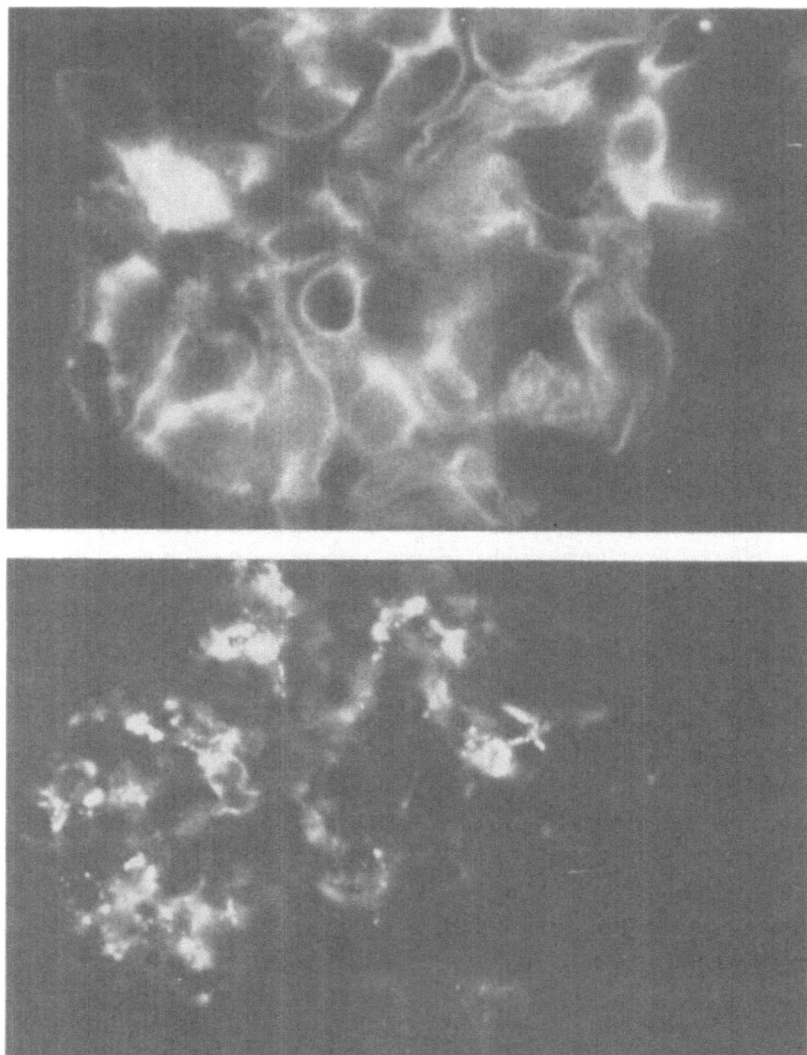

appropriate antigen to form IC's in situ. They suggested that this attachment of antibody to glycosylated collagen might explain the observation of linear protein deposition seen along the glomerular basement membrane in diabetes mellitus [28] and might also help to explain the glomerular IC's reported in this disease [29]. Given our previous observations on the immunoabsorbative capacity of glomerular bound RF it was therefore of interest to see whether non specific attachment of RF to glomerular basement membrane by virtue of charge alone would preserve the ability to bind IC's in situ. Cationisation of RF positive and RF negative human IgM was carried

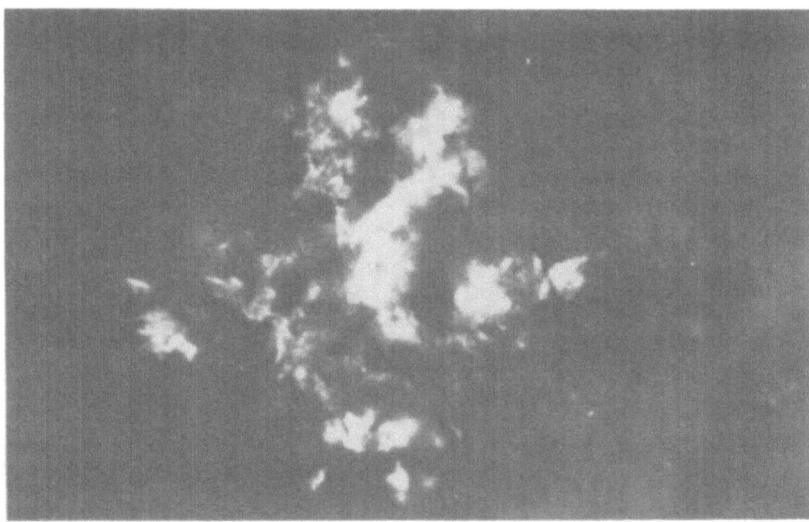

Figure 3, 4, 5. Glomeruli from mice injected with cationised human IgM with positive rheumatoid factor activity (dose: 14 mg/100 g body wt.). Stained with FAB FITC goat antihuman IgM. Fig. 3, 12 hours after injection of IgM, showing linear staining. Fig. 4, 36 hours after injection showing disruption of linear staining. Fig. 5, 4 days after injection showing clearance of IgM into the mesangium (all at ×500 original magnification).

out by the method described for immunoglobulin by Gauthier et al. [22] and produced a final IgM product with a pI between 9 and 9.5 on isoelectric focusing. RF activity in the RF positive IgM was little reduced from the starting sheep cell agglutination titre, the final titre being 1/1024 at a concentration of IgM of 7 mg/ml. The control RF negative cationic preparation was adjusted to the same concentration.

Injection of cationic IgM IV in a dose of 14 mg/100 g body wt. of mouse produced a linear deposition of human IgM along the basement membrane in mice killed 12 hrs after injection (Fig. 3) for both RF positive and negative preparations. Mice killed at 24 hr intervals over the next 4 days showed a similar progression of events in both groups with the linear staining becoming disrupted by 36 hrs (Fig. 4) and with clearance into the mesangium over the next two days of most of the IgM (Fig. 5). Staining for the presence of mouse immunoglobulin revealed no definite staining at any time point in the RF negative group. However in the RF positive group finely granular staining for mouse Ig became evident in the capillary walls at 35 hrs with clearance into the mesangium at a similar rate to the IgM over the next two days (Fig. 6, 7) suggesting that the IgM with RF activity was binding endogenously produced circulating IC's. Transient proteinuria was noted in both RF positive and negative groups following cationised IgM injection presumably due to neutralisation of the normal charge barrier on

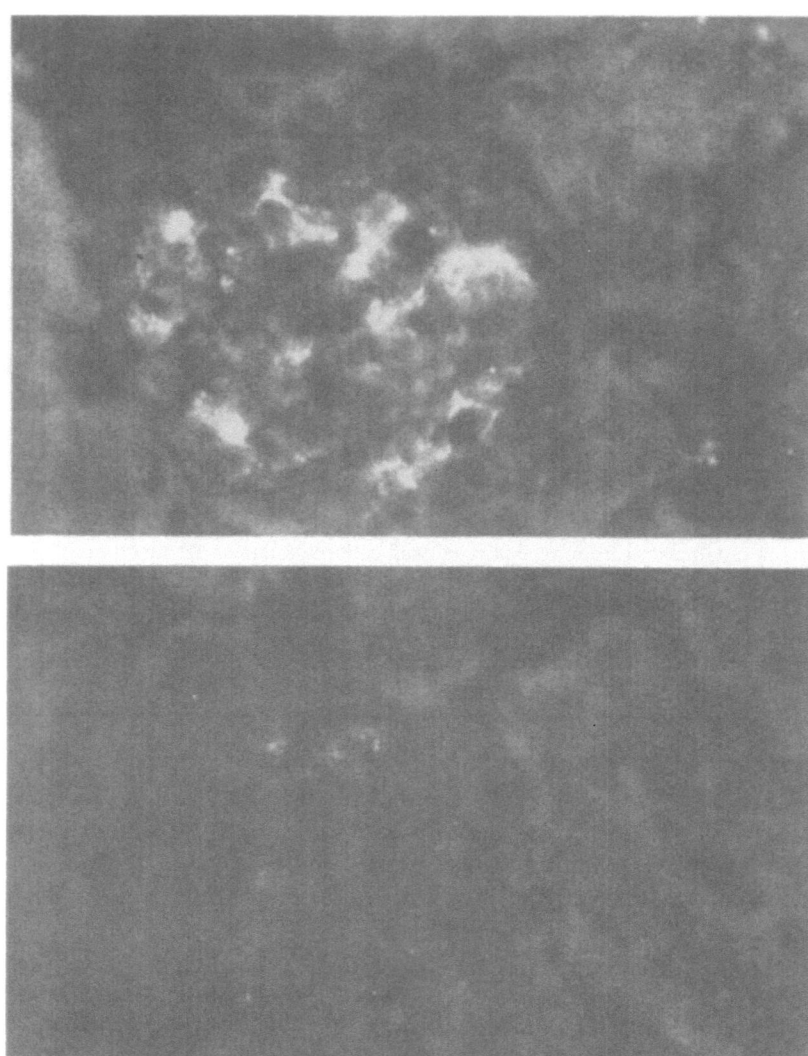

Figure 6, 7. Staining for mouse immunoglobulin in glomeruli from animals given either I.V. cationised human IgM rheumatoid factor 48 hours previously (Fig. 6) or I.V. cationised human IgM without rheumatoid factor activity (Fig. 7). Note the particulate staining for mouse immunoglobulin in the RF positive mouse with no staining in the RF negative animal (original magnification × 500).

the basement membrane [30]. Animals given non cationised (pI 6–7.5) RF positive or negative IgM showed no significant staining on the glomeruli. IV injection of small quantities of BSA-rabbit antiBSA IC's into mice 6 hours after injection of either RF positive or negative cationic IgM showed a small mesangial deposition of complex components in the RF negative group with

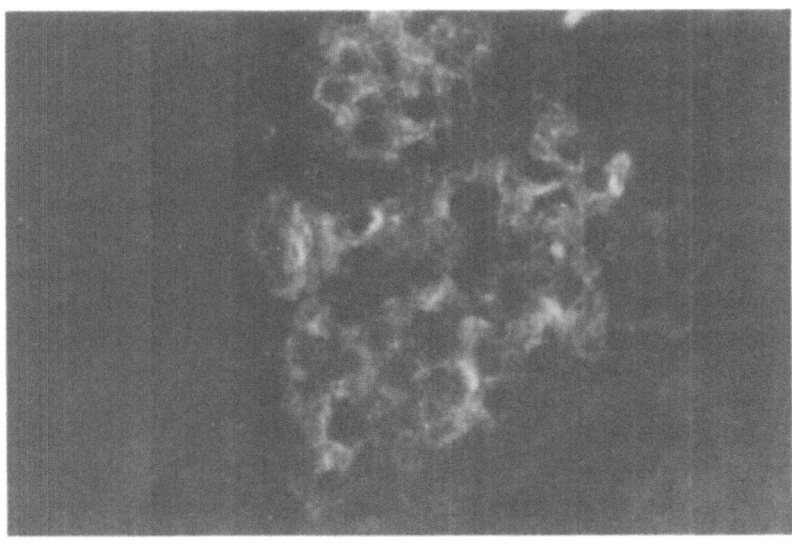

Figure 8. Staining for rabbit immunoglobulin in the glomerulus of a mouse given I.V. cationised human IgM rheumatoid factor followed 6 hours later by I.V. BSA-rabbit antiBSA immune complexes. Note diffuse mesangiocapillary distribution of particulate staining for rabbit immunoglobulin. Animals given rheumatoid factor negative cationic IgM followed by immune complexes gave less pronounced staining confined to the mesangium and similar to Fig. 1 (original magnification × 500).

a much enhanced deposition along capillary walls and in the mesangium from the RF positive group (Fig. 8, Table 3). Similar results were obtained when heat aggregated human IgG was substituted for immune complexes (Table III).

These results [30] would indicate that RF when bound in a non specific charge related manner to the basement membrane is still capable of acting

Table III. Staining patterns and intensity following injection of BSA-antiBSA immune complexes or heat aggregated human immunoglobulin into mice given prior injections of cationised rheumatoid factor (RF)+ or cationised RF− human IgM.

Group	Mean glomerular staining intensity (+sd)	Pattern deposition
BSA-antiBSA (rabbit) immune complexes	For rabbit Ig	
A Cationised IgM RF+	2.9±0.6	Capillary & Mesangial
B Cationised IgM RF−	0.73±0.4	Mesangial only
Heat aggregated human Ig	For human IgG	
A Cationised IgM RF+	2.6±0.7	Capillary & Mesangial
B Cationised IgM RF−	0.8±0.5	Mesangial only

as an immunoabsorbent and binding IC's by their antibody component regardless of the antigen constituent.

Conclusion

IgM rheumatoid factor in the glomerulus whether attached to previously formed immune complexes or attached by non immunologic mechanisms is clearly able to act as an immunoabsorbent and bind circulating immune complexes. The demonstration of antiglobulin activity in the glomerulus in a number of human renal diseases suggests an involvement in the pathogenesis, perhaps by perpetuating the process in a way that no longer involves the antigen which provided the initial stimulus. The ability of IgM RF to attach to the basement membrane in a non specific manner whilst still retaining its antiglobulin activity might indicate that under some circumstances primary deposition of antibody could be the initiating event in the localisation or formation of immune complexes.

References

1. Meltzer M, Franklin EC, Elias K. et al.: Cryoglobulinemia-a clinical and laboratory study. II. Cryoglobulins with rheumatoid factor activity. Am J Med 40:837, 1966.
2. Edelman GM, Kunkel HG and Franklin EC: Interaction of the rheumatoid factor with antigen-antibody complexes and aggregated gamma globulin. J Exp Med 108:105, 1958.
3. Agnello V: Detection of immune complexes. In Manual of Clinical Immunology. Rose NR and Freeman H (Ed) Washington. American Society for Microbiology, p 669, 1976.
4. Rossen RD, Rickaway RH, Reisberg MA et al.: Renal localisation of antiglobulins in glomerulonephritis and after renal transplantation. Arthritis Rheum 20:257, 1977.
5. McIntosh RM, Rabideau D, Allen JE et al.: Acute post streptococcal glomerulonephritis in Maracaibo. II. Studies on the incidence, nature and significance of circulating anti-immunoglobulins. Ann Rheum Dis 38:257, 1979.
6. Rodriguez-Iturbe B, Rabideau D, Garcia R et al.: Characterisation of the glomerular antibody in acute post streptococcal glomerulonephritis. Ann Int Med 92:478, 1980.
7. Maggiore Q, Bartolomeo F, L'Abbate A et al.: Glomerular localisation of circulating antiglobulin activity in essential mixed cryoglobulinemia with glomerulonephritis. Kidney Int 21:387, 1982.
8. Cormick JN, Day J, Morris CJ et al.: The potentiating effect of rheumatoid arthritis serum on the immediate phase of nephrotoxic serum nephritis. Clin Exp Immunol 4:17, 1969.
9. Zanetti M and Druet P: Heymann's nephritis as a model of glomerulonephritis mediated by antibodies to immunoglobulins. Clin Exp Immunol 41:189, 1980.
10. Sindrey M, Barrat J, Hewit J et al.: Infective endocarditis-associated glomerulonephritis in rabbits-evidence of a pathogenetic role for antiglobulins. Clin Exp Immunol 45:253, 1981.
11. Floyd-M and Tessar JT: The role of IgM rheumatoid factor in experimental immune vasculitis. Clin Exp Immunol 26:165, 1979.
12. Davis JS: A hypothetical common mechanism in systemic lupus erythematosus and rheumatoid arthritis. Arthritis Rheum 9:631, 1966.

13. Van Snick L, Van Roost E and Markowetz B: Enhancement by IgM rheumatoid factor of in vitro ingestion by macrophages and in vivo clearance of aggregated IgG or antigen-antibody complexes. Eur J Immunol 8:279, 1978.

14. Ford PM and Kosatka I: The effect of human IgM rheumatoid factor on renal immune complex deposition in passive serum sickness in the mouse. Immunol 46:761, 1982.

15. Ford PM and Kosatka I: In situ reactivity of human IgM rheumatoid factor with glomerular immune complexes in experimental chronic serum sickness. Arthritis Rheum (suppl) 25:137, 1982.

16. Stollar BD, Staedecker MJ and Morecki S: Comparison of the inactivation of IgM and IgG complement fixation sites by acid and base. J Immunol 117:1387, 1976.

17. Couser WB, Steinmuller DR, Sillmont MM et al.: Experimental glomerulonephritis in the rat induced by antibodies directed against tubular antigens. Lab Invest 38:502, 1978.

18. Ford PM and Kosatka I: In situ formation of antigen antibody complexes in the mouse glomerulus. Immunol 48:473, 1979.

19. Couser WG and Salant DJ: In situ immune complex formation and glomerular injury. Kidney Int 17:1, 1980.

20. Ford PM and Kosatka I: In situ immune complex formation in the mouse glomerulus: reactivity with human IgM rheumatoid factor and the effect on subsequent immune complex deposition. Clin Exp Immunol 51:285, 1983.

21. Gallo G, Caulin-Glaser T and Lamm ME: Charge of circulating immune complexes as a factor in glomerular basement membrane localisation in mice. J Clin Invest 67:1305, 1981.

22. Gauthier VJ, Mannik M and Striker GE: Effect of cationised antibodies in preformed immune complexes on deposition and persistance in renal glomeruli. J Exp Med 155:460, 1982.

23. Ward HJ, Cohen AH and Border WA: In situ formation of subepithelial immune complexes in the rabbit glomerulus: requirement of a cationic antigen. Nephron 36:257, 1984.

24. Jalkanen M and Jalkanen S: Immunological detection of proteins after isoelectric focusing in thin layer agarose gel: a specific application for the characterisation of immunoglobulin diversity. Clin Lab Immunol 10:225, 1983.

25. Sela M and Mozes E: Dependance on the chemical nature of antibodies on the net electrical charge of antigen. Proc Nat Acad Sci 55:445, 1966.

26. Ebling F and Hahn BH: Restricted subpopulations of DNA antibodies in kidneys of mice with systemic lupus. Comparison of antibodies in serum and renal eluates. Arthritis Rheum 23:392, 1980.

27. Brownlee M, Pongor S and Cerami A: Covalent attachment of soluble proteins by nonenzymatically glycosylated collagen. J Exp Med 158:1739, 1983.

28. Cavallo T, Pinto JA, Abbott LC et al.: Immune complex disease complicating diabetic glomerulosclerosis. Lab Invest 48:13A, 1983.

29. Barnes JL, Radnick RA, Gichrist EP et al.: Size and charge selective permeability defects induced in the glomerular basement membrane by a polycation. Kidney Int 25:11, 1984.

30. Ford PM and Kosatka I: Cationised IgM rheumatoid factor: in vivo glomerular localisation and immunoabsorptive capacity in the mouse. Clin Exp Immunol 62:150, 1985.

6. Anti-Idiotypic Antibodies in Glomerulonephritis and in Tubulointerstitial Nephritis Models of Immune Renal Injury

CURTIS B. WILSON, KYM M. BANNISTER,
FRANCISCO M. MAMPASO, THOMAS R. ULRICH and
MAURIZIO ZANETTI

The idiotype-anti-idiotype system

The recognition that the structural variations in immunoglobulin molecules necessitated by their antigenic specificity rendered molecules antigenic led to the concept of idiotypy [1, 2]. Accordingly, the uniqueness of the antigen binding site of the immunoglobulin molecule itself was able to subsequently stimulate the host immune system. Autoantibodies, called anti-idiotypes, then form which are specific for the idiotypic differences on the original antibody population. In some instances, the anti-idiotypes that form can mimic the original antigenic determinant, producing an internal image [3, 4] which may be useful as an antigenic stimulus in instances where the original antigen may itself be difficult to obtain or, in some instances, may be infectious in nature [5–7]. In other situations, the internal image may have deleterious effects as will be discussed shortly.

There is now considerable experimental evidence that the concept of idiotype and auto-anti-idiotypic antibody formation is important in the overall regulation of the immune response [8, 9]. The regulatory idiotype reaction is based upon recognition between idiotype and complementary anti-idiotype, both in the form of free antibody molecules and surface-bound immunoglobulin in the case of B lymphocytes and perhaps cellular receptors on T lymphocytes [10]. Immunization then leads to the production of antibody, with the generation of anti-idiotypes and potentially anti-anti-idiotypes based on the idiotypic antigenicity of each generation of antibody. Because of the complementarity between idiotype and anti-idiotype sites, the cycles of anti-anti-idiotype production are probably self-limited. Experimental manipulations of the idiotype network can lead to stimulatory or suppressive responses in immunologic reactions. Induction of anti-idiotypic immunity can lead to specific immunosuppression, and it is possible to induce tolerance to histocompatibility antigens with subsequent modulation of organ rejection with these methods [11].

The existence of cross-reacting idiotypes on the variable regions of autoantibody molecules indicate that some idiotypic determinants are highly conserved [12]. For example, in autoantibody formation such as human rheumatoid factor, certain idiotypes are encoded by closely related variable region genes. The commonality in idiotype suggests that studies of the idiotype network may be of value in understanding events involving self-recognition and the induction of autoimmune phenomena. The discrimination between self and non-self which takes place in the context of the major histocompatibility complex probably depends upon active control processes. These processes may, in part, be related to regulation by idiotype-anti-idiotype expression. In this regard, some of the regulatory events may be based on preferential use of certain idiotypes termed regulatory idiotypes [13]. These may be selected through genetic or environmental pressures to act as regulators of autoimmune responses. Conversely, as noted above, anti-idiotypic antibodies, via the internal image concept, may stereochemically mimic self-antigens. This has been identified with anti-hormone autoantibodies with which the subsequent anti-idiotypic antibody, through its internal image, may resemble the hormone and be capable of mimicking the hormone's biologic function at the level of the appropriate cellular receptor [14]. Interestingly, in terms of autoimmune reactions, it has been shown that rats and mice can be induced to develop autoantibodies to thyroglobulin in the absence of specific antigen administration if they are immunized with anti-anti-thyroglobulin (anti-idiotype antibodies) [15, 16]. This and other examples of internal image anti-idiotypes could lead to the repeated stimulation of autoantibody formation.

Idiotype-anti-idiotype reactions in immune mediated renal injury

Current concepts of the generation of immunologically mediated renal disease center on the formation of antibodies that react directly with tissue-fixed antigens, either present as structural components of the kidney or as material trapped there from the circulation [17]. Antibodies may also combine in dynamic equilibrium with soluble antigens in the vascular compartment to form complexes that subsequently accumulate and reassociate within various areas in the kidney. Since both situations require the generation of a sustained antibody response, either to self, cross-reacting, or foreign antigen, anti-idiotypes could play an important role in the development and/or persistence of the immune response essential for the immunopathologic manifestations of the disease.

Idiotype-anti-idiotype reactions can be considered in two major ways as they may apply to immune renal injury [18]. These include the role of anti-idiotypic antibody reactions in the control of nephritogenic immune responses, and the converse, namely the possible contribution of auto-anti-idiotypic antibodies in the generation of nephritogenic immune deposits within the glomeruli and potentially elsewhere within the kidney. To study the first issue, anti-idiotypic antibodies were used to help dissect the contribution of the relevant anti-tubular basement membrane (TBM) antibody response in the generation of tubulointerstitial nephritis in the rat. To examine the possible contribution of anti-idiotypic antibodies to the generation of immune deposits and renal injury, auto-anti-idiotypic antibodies were sought in immune deposits in chronic serum sickness in rabbits.

The Role of Idiotype-Anti-Idiotype Reactions in the Control of Nephritogenic Immune Responses

Tubulointerstitial nephritis can be induced in Brown Norway (BN) rats by immunization with bovine TBM antigens in adjuvants [20]. This immunization induces circulating and kidney-bound anti-TBM antibodies. Complement fixation begins by day 8 and a polymorphonuclear leukocyte infiltration evolves, followed in 3–4 days by a mononuclear cell dominated interstitial infiltrate. The mononuclear infiltrate contains largely T cells and Ia^+ cells [21, 22]. Lymph node cells sensitized to solubilized bovine TBM antigens are demonstrable [22]. There is then evidence to suggest an interplay between cellular and humoral immunity in the generation of this lesion, although the individual contribution of the two arms of the immune system remain to be quantified. These questions arise because only minimal lesions are transferable with up to 45 ml of immune BN serum [23], or even subcapsular placement of immune BN cells [24]. Recently, transfer has been effected with immune lymph node cells after propagation with antigen in an IL-2 source [22]; however, these cells induce anti-TBM antibody production by the recipient, thereby again preventing distinction between humoral and cellular mechanisms.

To address the role of antibody, a series of studies has been done including the manipulation of the immune response with administration of auto-idiotypic antibody. When rats are immunized with particulate bovine TBM, they produce anti-TBM antibodies that react with both particulate and collagenase solubilized (CS) TBM from both bovine and BN rat TBM sources [25]. In the serum, the reaction with bovine TBM antigens is greater than with the BN counterparts. A specific concentration (serum to eluate ratio) of anti-BN TBM antibody can be recovered from kidney eluates of affected animals. Almost no concentration of anti-bovine TBM reactivity is found in the eluates. Of the anti-BN TBM antibodies recovered from the eluates, about 70% of the reactivity is directed toward antigens in the non-collagenous portion of the TBM represented by the BN CS TBM antigen.

The reactive antigen in this mixture is a 42–45 kD material, and similar sized reactive fragments are present in both bovine and BN collagenase extracts [23, 25]. Of interest, the reactive antigen in human anti-TBM nephritis which cross-reacts with the BN kidney TBM is also of a similar size, as demonstrated some years ago in our laboratory.

To analyze the significance of the anti-BN CS TBM antibody recovered from the kidneys of these rats, a heterologous anti-idiotypic antibody was used to modulate the nephritogenic immune response. Previous work by Brown et al. [26] had used anti-idiotypic antibodies to modify anti-TBM antibody-associated tubulointerstitial nephritis in guinea pigs. Similarly, Neilson et al. [27], in the rat, attained attenuation of tubulointerstitial nephritis by inducing an active state of anti-idiotypic immunity by administering TBM antigen-reactive T cells.

The anti-idiotypic antibodies were prepared in rabbits by immunization with BN anti-TBM IgG eluted and purified from nephritic BN rat kidneys. The rabbit antibody was made idiotype specific by absorption with BN IgG-coated columns, and was also absorbed with BN kidney homogenate [28]. The anti-idiotypic reactivity was tested by fluid phase double antibody radioimmunoassay using the radiolabeled rat anti-TBM antibody IgG idiotype as the probe. Using such an assay, reactivity could be demonstrated with the idiotype but not with normal BN IgG or purified rat anti-thyroglobulin antibody as controls. Similarly, no reactivity was found within preimmune rabbit serum. The reactivity of the anti-idiotype was suggested to be at or near the antigen binding site because unlabeled idiotype was successful in inhibiting the anti-idiotype radioimmunoassay in a dose response fashion. Since the inhibition was incomplete, it was suggested that some heterogeneity in the anti-TBM antibody idiotype population was present. The controls were unable to inhibit the reaction. The anti-idiotypic antibody did not react with renal bound BN anti-TBM antibody when studied by indirect immunofluorescence, again suggesting that the idiotype and antigen binding sites were closely associated.

Of interest, F(ab')$_2$ fragments of the rabbit anti-idiotypic antibody were reactive with the surface of a small percentage of splenic lymphocytes from bovine TBM immunized BN rats but not from rats given a variety of other immunizations [28]. The surface staining could be largely inhibited by prior treatment of the spleen cells with BN CS TBM antigen, again indicating the idiotypic site was in or near the antigen binding site. The stained cells were largely B cells based on panning experiments to remove B cells from the population. No idiotype-positive cells were found in the renal interstitial infiltrates by indirect immunofluorescence on renal tissue sections. This may reflect the low number of B cells present in the infiltrate population.

The effects of the anti-idiotypic antibody on the anti-TBM antibody response and induction of tubulointerstitial nephritis were studied by intravenous administration of the antibody 48 hrs before the usual immunization to induce BN rat tubulointerstitial nephritis [28]. Normal rabbit serum or saline served as controls. The anti-idiotypic antibody treatment resulted in no demonstrable effect on the anti-bovine particulate or anti-bovine CS TBM antibody responses, with results comparable to those seen in rats given the control injections. On the other hand, the anti-BN TBM response to BN CS TBM antigens was selectively and significantly blunted, especially early in the course of the immune response. The extent to which the anti-BN CS TBM antibody response was diminished by the anti-idiotypic antibody treatment could be correlated with the impairment of induction of the BN rat tubulointerstitial nephritis. Rats forming less than 3 μg/ml of this antibody were protected compared to the controls or treated rats forming greater amounts (greater than 3 μg) of anti-BN CS TBM antibody.

The importance of the anti-BN CS TBM antibody in this model has been further confirmed in recent studies. When TBM antigen-negative Lewis rats are immunized with TBM antigen-positive renal basement membrane, two interesting things happen. First, the Lewis rats develop an unique kind of nodular granulomatous tubulointerstitial nephritis. This lesion appears to have a cellular mechanism and is easily transferable to other Lewis rats with Lewis lymphoid cells, which can be demonstrated to be sensitized to the BN antigen [29]. The second interesting feature, and the one relevant to the present discussion, is that Lewis rats also make a very high titer of alloantibody responsive to BN rat TBM antigens, of which anti-BN CS TBM antibody is a prominent component [23]. As little as 3 ml of this alloreactive antibody can transfer tubulointerstitial nephritis to BN rats within 24–30 hrs. In kinetic studies, the binding of this Lewis anti-BN TBM antibody slowly increases over 6 days. This is in contrast to fixation of antibodies such as those reactive with the glomerular basement membrane, in which binding is very rapid, occurring over minutes and reaching a maximum within a few hours after administration. It can be calculated that about 170 μg of antibody fixation per gram of kidney is required for induction of tubulointerstitial inflammation after this transfer [23]. This is somewhat more than twice that needed for anti-GBM antibody fixation to induce inflammation in rat glomeruli [30]. As might be expected, the transferred lesion in the BN rat is complement dependent [23], as is a major portion of the actively induced disease (Ulich, T.R., Bannister, K.M., and Wilson, C.B., in preparation), again suggesting a role for antibody in this particular model.

The use of anti-idiotypic immunity, then, has provided supportive evidence for demonstrating the role of antibody in induction of tubulointerstitial nephritis in the rat. One could logically ask if anti-idiotypic antibodies are normally involved in the control of the anti-TBM antibody response in this model. In this regard, auto-anti-idiotypic antibodies have not been demonstrated in these rats as yet. Neilson et al. [31] have recently suggested that the production of auto-anti-idiotypes is limited by cyclophosphamide-sensitive suppressor cell set that develops in rats after immunization. In a somewhat different murine TBM tubulointerstitial nephritis model, Neilson et al. [32], have published data suggesting that an idiotype-positive suppressor T cell system can be used to modulate the disease process. Although the anti-idiotype studies and recent transfer studies clearly demonstrate a role for antibody in the BN tubulointerstitial nephritis model, any additional contribution of cellular immunity remains to be quantified. In another anti-basement membrane antibody response to glomerular basement membrane antigens associated with mercuric chloride toxicity in BN rats, anti-idiotypic immunity has been suggested to play a role in the transient anti-glomerular basement membrane antibody response [33].

The idiotype network has been used experimentally to modify the systemic lupus erythematosus (SLE)-like disease of the NZB/W F_1 hybrid mice [34]. By treating 4–6 wk old mice with repeated injections of a monoclonal antibody to double stranded DNA, specific suppression of autoantibodies to double but not single stranded DNA was identified [35]. The suppressive effect was associated with the appearance of antibodies to the idiotype of the immunizing anti-DNA monoclonal antibody. The mice were partially protected from proliferative nephritis. In additional experiments by the same group [36], treatment of 20 wk old mice with a monoclonal anti-idiotypic antibody significantly delayed the onset of glomerulonephritis with a corresponding improvement in the survival rate over that in controls.

It is then clear that at least some auto-antibodies can be controlled experimentally using anti-idiotypic immunity. In spite of the fact that humoral autoimmune responses are usually polyclonal, it has been clearly demonstrated that autoantibodies do share idiotypy, even when they recognize different epitopes on the same antigen [37–39]. Thus it may be possible to down regulate idiotype-bearing autoreactive antibody clones via this complementarity. Whether suppression of the nephritogenic autoantibody formation is via functional inactivation of B lymphocytes or through the activation of T suppressor cells has not been fully determined. The true value of anti-idiotypic antibody immunosuppression in terms of therapeutic potential in human nephritogenic antibody responses remains the subject of future research endeavors.

Idiotype-Auto-Anti-Idiotype Reactions Contributing to Immune Complex Forms of Renal Injury

We now will turn to a discussion of idiotype anti-idiotype reactions in experimental immune complex types of glomerular injury. The concept that idiotype anti-idiotype antibody reactions could contribute to immune deposits and subsequently to the phlogogenic stimulus responsible for the renal damage produced by these deposits is a concept with some experimental support [40]. Anti-idiotypic antibodies are a natural occurrence during any immune response, and idiotype-anti-idiotype complexes would be expected to be a normal sequela. Naturally occurring idiotype-anti-idiotype complexes have been found in the serum of health subjects [41]. In mixed cryoglobulinemia, the IgM fraction has been shown to contain idiotype-anti-idotype complexes [42]. The natural formation of circulating idiotype-anitidiotype complexes has also been defined in BALB/c mice immunized with pneumococcus vaccine which bears phosphorycholine as a major antigenic determinant [43]. A similar immune response occurs when the mice are infected with *Trypanosoma brucei brucei* [44]. BALB/c mice produce antiphosphorycholine antibodies expressing the cross-reacting idiotype termed T-15. In this system, idiotype-anti-idiotype immune complexes can be found. The possible pathogenic role of the idiotype-anti-idiotype complexes has been the subject of several studies. Using the phosphorycholine system, the generation of idiotype-anti-idiotype complexes in the kidney was demonstrated after polyclonal B cell activation using bacterial lipopolysaccharide [45]. Elutions and immunofluorescence studies confirmed the presence of anti-idiotype-bearing immunoglobulins and anti-idiotypic antibodies within the glomeruli of mice treated with lipopolysaccharide. In our own studies using chronic serum sickness in rabbits, auto-anti-idiotypic antibodies were also found in glomeruli, as will be described shortly.

First, it should be stressed in thinking about immune complex formation and tissue deposition that the dynamics of antigen-antibody reactions with interchange of antigen or antibody with previously deposited complexes must always be kept in mind [17]. Rheumatoid factors and complement activation may also affect the dynamics of the interaction. The latter, in some instances, may favor immune complex solubilization. Auto-anti-idiotypic antibodies could conceivably also contribute. The evidence for dynamic interchange of antigen and antibody within glomerular immune deposits is severalfold. Glomerular immune complex deposits can be quantitatively dissolved by antigen excess treatment [46]. We have recently shown that antigen and antibody interchange within glomerular immune deposits can be quantitatively shown to relate to the antigen:antibody ratio that has been present in the environment of the deposits prior to exposure to either antigen or antibody (Wilson, C.B., in preparation). In this situation, complexes having been in antibody excess preferentially interchange better with antigen than with antibody, and complexes in antigen excess interact better with antibody than antigen. We have also shown by transplanting normal kidneys into rabbits with chronic serum sickness, and then subsequently exposing the two kinds of kidneys to the same circulating load of immune complex material, that radiolabeled bovine serum albumin (BSA) containing immune complexes selectively localizes in the rabbit's own nephritic kidney (Ward, D.M., Lee, S., and Wilson, C.B., submitted). This demonstrates the probable effects of local factors, presumably via antigen-antibody dynamic interaction, leading to the continuing accumulation of immune complexes preferentially once immune complex localization begins.

To study the role of auto-anti-idiotypic antibodies in the chronic serum sickness model, inbred III/J rabbits were chosen to avoid problems in interpretation due to immunoglobulin allotypes [47]. Rabbits were immunized daily with BSA in amounts appropriate to match their antibody production as measured weekly by the P80 radioactive precipitin method. Serum was obtained on day 15 for preparation of anti-BSA idiotype. This idiotype was used to induce a control homologous anti-idiotypic antibody. The idiotype was also used as an enzyme-linked probe to detect anti-idiotypic antibody using an ELISA technique. The donor of the idiotype was continued on daily immunization until nephritis developed and its serum and kidney eluates were tested for auto-anti-idiotypic antibody reactivity. The anti-BSA idiotype was isolated by affinity chromatography and cleared of any BSA and BSA-anti-BSA complexes. $F(ab')_2$ fragments were made from the idiotype and used throughout the experiment. The anti-idiotypic antibody prepared by immunization with these $F(ab')_2$ fragments was rendered idiotype specific by absorption with homologous preimmune serum. The idiotype binding site appeared to be outside the antigen binding site because excess BSA did not inhibit the reaction of the anti-idiotype. The anti-idiotype also did not bind BSA. Cross-reactive anti-idiotypes were found among other BSA-immunized III/J rabbits. Auto-anti-idiotypic antibodies became detectable in the circulation by 27 days of BSA immunization. The auto-anti-idiotype was detected using a solid phase radioimmunoassay in which wells were coated with $F(ab')_2$ fragments of the idiotype. Any bound anti-idiotype was detected with radiolabeled Fc-specific anti-rabbit immunoglobulin antibody. The auto-anti-idiotypic antibody reactivity was much less than the syngeneic anti-idiotype binding produced by immunizing other III/J rabbits with the $F(ab')_2$ idiotype fragment. An acid renal eluate was prepared from the nephritic kidneys of a III/J rabbit 35 days after immunization. Any contaminating BSA and unassociated BSA-containing immune complexes were removed by passage through a Blue/Sepharose/CM-6B column. An IgG fraction was obtained from the eluate by sucrose density gradient and ultracentrifugation under acid conditions to further reduce contamination with BSA-containing immune complexes. Finally, a blocking step was included in the ELISA assay to rule out binding of the anti-BSA idiotype probe to any residual BSA in the eluate that may have evaded the other purification steps. This was done by using a rat anti-BSA antibody to block the wells prior to probing with the anti-BSA idiotype. Using this assay system, it was then possible to demonstrate that the eluted immunoglobulin reacted with the anti-BSA idiotype probe even after blocking with the rat anti-BSA antibody, demonstrating the presence of an auto-anti-idiotype within the eluate.

Autologous anti-idiotypic antibodies can appropriately be added to the growing list of factors that may influence the dynamics of glomerular immune complex formation, rearrangement, and resolution. The phlogogenic role of auto-anti-idiotypic antibodies incorporated into the glomerular immune complex deposit is unknown. It is of interest that 4–6 wks of daily exposure to circulating immune complexes are needed before glomerular immune complex accumulation rapidly accelerates and proteinuria begins in this model [46]. The late appearance of auto-anti-idiotypic antibody coincides temporally with this change in pathogenicity of the daily immune complex load, and may in some way contribute to the accelerated accumulation.

Summary

The recognition of antigenic structurally determined differences among antibody molecules led to the identification of the idiotype-anti-idiotype network important in the regulation of the immune system. The idiotype network can influence immunologically induced immune renal injury in at least two very different ways, either by influencing the specific nephritogenic immune response or by directly contributing to immune deposition. This discussion will review studies we have done to address these two issues. First, the anti-idiotypic control of the immune response was used to help identify the importance of the particular anti-tubular basement membrane antibody immune response involved in the induction of experimental tubulo-interstitial nephritis in rats. Second, the production of auto-anti-idiotypic antibodies was studied in experimental chronic serum sickness in rabbits and the contribution of these antibodies to the glomerular immune deposit was established. In the latter model, the anti-idiotypic antibody may be important in influencing the dynamics of immune complex formation, tissue accumulation and rearrangement, and may add to the phlogogenic potential of the immune complex deposition.

Acknowledgments

This is publication No. 4176-IMM from the Department of Immunology, Scripps Clinic and Research Foundation, La Jolla, California 92037. This work was supported in part by United States Public Health Service Grants AI07007, AM20043, AM32353, AG04342, T32-AG00080, and Biomedical Research Support Grant RRO-5514. Dr. Bannister was the recipient of a fellowship from the National Kidney Foundation.

References

1. Oudin J and Michel M: Une nouvelle forme d'allotypie des globulines du sérum de lapin apparamment liée à la fonction et a la spécificité anticorps, CR Acad Sci 257:805–808, 1963.
2. Kunkel HG, Mannik M and Williams RC: Individual antigenic specificity of isolated antibodies. Science 140:1218–1219, 1963.
3. Lindenmann J: Speculations on idiotypes and homobodies. Ann Immunol (Paris) 125: 373–389, 1974.
4. Jerne NK: Towards a network theory of the immune system. Ann Immunol (Paris) 125:373–389, 1974.
5. Nisonoff A and Lamoyi E: Hypothesis. Implications of the presence of an internal image of the antigen in anti-idiotypic antibodies: Possible application to vaccine production. Clin Immunol Immunopathol 21:397–406, 1981.
6. Sacks DL, Esser KM and Sher A: Immunization of mice against African trypanosomiasis using anti-idiotypic antibodies. J Exp Med 155:1108–1119, 1982.
7. Uytdehaag FGCM Osterhaus ADME: Induction of neutralizing antibody in mice against poliovirus type II with monoclonal anti-idiotypic antibody. J Immunol 134:1225–1229, 1985.
8. Jerne NK: Idiotypic networks and other preconceived ideas. Immunol Rev 79:5–24, 1984.
9. Bona CA and Pernis B: Idiotypic networks. In: Fundamental Immunology. Ed. WE Paul. Raven Press, New York, pp 577–592, 1984.
10. Eichmann K: Expression and function of idiotypes on lymphocytes. Adv Immunol 26: 195–254, 1978.
11. Binz, H and Wigzell H: Successful induction of specific tolerance to transplantation antigens using autoimmunisation against the recipient's own, natural antibodies. Nature 262: 294–295, 1976.
12. Zanetti M: Idiotype network and its relevance to autoimmune diseases. Functional considerations. In: Concepts in Immunopathology, Vol. 3. Eds. Cruse JM and Lewis RE, Jr. Karger, New York, in press, 1985.
13. Paul WE and Bona C: Regulatory idiotypes and immune networks: A hypothesis. Immunol Today 3:230–234, 1982.
14. Strosberg AD: Auto-idiotype and anti-hormone receptor antibodies. Springer Semin. Immunopathol 6:67–78, 1983.
15. Zanetti M and Rogers J: Induction of autoreactivity by anti-idiotypic antibodies. In: Regulation of the Immune System, Vol. 18. Eds. Sercarz E, Cantor H and Chess L. Alan R. Liss, New York, pp 893-907, 1984.
16. Zanetti M and Katz DH: Self recognition, autoimmunity and internal images. In: Current Topics in Microbiology and Immunology. Eds. Koprowski H and Melchers F. Springer-Verlag, New York, in press, 1985.
17. Wilson CB and Dixon FJ: The renal response to immunological injury. In: The Kidney, 3rd Edition. Brenner BM and Rector FC, Jr. (Eds) Saunders, Philadelphia, pp 800–889, 1986.
18. Zanetti M and Wilson CB: A role for anti-idiotypic antibodies in immunologically mediated nephritis. Am J Kidney Dis, in press, 1986.

19. Neilson EG and Zakheim B: T cell regulation, anti-idiotypic immunity, and the nephritogenic immune response. Kidney Int 24:289–302, 1983.
20. Lehman DH, Wilson CB and Dixon FJ: Interstitial nephritis in rats immunized with heterologous tubular basement membrane. Kidney Int 5:187–195, 1974.
21. Mampaso FM and Wilson CB: Characterization of inflammatory cells in autoimmune tubulointerstitial nephritis in rats. Kidney Int 23:448–457, 1983.
22. Ulich TR, Bannister KM and Wilson CB: Tubulointerstitial nephritis induced in the Brown Norway rat with chaotropically solubilized bovine tubular basement membrane: The model and the humoral and cellular responses. Clin Immunol Immunopathol 36:187–200, 1985.
23. Bannister KM and Wilson CB: Transfer of tubulointerstitial nephritis in the Brown-Norway rat with anti-tubular basement membrane antibody: quantitation and kinetics of binding and effect of decomplementation. J Immunol, in press, 1985.
24. Lehman DH and Wilson CB: Role of sensitized cells in antitubular basement membrane interstitial nephritis. Int Archs Allergy Appl Immunol 51:168–174, 1976.
25. Zanetti M and Wilson CB: Characterization of anti-tubular basement membrane antibodies in rats. J Immunol 130:2173–2179, 1983.
26. Brown CA, Carey K and Colvin RB: Inhibition of autoimmune tubulointerstitial nephritis in guinea pigs by heterologous antisera containing antiidiotype antibodies. J Immunol 123:2101–2107, 1979.
27. Neilson EG and Phillips SM: Suppression of interstitial nephritis by auto-anti-idiotypic immunity. J Exp Med 155:179–189, 1982.
28. Zanetti M, Mampaso F and Wilson CB: Anti-idiotype as a probe in the analysis of autoimmune tubulointerstitial nephritis in the Brown Norway rat. J Immunol 131:1268–1273, 1983.
29. Bannister KM, Ulich TR and Wilson CB: Cell-mediated autoimmune tubulo-interstitial nephritis (TIN) in the Lewis (LEW) rat. Kidney Int (Abstr.) 27:205, 1985.
30. Unanue ER and Dixon FJ: Experimental glomerulonephritis. V. Studies on the interaction of nephrotoxic antibodies with tissues of the rat. J Exp Med 122:697–714, 1965.
31. Neilson EG, McCafferty, E, Phillips SM, Clayman MD and Kelly CJ: Anti-idiotypic immunity in interstitial nephritis. II. rats developing anti-tubular basement membrane disease fail to make an anti-idiotypic regulatory response: the modulatory role of an RT 7.1$^+$, OX 8− suppressor T cell mechanism. J Exp Med 159:1009–1026, 1984.
32. Neilson EG, McCafferty E, Mann R, Michaud L and Clayman M: Tubular antigen-derivatized cells induce a disease-protective, antigen-specific, and idiotype-specific T cell network restricted by I-J and Igh-V in mice with experimental interstitial nephritis. J Exp Med 162:215–230, 1985.
33. Chalopin JM and Lockwood CM: Autoregulation of autoantibody synthesis in mercuric chloride nephritis in the Brown Norway rat. II. Presence of antigen-augmentable plaque-forming cells in the spleen is associated with humoral factors behaving as auto-anti-idiotypic antibodies. Eur J Immunol 14:470–475, 1984.
34. Hahn BH: Suppression of autoimmune diseases with antiidiotype antiidiotypic antibodies: Murine lupus nephritis as a model. Springer Semin Immunopathol 7:25–34, 1984.
35. Hahn BH and Ebling FM: Suppression of NZB/NZW murine nephritis by administration of a syngeneic monoclonal antibody to DNA. Possible role of anti-idiotypic antibodies. J Clin Invest 71:1728–1736, 1983.
36. Hahn BH and Ebling FM: Suppression of murine lupus nephritis by administration of an anti-idiotypic antibody to anti-DNA. J Immunol 132:187–190, 1984.
37. Andrejewski C Jr, Rauch J, Lafer E, Stollar BD and Schwartz RS: Antigen-binding diversity and idiotype cross-reactions among hybridoma autoantibodies to DNA. J Immunol 126:226–231, 1980.
38. Zanetti M, DeBaets M and Rogers J: High degree of idiotypic cross-reactivity among murine monoclonal antibodies to thyroglobulin. J Immunol 131:2452–2457, 1983.

39. Hahn BH and Ebling FM: A public idiotypic determinant is present on spontaneous cationic IgG antibodies to DNA from mice of unrelated lupus-prone strains. J Immunol 133:3015-3019, 1984.
40. Goldman M, Renversez JC and Lambert PH: Pathological expression of idiotypic interactions: Immune complexes and cryoglobulins. Springer Semin Immunopathol 6:33-49, 1983.
41. Morgan AC Jr, Rossen RD and Twomey JJ: Naturally occurring circulating immune complexes: Normal human serum contains idiotype-anti-idiotype complexes dissociable by certain IgG antiglobulins. J Immunol 122:1672-1680, 1979.
42. Geltner D, Franklin EC and Frangione B: Anti-idiotypic activity in the IgM fraction of mixed cryoglobulins. J Immunol 125:1530-1535, 1980.
43. Rose LM and Lambert PH: The natural occurrence of circulating idiotype-anti-idiotype complexes during a secondary immune response to phosphorylcholine. Clin Immunol Immunopathol 15:481-492, 1980.
44. Rose LM, Goldman M and Lambert PH: Simultaneous induction of an idiotype, corresponding anti-idiotypic antibodies, and immune complexes during African trypanosomiasis in mice. J Immunol 128:79-85, 1982.
45. Goldman M, Rose LM, Hochmann A and Lambert PH: Deposition of idiotype-anti-idiotype immune complexes in renal glomeruli after polyclonal B cell activation. J Exp Med 155:1385-1399, 1982.
46. Wilson CB and Dixon FJ: Quantitation of acute and chronic serum sickness in the rabbit. J Exp Med 134:7s-18s, 1971.
47. Zanetti M and Wilson CB: Participation of auto-anti-idiotypes in immune complex glomerulonephritis in rabbits. J Immunol 131:2781-2783, 1983.

7. Experimental analysis of the generation of pathogenic immune complexes resulting from immonoblogulin interactions

P.H. LAMBERT, S. IZUI, Y. GYOTOKU, M. ABDELMOULA
and F. SPERTINI

Immune complexes (IC) resulting from specific interactions between immunoglobulin molecules probably represent the most important source of IC.

In the last few years, a number of experimental models have been developed in mice allowing us to analyze the potential pathogenic effect of such IC. First, some strains with spontaneous antibodies and by a massive cryoglobulinemia. Second, mice undergoing polyclonal B cell activation after injection of LPS or during parasitic infections may develop idiotype-anti-idiotype IC. In these two situations, it has been possible to evaluate the pathogenic potential of IC resulting from interactions between immunoglobulin molecules.

I. Generation of pathogenic IC resulting from Ig interactions in mice bearing the 1pr gene

Recently, high levels of rheumatoid factor (RF) have been found in a murine strain, MRL-1pr/1pr. These mice, in addition to lupus-like syndrome, spontaneously develop serologic and pathologic abnormalities that closely resemble those in patients with Rheumatoid arthritis (RA) [1]. Their sera contain not only RF but also intermediate-sized IC [2] similar to those found in the sera and synovial fluids of some patients with RA. MRL-1pr/1pr mice develop large amounts of cryoglobulins which parallel the production of RF [1]. The availability of such a murine strain provides a unique opportunity to analyze the role of RF for the formation of IC and cryoglobulins and eventually for the development of tissue lesions.

The autosomal recessive mutant gene, 1pr, was first observed in the 12th generation of brother × sister mating, while developing the MRL strain from a series of crosses involving strains AKR/J, C57BL/6J, C3H/Di and LG/J [3]. The expression of this 1pr gene in MRL mice (MRL-1pr/1pr) leads to massive generalized lymph node enlargement due to the proliferation of T cells. Such lymphadenopathy is notably associated with early onset of fatal systemic lupus erythematous (SLE) with 50% mortality at 5.5 mo of age, while MRL$-+/+$ mice lacking the lpr mutation have no lymphoproliferation and develop SLE in their second year of life. Thus, lpr gene product(s) may be capable of turning the late onset of SLE into an early, acute, fatal disease. To further study the role of the lpr/lpr gene on the development of autoimmune disease, the lpr gene was transferred from the MRL strain to three different non-autoimmune strains such as C3H/HeJ (C3H), C57BL/6J (B6) and AKR/J by multiple cross-intercross matings followed by brother × sister inbreeding. In the presence of the lpr gene, the C3H, B6 and AKR strains were able to produce spontaneously different kinds of autoantibodies including antibodies to double-stranded DNA, single-stranded DNA, thymocytes and a serum glycoprotein, gp70 [4]. Although levels and types of autoantibodies induced by the lpr gene were quite different among the strains, it is clear that the action of the lpr gene on the development of autoantibody response does not require the particular abnormalities of the MRL genome. Clearly, the lpr gene not only accelerates the progression of autoimmune disease inherent in the MRL background but also initiates the autoimmune response in mice without the predisposition to SLE. The difference in expression of autoantibody formation among the strains bearing the lpr gene is certainly a reflection of the difference in the background genome of the strain.

IgM RF could be relatively easily induced in various strains of mice as a result of polyclonal B cell activation [5] or of a secondary immune response against IgG-containing IC [6, 7]. Spontaneous production of IgM RF has been also described in a colony of the murine strain 129/Sv [8]. Such a production has not been associated with any apparent pathological changes. In contrast, MRL-lpr/lpr mice have been shown to produce high titers of IgG RF as well as IgM RF. Since only MRL-lpr/lpr mice among the SLE-prone mice develop arthritic changes resembling RA [1], IgG RF may be related to the development of the arthritic lesions found.

The presence of intermediate-sized IgG RF-containing IC in sera from MRL-lpr/lpr mice was first suggested by the presence of a unique interaction between two different individual MRL mouse sera: one serum forms a precipitin line in gels with another serum from a different mouse [2]. Intermediate-sized complexes of IgG, sedimenting between 7S and 19S and presumably containing IgG RF, were found to be reactants causing these precipitin interactions. Recently, such IgG RF IC were isolated from sera from MRL-lpr/lpr mice by affinity chromatography with agarose-mouse IgG columns. Apparently, IgG RF isolated from MRL-lpr/lpr mice underwent concentration dependent self-association similar to those from patients with RA [9].

In order to facilitate the detection of IgG RF, particularly those which had already formed IC, a new radioimmunoassay (RIA) has been developed. In this RIA, sera are first treated with acetate buffer pH 3.5 for 1 h at 37 °C and for 2 h at room temperature to dissociate RF IC present in the sera. ^{125}I-labelled mouse IgG (MGG) is added before adjusting to pH 7.2 with Tris, and the mixture is then incubated overnight at 4 °C. ^{125}I-MGG bound to RF is precipitated with 7% polyethylene glycol, which would not precipitate free ^{125}I-MGG. As control, sera are incubated with ^{125}I-MGG under neutral pH condition. Using this acid treatment the binding activity to ^{125}I-MGG was enhanced in sera from MRL-lpr/lpr mice. However, only a slight increase was observed in sera from non-autoimmune strains of mice such as C57BL/6, BALB/c or C3H. Sucrose density gradient analysis have demonstrated that the significant binding activity to ^{125}I-MGG was only detectable in intermediate fractions but not in 19S and 7S fractions. This indicates that almost all the IgG RF in sera were present as IgG-IgG RF IC.

Among several SLE-prone autoimmune mice, MRL-lpr/lpr mice are the only strain that spontaneously develop high titers of RF. The fact that MRL − +/+ mice lacking the lpr gene failed to develop RF suggests that the lpr gene enhances the production of RF similar to other autoantibodies such as anti-DNA or anti-serum gp70 antibodies. Further, C3H and B6 mice without apparent background for autoimmune diseases were shown to produce high titers of RF when the lpr gene was transferred from the MRL strain to these strains of mice. This further supports that this autoimmune response is not a unique product of the MRL genome, and the production of RF may be closely associated with the expression of the lpr gene.

Several strains of mice which spontaneously develop SLE-like syndrome also form significant amounts of cryoglobulins and the highest level have been found in MRL-lpr/lpr mice. Cryoglobulins have also been demonstrated in C3H and B6 mice bearing the lpr gene. It is significant that the sole or major components of cryoglobulins from lpr mice are immunoglobulins and that the concentration of IgG in cryoglobulins was 30 times greater than the concentration of IgM. Furthermore, the IgG3 subclass was markedly enriched in cryoglobulins as compared with other IgG subclasses and IgM.

Of interest, we have recently found that 18 monoclonal IgG RF derived from MRL-lpr/lpr mice were all IgG3. Further, BALB/c mice injected with some hybridomas secreting IgG3 RF developed substantial amounts of cryoglobulins in ascites and sera. These results suggest that the IgG3 RF represents the major source of cryoglobulins occurring in lpr mice. In addition, it was seen that normal mice bearing one of the IgG3-RF hybridomas developed extensive pathological manifestations within a few days, including peripheral vasculitis and glomerulonephritis. This observation provide a good basis to study the pathogenesis of cryoglobulin-associated lesions.

The exact molecular nature of Ig interactions responsible for cryoglobulin formation remains unclear. IgG3 RF may have a tendency to form larger sized self-associating RF complexes because these complexes would not be subjected to complement-dependent solubilization. IgG3 can also relatively easily form microaggregates [10] and this physicochemical characteristic would certainly facilitate the precipitation of IgG3 RF complexes at 4 °C. Obviously, more sophisticated biochemical and immunochemical analysis on immunoglobulins in cryoglobulins from mice receiving monoclonal IgG3 RF would help elucidate the molecular mechanisms responsible for the formation of cryoglobulins.

II. Generation of pathogenic IC resulting from idiotypic interactions

Interactions between immunoglobulin molecules occurring through complementary sites in hypervariable regions have been observed during natural immune responses and polyclonal B cell activation and have been shown to contribute to the generation of soluble or cryoprecipitable complexes.

There is evidence that auto-anti-idiotypic antibodies may occur during the course of an immune response, with a specificity for the major idiotypic determinants of the antibodies resulting from this immune response. The reaction of anti-idiotypic antibodies with immunoglobulin molecules bearing corresponding idiotypes leads in such situations, to the formation of idiotype-anti-idiotype immune complexes [11]. Some conditions are characterized by repeated antigenic stimulations. It is possible that, in these situations, the frequent reinduction of antigen-specific antibodies and of their corresponding anti-idiotypic of antibodies could result in the formation of pathogenic idiotype-anti-idiotype complexes. The occurrence of circulating idiotype-anti-idiotype immune complexes does not depend directly on the presence in the circulation of a given antigen and thus idiotypic interactions leading to the formation of immune complexes may persist after elimination of the antigen inducing the initial immune response.

The possible role of idiotypic interactions in the pathogenesis of IC diseases was particularly studied in experimental situations where pathogenic IC were formed in association with polyclonal B cell activation. Indeed, the non-specific triggering of the B cell repertoire induced by B cell mitogens, such as bacterial lipopolysaccharides, or naturally occurring in the course of certain parasitic diseases (African trypanosomiasis, malaria) is often associated with the generation of circulating immune complexes [12, 13] and with the development of immune complex-mediated tissue lesions. In these situations, a wide variety of antibodies is produced, including antibodies directed against certain haptens, heterologous proteins, and also certain autoantigens. Thus, we have investigated whether polyclonal B cell activation could trigger the production of auto-anti-idiotypic antibodies and, if so, whether the reaction of these antibodies with immunoglobulin molecules bearing corresponding idiotypic specificities could lead to the formation of idiotype-anti-idiotype immune complexes. To test this hypothesis, polyclonal B cell activation was induced in BALB/c mice by injection of bacterial LPS, and the spleens of these mice were assayed for antibody-producing cells to phosphorylcholine (PC), to TEPC-15 myeloma protein (anti-PC), and to other myeloma proteins [14]. We found that LPS injection results in a triggering of both anti-PC and anti-TEPC-15 antibody producing cells. Anti-PC antibodies could be detected in the circulation and the majority of these antibodies was found to bear the T15 idiotype. The simultaneous production of anti-T15 idiotype antibodies were shown to lead to the formation of idiotype-anti-idiotype immune complexes. It is clear that T15 idiotype immune complexes represent only a fraction of the immune complexes formed in BALB/c mice after LPS injection or during experimental trypanosomiasis. However, polyclonal B cell activation is known to stimulate a wide variety of B cell clones and one may consider that a certain proportion of these clones produced antibodies able to react with idiotypic determinants of immunoglobulins produced by other clones that have been simultaneously triggered.

Immune complexes formed after injection of bacterial LPS in mice are responsible for the development of an immune complex glomerulonephritis. Therefore, BALB/c mice were studied for a possible renal deposition of T15 idiotype-anti-T15 idiotype immune complexes after injection of bacterial LPS [15]. Using immunofluorescence, we first investigated whether rabbit anti-T15 idiotype antibodies could detect T15 idiotype-bearing immunoglobulins within the immune complexes deposited in the renal glomeruli. From day 6 to day 28 after LPS injection, rabbit anti-T15 idiotype antibodies were found to react with molecules deposited in a granular fashion in the glomeruli, suggesting a glomerular deposition of immunoglobulins bearing the T15 idiotype. Further evidence for a glomerular deposition of T15 idiotype-anti-T15 idiotype immune complexes was obtained by the analysis of kidney eluates from mice injected 18 days earlier with LPS. An idiotype specific reaction of the eluates with the TEPC-15 myeloma protein was seen, indicating the presence of anti-T15 idiotype antibodies in the kidney eluates. Therefore, the potential role of idiotypic interactions in the pathogenesis of renal lesions should certainly be considered.

Similar idiotypic interactions may also be involved in the generation of cryoglobulins. Thus, in mice infected with Plasmodium yoelli, the peak of parasitemia (days 8–12) was associated with a five to six fold increase of Ig levels, with the occurrence of circulating IC and with the presence of cryoglobulins in serum. These cryoglobulins consisted mainly of IgM and IgG3, including trace amounts of anti-malaria antibodies [16]. Cryoglobulins were dissociated by ultracentrifugation on acid sucrose gradients and the reactivity of their Ig components was analyzed. The majority of IgG molecules of such cryoglobulin fractions could reassociate with the corresponding IgM fractions but acid-treated IgG from normal mouse serum did not react with these IgM. These mice also produced a variety of anti-immunoglobulin antibodies. It is conceivable that cryoglobulins would contain the most avid idiotype-anti-idiotype pairs, possibly involving anti-malarial antibodies.

Acknowledgement

This work was supported by the Swiss National Foundation (grant no 3.826.0.83 and 3.621.0.84) and by the Swiss Confederation on the proposal of the 'Commission Fédérale des Maladies Rhumatismales'.

References

1. Andrews BS, Eisenberg RA, Theofilopoulos AN, Izui S, Wilson CB, McConahey PJ, Murphy ED, Roths JB, Dixon FJ: Spontaneous murine lupus-like syndromes. Clinical and immunopathological manifestations in several strains. J Exp Med 148:1198–1215, 1978.
2. Eisenberg RA, Thor LT, Dixon FJ: Serum-serum interactions in autoimmune mice. Arthritis Rheum 22:1074–1081, 1979.
3. Murphy ED, Roths JB: Autoimmunity and lymphoproliferation: induction by mutant gene lpr, and acceleration by a male-associated factor in strain BXSB mice. "Genetic Control of Autoimmune Disease" NR Rose, PE Bigazzi and NL Warner, eds, Elsevier/North Holland, New York, 207–219, 1978.
4. Izui S, Kelley VE, Masuda K, Yoshida H, Roths JB, Murphy ED: Induction of various autoantibodies by mutant gene lpr in several strains of mice. J Immunol 133:227–233, 1984.
5. Izui S, Eisenberg RA, Dixon FJ: IgM rheumatoid factors in mice injected with bacterial lipopolysaccharides. J Immunol 122:2096–2102, 1979.
6. Nemazee AA, Sato VL: Induction of rheumatoid antibodies in mouse. Regulated production of autoantibody in the secondary humoral response. J Exp Med 158:529–545, 1983.
7. Van Snick JL, Gulie P: Rheumatoid factors and secondary immune responses in the mouse. I. Frequent occurrence of hybridomas secreting IgM anti-IgGl autoantibodies after immunization with protein antigens. Eur J Immunol 13:890–894, 1983.
8. Van Snick JL, Masson PL: Age-dependent production of IgA and IgM autoantibodies against IgG2a in a colony of 129/Sv mice. J Exp Med 149:1519–1530, 1979.
9. Nardella FA, Teller DC, Izui S, Mannik M: Self-associating IgG rheumatoid factors in MRL/1 autoimmune mice. Arthritis Rheum 27:1165, 1984.
10. Grey HM, Hirst JW, Cohn M: A new mouse immunoglobulin IgG3. J Exp Med 133:289–304, 1971.
11. Rose LM, Lambert PH: The natural occurrence of circulating idiotype-anti-idiotype complexes during a secondary immune response to phosphorylcholine. Clin Immunol Immunopathol 15:481–492, 1980.
12. Lambert PH, Berney M, Kazyumba G: Immune complexes in serum and in cerebrospinal fluid in African trypanosomiasis. Correlation with polyclonal B cell activation and with intracerebral immunoglobulin synthesis. J Clin Invest 67:77–85, 1981.

13. Ramos Niembro F, Fournié G, Lambert PH: Induction of circulating immune complexes and their renal localization after acute or chronic polyclonal B cell activation in mice. Kidney Int. 31 (suppl 11): pp S-29 S-38, 1982.
14. Rose LM, Goldman M, Lambert PH: The production of anti-idiotypic antibodies and of idiotype-anti-idiotype immune complexes following polyclonal activation induced by bacterial LPS. J Immunol 128:2126–2133, 1982.
15. Lambert PH, Morel PA, Renversez JC, Goldman M: Idiotypic interactions and immune complexes in infectious diseases. Progress in Immunology V, 1343–1346, Y Yamamura and T Tada eds, Academic Press, Japan, 1983.

Discussion Part II

WILSON: Dr Naish, as regards rabbits with RF bound in their kidneys, did they have a different kind of histologic lesions? Is there any association with pathogenicity or phlogogenicity in the rabbits that do or do not have this material bound in their kidneys?

NAISH: There was a higher degree of proteinuria, of inflammatory reaction within the glomeruli (polymorphs infiltration) and of deposited immunoglobulins, but it wasn't terribly dramatic though.

MAGGIORE: Dr Naish, did you look for the development of cryoglobulinemia in your rabbits? Did the rabbits treated with penicillin have less proteinuria than the untreated ones and finally, did you try to separate the IgM component in the acid eluate on Sephadex G-200 column and then test it for antiglobulin activity?

NAISH: We did not try to do this experiment because we were actually dealing with a very small amount of material. I take your point that it would be something very much worth doing. We did not look for cryoglobulinemia and the proteinuria disappeared rapidly in the penicillin-treated animals.

PETERS: One comment directed to dr Ford, who showed very elegantly that IgM RF in the kidneys could, under certain circumstances, bind to deposited immune complexes: I think that in real life the sequence of events is much more complicated since it is unlikely that you have this clean system where you have RF bound in the kidney and not any RF present in the circulation: the influence of the RF in the kidney should depend upon how successfully it competes with RF in the circulation, for whatever effect it will have on the distribution of rheumatoid complexes. It is not to say that this model that is described is unimportant, I just want to draw attention to the complexity of the physiologic system that might arise under these circumstances.

FORD: I take your point. When we injected the RF first, it did not prevent the complex from depositing in the glomerulus: one of the features of the RF is that it reacts better with immunoglobulins when they are present on surfaces than when they are suspended in solution. By depositing the complexes you probably increase the reactivity of the RF: we certainly showed that RF would not prevent the complexes from depositing but would react with them, once deposited.

BONA: Dr Ford, I wonder if this phenomenon that you describe is not restricted to a certain population of RFs, because, both in humans and in mice, analyzing the specificity of the RFs you can observe that some are specific only for allotypes like Gm allotypes in humans or gamma 2 a allotypes in mice. There are also RFs which are specific for determinants shared by various subclasses of IgG and finally a third category specific for determinants of immunoglobulins from many species.

FORD: The reason why we used that preparation was indeed because it reacted with immunoglobulins from many species and therefore allowed us to use a number of antibodies from different species as markers in the experiments: we weren't confined to using human immunoglobulins. I take your point though, that there are RF with more restricted reactivity, but in many respects it may be more relevant in this type of study to use a poly-clonal polyspecific antibody rather than a monoclonal one with very re-stricted reactivity. Our RF was after all obtained from patients with clinical illness.

WILLIAMS (London): I'm sure that dr Ford has thought of the dr Naish's experiment which parallels his own- and that is patients with rheumatoid arthritis that have a large amount of circulating rheumatoid factor in whom glomerulonephritis is uncommon. The question really is: does he have any information on the distribution of isoelectric point of RF in patients with rheumatoid arthritis in general, or in particular in those few patients who do get that form of rheumatoid arthritis? And, secondly has he or indeed any-body looked at overtly normal kidneys from patients with rheumatoid arthritis to see if they have IgM-RF deposited therein?

FORD: When you talk about the interaction of the RF and the immune complex in this sort of system, somebody always raises the question of rheumatoid arthritis, which indeed poses a problem as to the pathophysio-logic role of RF in that and other diseases. We did look at some sera from rheumatoid patients and isoelectric point was fairly neutral in the IgM of these patients. We haven't specifically looked at the glomeruli from rheu-matoid arthritis patients for RF activity.

GLASSOCK: I would like to focus on the question raised by dr Wilson at the end of his talk and ask the panelists, or anyone else, about the role of RF in complement mediated solubilization of immune complexes. Is there any active research in that area?

SCHIFFERLI (Geneve): Very little is known about the effect of comple-ment is the time of the reaction between RF and immune complexes *in vivo* in a soluble state. What we know is that RF enhances the formation of insoluble complexes even in the presence of complement. We don't know exactly how it does it. It could either block the effect of complement or perhaps it just increases the size of the complexes.

AGNELLO: We examined the question of whether RF blocked C1q bind-ing and found negative results. I have a question for dr Naish and dr Ford: were the aggregated IgG, used for the staining of the glomeruli, reduced and alkylated?

FORD: No.

AGNELLO: Then how do you rule out reactivity with C1q?

FORD: That was only one of the systems we used as a marker.

AGNELLO: It is an important control because you will find a large amount of C1q in most of those lesions.

SCHIFFERLI (Geneve): Dr Agnello, if you take C1q surely you have no interaction between IgM-RF and IgG. But under normal circumstances C1q is bound in a macromolecular complex with C1r and C1s. The whole C1 blocks the interaction between IgM-RF and IgG. That has been shown by Hällgran using latex particles covered with IgG.

NAISH: Dr Ford, did you find any evidence of inflammation in the glomeruli of those animals in which you orchestrated this enhancement of immune reactants?

FORD: No, we didn't. These are short-term experiments, of course, because our RF is a heterologous antibody and we want to stay within the period before the mouse mounts an antibody response against the human IgM. We did look at another system though, and that was chronic serum sickness in mice. When we took animals with an established but fairly mild chronic serum sickness and gave them RF, it localized in the glomeruli. They got an increased cellularity of the lesion but we weren't able to demonstrate any increase in proteinuria. You often have to do quite an extensive amount of damage in experimental mice to get significant degree of proteinuria without a decrease in EDTA clearance. And, again, the experiment had to be short-term because of the fact that the antibody was heterologous.

LAMBERT: Dr Wilson, did you study the relative clonality of your anti-TBM and anti-BSA antibodies in your model? If so, what would be the proportion of those antibodies recognized by your polyclonal anti-idiotypic antibody? We would also like to know whether the anti-idiotypes react with all your population of molecules reacting with TBM with BSA, or whether you pick up only some major idiotypes.

WILSON: We don't have any more information on this than I gave in the talk.

PETERS: Dr Wilson, following your observation on the late development of proteinuria in the chronic BSA model, I wonder whether you have considered giving the anti-idiotypes to animals, to see whether this does in fact induce proteinuria at an earlier stage.

WILSON: We have not done that with success. We were not able to work out the situation in which we could quantitate enough binding to make this distinction. It's not only the proteinuria that develops late, it is the immune complex accumulation itself that is delayed and develops late. The obvious beautiful experiment, if we had enough of this anti-idiotypic antibody, which in this situation is an auto-anti-idiotypic antibody and magnifies the problem, would be to give it at two or three weeks and see whether one could suddenly change the profile of the whole immune complex localization.

BONA: Let us start with specific questions and discuss together a very important point that was raised by dr Williams: are the rheumatoid factors and in general the auto-antibodies beneficial or deleterious?

MONTAGNINO (Milano): Dr Williams, dr Hahn and dr Ebling reported that the antibodies with anti-DNA activity in the mice with the worst renal lesions were those with the highest isoelectric points. You have found instead that in patients with glomerulonephritis IgG have the lowest isoelectric point. How do you explain this discrepancy?

WILLIAMS (London): I can't explain it as such. That simply has been found in a number of patients. Of course what we were looking at was in the circulation, not in the kidney.

MAGGIORE: In our previous studies we found that the presence of antiglobulins in the kidneys of patients with SLE and cryoglobulinemia was associated with the most severe forms of these diseases: I don't know if it was the antiglobulin to give this degree of severity, but anyway one can say it was not beneficial.

PETERS: Dr Lambert, in relation to the polyclonal activation generated by idiotypic-antiidiotypic reactions, you are arguing that this was the chance consequence of the clonal proliferation of two sets of molecules that happened to react with each other. I wondered why you chose that explanation rather than the conventional one of a response to a clonal proliferation with the generation of an antiidiotype.

LAMBERT: Yes, we choose to be non conventional. If you study antiidiotypes following an immune response induced by a classical antigen, you may observe a sequence ab1-ab2. In all experiments with polyclonal activation we found the two types of antibodies appearing at the same time, within really a few days, starting two days after the injection of the polyclonal activator.

PETERS: Did you look at the antibody forming cells to see whether they have got the same temporal relationship?

LAMBERT: In the reported experiment the antibody-forming cells were indeed measured.

BONA: I don't think that it is a really random process. In our system, in levan antigenic system, we found that the injection of minute amounts of antibodies against regulatory idiotopes activated clones producing antilevan and anti-galactan antibodies. This means that clones with completely different specificities were activated. The antibodies, which have been activated by anti-idiotypes are encoded by active VH genes deriving from the same VH germ line gene family. This means that the activation of clones with various specificities during infections is a complex phenomenon. Thus an ab1 polyclonally stimulated can elicit the synthesis of a complementary anti-idiotype. It is known that anti-idiotype antibodies administered in low amounts have an enhancing effect whereas in high amounts have a suppressive effect. These low amounts can stimulate the clones which are linked through the cross reactive regulatory idiotypes in a 'mini-network' made up of clones encoded by members of the same germ line gene family.

PETERS: Just a very general comment upon the question of whether things are good or bad, in terms of general immunological principles. Those factors that are good for circulating immune complexes to be cleared efficiently by the mononuclear phagocytic system are likely to be bad for the kidney in which immune complexes are localized. For example, the binding of C3b to the surface of an immune complex enhances its reaction with phagocytic cells and promotes its clearance. The binding of C3b to immune complexes in tissue enhances the reaction of inflammatory cells and increases the capacity of that complex to provoke inflammation. In relation to antiglobulins the same general principle can be applied. Thus the extent to which the generation of antiglobulins is protective or harmful depends very much on the predominant localization of the immune complexes, and in disease states both processes might be occurring simultaneously.

D'AMICO: In essential mixed cryoglobulinemia dr Maggiore and ourselves demonstrated the presence of large amounts of RF in the kidney in acute phase: nevertheless this is a nephritis with a rather benign prognosis in which, in general, there is no progression to chronic renal failure even if at the onset a severe acute exudative nephritis has occurred. This probably means that the renal deposition of RF is a harmful lesion in acute phase but not necessarily that it will lead to chronic irreversible stages.

NAISH: dr Lambert, did I understand you correctly to say that in those mice bearing the RF producing hybridomas who got the renal lesion, the renal lesion was really very short lived? If so, why do you think it was?

LAMBERT: The mice, not the lesions, were very short lived. You cannot keep the hybridomas very long. The mice died of cryoglobulinemia.

BONA: I would like to come back to beneficial vs pathological properties. We also have an experimental system like 129 SV mouse strain which developed a high amount of RF on aging, with deposition in the kidney without clinical symptomatology. Now, since one may ask why every immune response is associated with a production of rheumatoid factors, not only in the case of T-dependent antigen, but also after polysaccharide TI1 of TI2 injection, in my mind one beneficial effect can be just the clearing of antigen-antibody complex via promoting phagocytosis before deposition in kidney, a scavenger-like effect. The second aspect can be their real immunoregulatory effect. There are a few data which indicate for example that they can even exert an effect on the switching.

Part III. Classification of cryoglobulins and biochemical factors inducing, cryoprecipitation

8. Classification of Cryoglobulinemias

C. ZANUSSI, F. INVERNIZZI and P.L. MERONI

From a clinical point of view Brouet's classification of cryoglobulinemias, so widely accepted, has several limitations particularly because it cannot have a nosological meaning and also because of some technical aspects; in effect some cryoglobulins cannot be easily immunochemically classified: for example there are cryoglobulins consisting exclusively of polyclonal IgM or IgG [7]. But in order to discuss the problem of the classification of cryoglobulinemias we will present our case series; this collects also patients seen by Dr. M. Galli in the Clinic of Infectious Diseases of the University of Milan and by Dr. G. Monti in the Hospital of Saronno.

In Fig. 1 we have subdivided our series in essential and secondary forms. The percentage of the essential cryoglobulinemias (EMC), in which no underlying disease can be found at the moment of diagnosis, is similar to that described in other series [2, 3]. Among the secondary forms there is certainly a bias about the incidence of those related to renal diseases. This bias originates from the close prossimity of our Department to the nephrological unit. Waldenström's macroglobulinemia is the lymphoproliferative

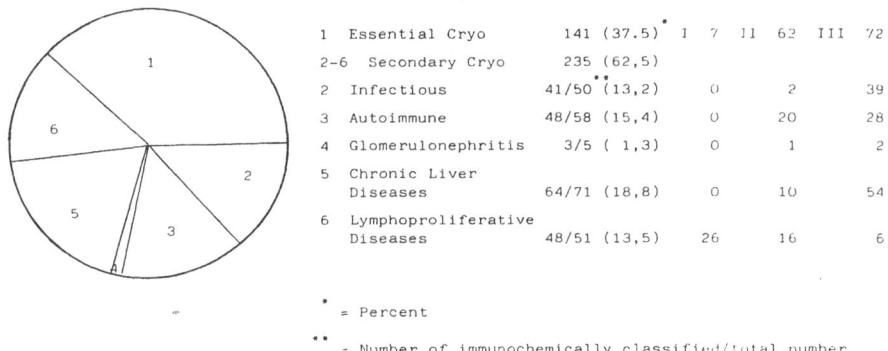

			I	II	III
1	Essential Cryo	141 (37.5)	7	62	72
2-6	Secondary Cryo	235 (62,5)			
2	Infectious	41/50 (13,2)	0	2	39
3	Autoimmune	48/58 (15,4)	0	20	28
4	Glomerulonephritis	3/5 (1,3)	0	1	2
5	Chronic Liver Diseases	64/71 (18,8)	0	10	54
6	Lymphoproliferative Diseases	48/51 (13,5)	26	16	6

* = Percent

** = Number of immunochemically classified/total number

Figure 1. Classification of 376 cryoglobulinemias (1966-1985).

96

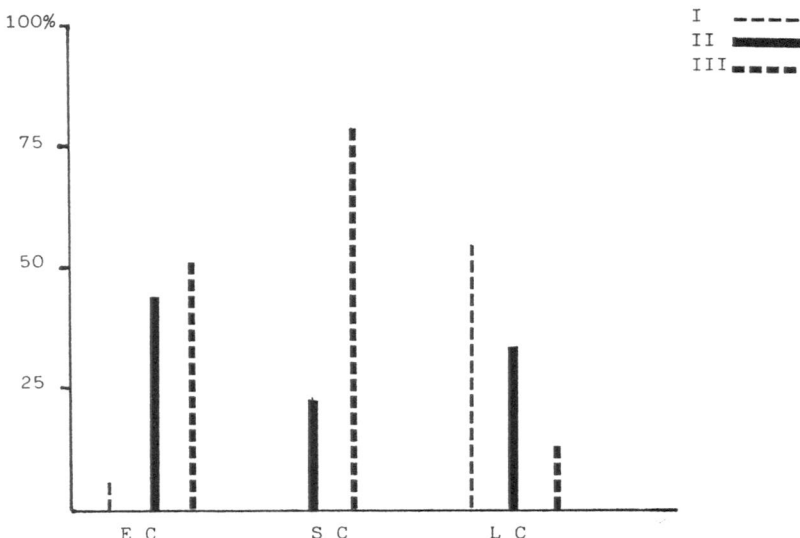

Figure 2. Immunochemical Classification of 345 Cryoglobulinemias.

disease most frequently associated with a cryoglobulinemia (17 patients), multiple myeloma is the next one (14 patients). In contrast to Brouet, the association between chronic lymphatic leukemia and cryoglobulinemia is not a common finding (7 patients).

In Fig. 2 we have reported the immunochemical classification of our series. In the first group are indicated the essential forms; in the second one all the secondary but for those secondary to a lymphoproliferative disease. We have set apart this group because it shares so different clinical and prognostic criteria [4] and because these cryoglobulins represent a paraproteinemic aspect of the abnormal immunoglobulin synthesis of a neoplastic cell; on the other hand this cryoglobulin sometimes may show an auto-antibody activity against, for example, lipoproteins.

It is possible to see the considerable overlapping in the distribution of the immunochemical types among the three groups and this proves our previous assumption of an unreliability of Brouet's criteria for a clinical classification.

Studying the evolution of EMC we have observed some interesting aspects. In the middle column of Fig. 3 we have indicated all our cases of EMC at the time of diagnosis; in the lateral ones the complications occurred and the evolution after the period considered, separating that of the type II cryoglobulinemias (left, from that of the type III (right). Basically we have to differentiate between the consequences of an immune complex disease and a particular type of evolution of the cryoglobulinemia. To the first belong the appearance of a glomerulonephritis, or of an hepatopathy; to the second one the evolution in an overt autoimmune disease (only Sjögren syndrome, nev-

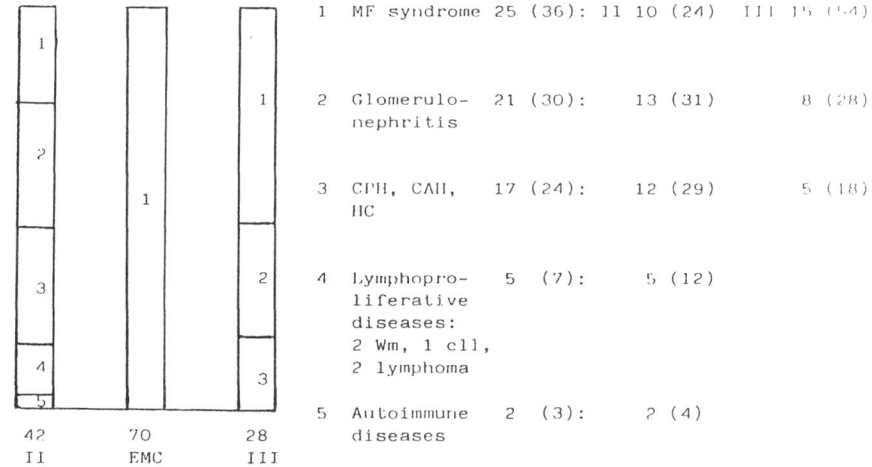

1	MF syndrome	25 (36):	11	10 (24)	III	15 (54)
2	Glomerulo-nephritis	21 (30):		13 (31)		8 (28)
3	CPH, CAH, HC	17 (24):		12 (29)		5 (18)
4	Lymphopro-liferative diseases: 2 Wm, 1 cll, 2 lymphoma	5 (7):		5 (12)
5	Autoimmune diseases	2 (3):		2 (4)

Figure 3. Follow-up in 70 EMC (4 years).

er SLE in our series) or in a lymphoproliferative disease (2 Waldenström's macroglobulinemia, 1 cll, 2 non-Hodgkin lymphoma). The important thing that the figure shows is the different evolution between crio type II and type III; and the difference is statistically significant: consider numbers 1 (cases

Table I. Spontaneous and PWM-induced differentiation into cytoplasmic immunoglobulin-positive cells and IgM and IgG synthesis of 1×10^6 normal and EMC peripheral blood mononuclear cells.

	cIg-positive cells $\times$ 10^3		IgM(ng/ml)		IgG(ng/ml)	
	PWM +	PWM −	PWM +	PWM −	PWM +	PWM −
Normal PBM	94±25.2	9±2.1	5170±1117	656±165	4116±1265	528±133
EMC PBM	18.55±8.4	9.1±4.2	1345±610	655±545	1333±545	435±399

Note. Values are the means ±SE of eight experiments.

Table II. Spontaneous and S. aureus-induced differentiation into cytoplasmic immunoglobulin-positive cells, and IgM and IgG synthesis of 1×10^6 normal and EMC peripheral blood mononuclear cells, and of 1×10^6 normal or EMC enriched B cells.

	cIg-positive cells $\times$ 10^3		IgM (ng/ml)		IgG (ng/ml)	
	S. aureus +	S. aureus −	S. aureus +	S. aureus −	S. aureus +	S. aureus
Normal PBM	39.62±12.1	9.12±1.12	3340±1062	430±181	1494±448	351±152
EMC PBM	14±8.05	9.31±6.09	270±73	210±70	246±108	200±61
Normal B	22.75±5.25	3.92±3.57	2860±1051	287±31	1395±495	312±108
EMC B	1.47±1.05	1.26±2.17	353±156	340±220	270±115	250±278

Note. Values are the means ±SE of six experiments.

98

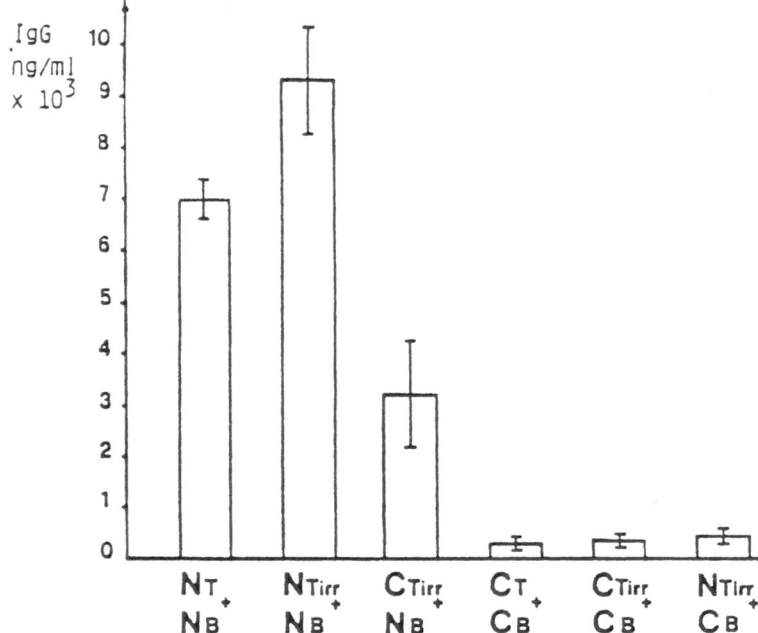

Figure 4. Pokeweed mitogen-induced IgG synthesis by normal and cryoglobulinemic B cells cocultered with irradiated and unirradiated T lymphocytes. (Enriched normal (N) and cryoglobulinemic (C) B cells 0.25×10^6 were cultures with 10^6 irradiated (irr) or unirradiated normal and cryoglobulinemic enriched T cells. Columns represent the means $\pm$SE of three experiments).

without any complication) and number 4 present only for type II. In conclusion the immunochemical type of EMC has in our series a prognostic meaning since those of type II seem to have a more severe course; for others [7] they belong to the plasma cell dyscrasia.

We have seen the peculiar clinical behaviour of EMC. Is it possible to find out a cellular correlation with these particular features? To do this we have studied the population of cells devoted to the Ig synthesis [5]. when we consider the ability of B cells from EMC patients to differentiate into cells containing cytoplasmic immunoglobulins and to synthesize IgG and IgM after PWM and S. aureus stimulated cultures, a functional defect of B cells comes into evidence (Tables I, II).

Coculture experiments were then carried out to determine if the reduced Ig synthesis could be reversed by normal lymphocyte populations. T cells suspension from normal and B cells populations from EMC patients, and vice versa, were cocultured. To exclude the possibility that an exaggerated EMC T ̄suppressor activity was responsible for the depression of PWM induced Ig synthesis by normal or cryoglobulinemic cells, coculture experiments with irradiated T cells were also carried out. As shown in Fig. 4

irradiated and unirradiated EMC T cells displayed comparable defective helper activity. Therefore the B cell defect coesists in EMC with an impaired T helper cell function.

However from the study of the IgM RF elaboration a different pattern is brought up into relief. As it can be seen in Table III the EMC peripheral blood lymphocytes and enriched B lymphocytes show a distinct advantage in this synthesis over normal cells both in basal conditions, and after stimulation with PWM and S. aureus [6].

The pattern resulting from these data appears peculiar to the EMC B and T cells, different from that of SLE, inasmuch as there is no polyclonal activation (this absence of a polyclonal activation in EMC reflects the meager

Table III. IgM RF elaboration by normal and cryoglobulinemic PBL and B ymphocytes.

	PWM	S. Aureus	Medium
PBL_n	12.4 ± 2.7	6.5 ± 1.7	3.5 ± 0.6
PBL_c	280.8 ± 129	101 ± 58	86.8 ± 62
B_n	1.6 ± 2.7	4.2 ± 3.1	2.1 ± 1.5
B_c	11.6 ± 4.5	143 ± 59	84.7 ± 30.9

Values are the mean ± SE of 8 experiments, and are expressed as ng IgM RF/10^6 cells.
PBL_n = normal peripheral blood lymphocytes
PBL_c = cryoglobulinemic peripheral blood lymphocytes
B_n = normal enriched B lymphocytes
B_c = cryoglobulinemic enriched B lymphocytes

Table IV. Classification of cryoglobulinemias according to our case series.

Cryo	Type	Cryocit %	Age	Sex	Evolution
Essential mixed	II ≃ III > I	1–15	30–49	F	MF syndrome (III > II) IC disease (II > III) lymphoproliferative disease (II)
Secondary Infectious Autoimmune Renal Liver diseases	III > II	< 1–10	that of underlying disease		that of underlying disease IC disease
Lymphoprolifera-tive diseases	I > II > III	5–> 15	> 45	F	that of underlying disease Hyperviscosity syndrome

auto-antibody production we have found). In conclusion it seems that EMC has not only a clinical picture which is distinct from known connective diseases, chronic infections, or clear-cut lymphoproliferative diseases, but also a distinct reactivity of B and T cells.

We propose here a mixed classification of the cryoglobuminemias, biochemical and clinical (Table IV); this classification is certainly useful and can have a certain degree of prognostic significance. In addition it shows that in the group of type II EMC, we certainly have a subset with the possibility of developing a lymphoproliferative desorder. The need to single out this group of patients at risk is not sufficiently overemphasized.

References

1. Brouet JC, Clauvel JP, Danon F, Klein M, Seligmann M: Biologic and clinical significance of cryoglobulins. A report of 86 cases. Am J Med 57:775–788, 1974.
2. Dammacco F, Guisci G, Silvestris F, Bonomo L: New clinical immunological trends in cryoglobulinemia. Ricerca Clin Lab 10:51–57, 1980.
3. Gorevic PD, Kassab HJ, Levo Y, Kohn R, Meltzer M, Prose P, Franklin EC: Mixed cryoglobulinemia. Clinical aspects and long-term follow-up. Am J Med 69:287–308, 1980.
4. Invernizzi F, Galli M, Monti G, Meroni PL, Granatieri C, Zanussi C: Secondary and essential cryoglobulinemias. Frequency, nosological classification and long-term follow-up. Acta Haematol 70:73–82, 1983.
5. Meroni PL, Barcellini W, De Bartolo G, Invernizzi F, Zanussi C: Abnormalities of in vitro immunoglobulin synthesis by peripheral blood lymphocytes from patients with essential mixed cryoglobulinemia. Clin. Immunol Immunopathol 33:245–257, 1984.
6. Meroni PL, Barcellini W, Sinico P: Manuscript in preparation.
7. Monteverde A, Allegra GC, Volta C, Zigrossi P, Bordin G: La crioglobulinemia mista: inquadramento clinico. Atti Seminari Medicina Interna, Punta Ala pp 163–170, 1985.
8. Winfield JB: Cryoglobulinemia. Human Pathology 14:350–354, 1983.

9. Intrinsic properties inducing precipitation of cryoglobulins

AN-CHUAN WANG and IRENE Y. WANG

General background

Cryoglobulins were initially discovered by Wintrobe and Buell [1] in 1933. These proteins precipitate or gel under reduced temperature, and the process is reversible when the precipitate or gel is warmed. Cryoglobulins are generally classified into three types [2]: type I includes monoclonal immunoglobulins containing one class or subclass of heavy (H) chain and/or one type or subtype of light (L) chain; type II contains mixed immunoglobulins with a monoclonal component possessing antibody activity toward polyclonal immunoglobulins; type III represents mixed polyclonal immunoglobulins without a monoclonal component and occasionally may also contain proteins other than immunoglobulins in the cryoprecipitate. All major immunoglobulin classes as well as Bence Jones proteins have been observed in each of the three types of cryoglobulins.

Cryoglobulins have been fascinating to protein chemists for many years. Why these proteins have reversible temperature-dependent precipitability whereas others don't represents a major scientific curiosity, and the answer to this question may generate important clues to a better understanding of protein behavior and function. In addition to basic sciences, cryoglobulins are also important to medical sciences. Cryoglobulinemia defines a disease condition in which a significant amount of cryoglobulin is detected in the patient's serum [3]. Patients commonly experience cold-induced cutaneous ulticaria, necrosis, and purpura. Cryoglobulins have also been found to associate with a wide spectrum of other diseases [3, 4]. Type I cryoglobulins are mainly found in patients with lymphoprolifeartive disorders or malignancies such as multiple myeloma, Waldenstrom's macroglobulinemia, Bence Jones proteinemia etc. Type II and Type III cryoglobulins are often found in patients with autoimmune, immune-complex, and/or infectious diseases (e.g. systemic lupus erythematous, rheumatoid arthritis, glomerulonephritis, vascular purpura, chronic hepatitis, etc.). Although cryoglobulins have drawn significant attention from the scientific community and have been studied intensively during the past 30 years, the factors responsible for the cold-induced precipitability remain to be identified. This article attempts to look into the intrinsic characteristics of cryoglobulins which might be relevant to the temperature-dependent precipitability, by comparing the amino acid composition and variable(V)-region amino acid sequence of certain type I cryoglobulins.

Possible mechanisms of cryoprecipitation

Many factors can influence the solubility of proteins; the most important ones are protein concentration, pH, ionic strength and temperature. The issues of pH and ionic strength will not be addressed in this article, because these are relatively constant under physiological conditions. However, concentrations of various serum proteins may differ from individual to individual and the temperature at which a certain cryoglobulin serum demonstrates protein precipitation is dependent on protein concentration. Generally speaking the higher the cryoglobulin concentration, the higher the temperature at which precipitation takes place. Therefore, a cryoglobulin that precipitates at a relatively higher temperature (e.g. 25 °C) at a high concentration (e.g. 20 mg/ml), upon dilution, would require a lower temperature to exhibit the same degree of precipitation.

The cold-induced precipitability appears to be an intrinsic characteristic of the cryoglobulin molecules, because practically all other serum proteins and vast majority of the immunoglobulins do not precipitate at low temperature. Generally, the overall tertiary structure (for Bence Jones proteins) or quaternary structure (for intact immunoglobulins) is important for cryoglobulins to maintain their cryoprecipitability. The separated Fc and Fab fragments, resulted from cleavage of individual cryoglobulins by papain digestion, usually lose the cold-induced precipitability [4–7]. However, there are exceptions, for example, the (Fab')$_2$ fragment obtained from pepsin digestion of an IgA cryoglobulin was shown to retain the cryoprecipitability [8].

Two mechanisms have been postulated to explain the temperature-dependent precipitation of cryoglobulins and pyroglobulins [9]. Formation of precipitation by mixed cryoglobulins (i.e. Type II or Type III) is believed to involve antigen-antibody reaction whereby cold-induced binding of antiglobulins (usually IgM rheumatoid factor) to epitopes of other immunoglobulin molecules leads to the formation of large insoluble aggregates [10, 11]. The phenomenon of cold-enhanced antigen-antibody reactions is not unique to mixed cryoglobulins; it is also observed in cold agglutinins [12, 13]. The mechanisms of a temperature-dependent antigen-antibody reaction, however, can not be easily applied to monoclonal cryoglobulins, which must involve diminished solubility of the cryoglobulin at reduced temperature [14]. Since the subject of gloublin-antiglobulin reaction will be addressed by Dr. Abraham in the next article, only the aspects regarding the molecular structure of cryoglobulins will be discussed in this article.

Content of serine in light chains of cryoglobulins

Cryoglobulins are not uniquely associated with any class or subclass of H chain or any type or subtype of L chains [2, 4, 9]. Therefore, the cryoprecipitability does not appear to be associated with constant (C) regions of the molecule. Indeed, of all the Fc fragments of cryoglobulins investigated thus far, none retains the ability to precipitate when cooled.

Both extrinsic (e.g. pH, ionic strength) and intrinsic factors can affect the solubility of proteins. Among the intrinsic factors, amino acid sequences and thus molecular conformation of the proteins probably have the greatest influence on their solubility. Polar and hydrophilic amino acid residues tend to be located at the surface of the molecules, whereas nonpolar and hydrophobic residues are generally buried in the anhydrous interior [9, 15]. Earlier studies in two laboratories indicated a decrease in tyrosine content in a monoclonal IgG [16] and a monoclonal IgM [17] cryoglobulins. However, a decrease in the number of tyrosine residues was not detected in many other cryoglobulins [18–21]. On the other hand, comparison of amino acid composition in L chains revealed that the content of serine is lower in monotypic cryoglobulins than in monoclonal immunoglobulins not precipitable at reduced temperature [18, 20–22]. The comparison involved kappa chains of at least eight type I cryoglobulins; three studied by Middaugh et al. [18] and five by Wang et al. [21, 22]. All eight had somewhat less serine than that of kappa chains of non-cryoprecipitable immunoglublins served as controls studied in parallel. The number of serine residues is presumably fewer in the V region, because only one gene encodes the C region of human kappa chains and the C allotypes do not differ in serine content [23]. The finding of lower serine content in cryoglobulins had led to considerable enthusiasm for the determination of V-region amino acid sequence of cryoglobulin L chains. It was disappointing that earlier NH_2-terminal amino acid sequence data of cryoglobulin L chains failed to find unusual substitutions involving serine inside the first framework and the first hypervariable region [21, 24–26]. In 1978 Chersi and Natali [19] reported the V-region amino acid sequence of a type I kappa Bence Jones cryoglobulin designated Ver. An updated sequence of Ver is listed in the 1983 issue of the book entitled *Sequences of Proteins of Immunological Interest* edited by Kabat et al. [27]. The updated sequence contains practically the entire V-region

Table 1. Comparison of V-region Amino Acid Content of Human Kappa Chains. Mean Solvent-Accessible Area, (A)*, of Amino Acids and Mean Fractional Area Loss, (f), as Calculated by Rose et al. [15] are Listed under Individual Amino Acids.

Number of Amino Acid Residues

	Lys	Gln	Glu	Glx	Asp	Asn	Asx	Arg	Pro	Ser	Thr	Gly	Ala	Tyr	His	Leu	Met	Trp	Val	Ile	Phe	Cys
Kappa(A)	110.3	74.0	72.3	73.2	60.9	62.2	61.6	93.8	53.7	44.2	46.0	25.2	31.5	59.1	46.7	29.0	30.5	41.7	23.5	23.0	28.7	13.9
Chain (f)	0.52	0.62	0.62	0.62	0.62	0.63	0.63	0.64	0.64	0.66	0.70	0.72	0.74	0.76	0.78	0.85	0.85	0.85	0.86	0.88	0.88	0.91
Ver	2	7	4	1	6	1	0	6	6	12	12	10	5	6	0	12	0	1	6	4	4	2
Wol	3	8	5	0	3	0	0	7	6	15	10	14	6	6	0	10	0	1	4	5	4	2
Sie	3	9	4	0	4	1	0	6	7	17	9	11	7	6	0	9	0	1	4	5	4	2
Pom	2	8	5	0	1	3	0	7	7	17	10	9	7	6	0	7	1	2	5	6	4	2
Lay	4	10	3	0	4	5	0	4	7	13	10	9	6	6	0	6	1	2	7	5	4	2
Ti	3	8	5	0	3	1	0	6	7	17	10	11	7	5	0	10	0	1	5	4	5	2
Tew	3	6	4	2	6	2	0	6	8	15	7	10	6	5	1	12	2	1	6	6	4	2
Mil	3	4	2	6	2	4	4	5	8	14	8	11	4	5	0	13	1	1	7	5	3	2
Nim	4	8	4	0	6	2	0	5	9	16	8	10	3	6	0	12	3	2	6	4	3	2
Cum	3	8	5	0	6	2	0	7	7	14	10	11	4	7	0	12	2	1	6	6	3	2
Fr	4	8	3	2	6	0	3	5	7	13	10	9	3	8	0	11	2	1	8	4	4	2
Len	6	9	4	0	4	4	0	4	6	18	8	8	6	9	0	9	1	2	6	5	3	2
Ou	3	1	0	10	2	0	5	5	6	18	12	9	6	6	1	7	1	1	3	6	5	2
Roy	6	9	2	0	8	2	0	3	6	12	11	10	6	4	0	8	1	1	4	7	7	2
Au	5	10	3	0	7	2	0	3	6	14	9	9	6	7	1	7	2	2	4	7	4	2
Rei	4	13	2	0	5	2	0	3	6	14	12	8	6	8	0	8	1	1	3	8	3	2
Hau	3	10	2	0	4	1	0	5	7	20	11	8	6	6	0	6	1	1	5	7	4	2
Gal	5	10	4	0	4	3	0	6	6	15	9	9	7	5	0	7	1	1	4	7	4	2
Scw	4	9	3	0	6	4	0	5	6	12	12	11	4	5	1	7	1	1	5	7	3	2
Wes	4	8	3	0	5	1	0	4	5	18	10	9	7	3	2	7	1	2	5	6	5	2
Eu	7	9	3	0	5	2	0	3	5	16	11	9	6	5	0	7	3	2	5	5	4	2
Den	4	9	4	0	5	1	0	5	5	17	12	9	5	6	0	7	1	2	3	6	5	2
Car	6	7	1	1	4	2	2	4	6	17	11	8	6	5	0	6	2	2	4	6	6	2
Bi	5	10	4	0	6	3	0	4	7	13	8	8	6	7	0	8	1	1	3	8	5	2
Ni	6	6	4	3	5	2	1	3	6	16	11	9	6	5	0	10	1	1	7	3	6	2
Ka	5	8	2	3	4	4	2	4	6	13	13	8	5	6	0	9	1	1	7	4	5	2
Kue	6	11	2	0	5	2	0	5	7	12	13	7	6	7	0	7	2	3	3	7	4	2

* Mean Solvent-accessible Area, (A), in square Angstroms. The values of (A) and (f) for Asx and for Glx are taken as the average of Asn and Asp, and of

sequence of Ver. The uncertain sequences are: (a) at positions 26 and 27 which have a Ser and a Glu residue, (b) at positions 30 to 32 which contains one residue each of Asn, Ser, and Gln, and (c) at positions 39 to 43 which have one residue each of Arg, Pro, Gly, Glx, and Ser based on the data reported in the reference [19].

The sequence information on Ver allows a direct comparison of the complete V-region amino acid sequence of a monoclonal kappa cryoglobulin with those of other human kappa chains available in the literature. The complete V-region amino acid sequences of a total of 27 human monotypic kappa chains have been reported [27]. Based on the sequence information on these 27 chains, the actual numbers of amino acid residues of their V regions are counted and listed in Table I. Table II focuses on the comparison between the number of serine residues in the V-region of these kappa chains in terms of cryoprecipitability and V-region subgroup designation. It is immediately noticeable that Ver kappa chain has only 12 V-region serine residues; at the lowest end of all kappa chains compared. The number of the V-region serine residues in kappa chains of 22 non-cryoglobulins ranges from 12 to 20 with a mean of 15.18 and a standard deviation of ± 2.23 (Table III). Therefore, the content of serine in the monoclonal cryo Bence

Table II. Subgroup Classification and Number of Serine Residues in the Variable Region of Sequenced Human Monotypic Kappa Chain.* Please see Kabat et al. [27] for sequence information.

Cryo or non-cryo	Protein	V-region subgroup	Number of Ser	Cryo or non-cryo	Protein	V-region subgroup	Number of Ser
Monoclonal cryo	Ver	$V_\kappa III$	12	Noncryo	Ou	$V_\kappa I$	18
				Non cryo	Roy	$V_\kappa I$	12
Mixed cryo	Wol	$V_\kappa III$	15	Non cryo	Au	$V_\kappa I$	14
Mixed cryo	Sie	$V_\kappa III$	17	Non cryo	Rei	$V_\kappa I$	14
Mixed cryo	Pom	$V_\kappa III$	17	Non cryo	Hau	$V_\kappa I$	20
Mixed cryo	Lay	$V_\kappa I$	13	Non cryo	Gal	$V_\kappa I$	15
				Non cryo	Scw	$V_\kappa I$	12
Non Cryo	Ti	$V_\kappa III$	17	Non cryo	Wes	$V_\kappa I$	18
				Non cryo	Eu	$V_\kappa I$	16
Non cryo	Tew	$V_\kappa II$	15	Non cryo	Den	$V_\kappa I$	17
Non cryo	Mil	$V_\kappa II$	14	Non cryo	Car	$V_\kappa I$	17
Non cryo	Nim	$V_\kappa II$	16	Non cryo	Bi	$V_\kappa I$	13
Non cryo	Cum	$V_\kappa II$	14	Non cryo	Ni	$V_\kappa I$	16
Non cryo	Fr	$V_\kappa II$	13	Non cryo	Ka	$V_\kappa I$	13
				Non cryo	Kue	$V_\kappa I$	12
Non cryo	Len	$V_\kappa IV$	18				

* Include only chains for which complete variable-region amino acid sequence have been determined.

Jones protein Ver is appreciably lower than that in other human kappa chains.

Human kappa chains are classified into four subgroups, i.e. $V_\kappa I$ to $V_\kappa IV$, based on degree of amino acid sequence homology at the framework regions [27]. Ver belongs to the $V_\kappa III$ subgroup. The four subgroups do not appear to differ greatly in their serine content (Table IV). Johnston et al. [25] and Ledford et al. [28] noticed a preferential association of $V_\kappa III$ L chains with mixed cryoglobulins having anti-globulin activity. These authors investigated a total of 15 IgM(κ) mixed cryoglobulins, and the NH_2-

Table III. Apparent difference in number of several amino acid residues of protein Ver as compared with the average number of corresponding residues of other monoclonal immunoglobulins listed in Table I. Proteins are grouped according to their cryoprecipitability.

		Classification		
		Monoclonal cryoglobulin (Ver)	Mixed cryoglobulin	Non cryo-precipitable immunoglobulin
No of proteins		1	4	22
Number of residues	SER	12	15.50 ± 1.91*	15.18 ± 2.23
	LYS	2	3.00 ± 0.82	4.50 ± 1.26
	MET	0	0.50 ± 0.58	1.27 ± 0.70
	ILE	4	5.25 ± 0.48	5.82 ± 1.40
	LEU	12	8.00 ± 1.83	8.64 ± 2.16
	THR	12	9.75 ± 0.50	10.27 ± 1.69

* Mean $\pm$ Standard Deviation.

Table IV. Apparent difference in number of several amino acid residues of protein Ver as compared with the average number of corresponding residues of other monoclonal immunoglobulins listed in Table I. Proteins are grouped according to the V-region subgroup of their L chains.

		Subgroup				
		Ver ($V_\kappa III$)	$V_\kappa III$	$V_\kappa I$	$V_\kappa II$	$V_\kappa IV$
No of proteins		1	5	16	5	1
Number of residues	SER	12	15.60 ± 2.19	15.00 ± 2.50*	14.40 ± 1.14	18
	LYS	2	2.60 ± 0.55	4.82 ± 1.17	3.40 ± 0.55	6
	MET	0	0.20 ± 0.45	1.13 ± 0.50	2.00 ± 0.71	1
	ILE	4	4.40 ± 0.84	6.19 ± 1.34	5.00 ± 1.00	5
	LEU	12	9.60 ± 1.82	7.31 ± 1.08	12.00 ± 0.71	9
	THR	12	10.20 ± 1.10	10.94 ± 1.44	8.60 ± 1.34	8

* Mean $\pm$ Standard Deviation.

terminal sequence of kappa chains of these proteins did not show a lower number of serine. Four of the proteins (i.e. Wol, Sie, Pom and Lay in Table II) compared in this paper are IgM(κ) type II mixed cryoglobulins and the content of serine in their kappa chains does not differ much from the average of the other non-cryoglobulin kappa chains (Table III). These four mixed cryoglobulins also show preferential association with the $V_\kappa III$ subgroup, since three of them belong to the $V_\kappa III$ subgroup (Table II). The cryoprecipitation of monoclonal and of mixed cryoglobulins may involve different mechanisms. The cryoprecipitation of the latter is likely due to cold-induced or cold-enhanced antigen-antibody reactions, whereas that of the former may be due to intrinsic chemical characteristics, e.g. reduced serine content in the V-region.

Obviously, a low content of serine alone will not be enough to explain cryoprecipitability, because three non-cryoglobulins listed in Table II also have low serine content. Perhaps serine is needed at certain key positions, and its absence in such positions could lead to low solubility of the protein molecule at low temperature. All kappa chains have an extremely hydrophilic stretch of amino acids inside the third framework region. This stretch covers positions 63 to 70 and has a nearly invariable sequence of Ser-Gly-Ser-Gly-Ser-Gly-Thr-Asp. To date, sequences at this stretch have been reported for 33 other human kappa chains in addition to protein Ver [27]. Serine occurs in 31 out of the 33 proteins at position 63, and 30 out of the 33 proteins at position 65. At position 66, 32 out of the 33 proteins have a glycine residue. None of the 33 proteins has more than one substitution at these three positions. It is highly unusual that Ver has three substitutions in this stretch; threonine at position 63, arginine at position 65, and alanine at position 66 [19].

While the comparison made above is interesting, its significance remains to be evaluated by further studies. A direct approach would be the determination of complete V-region amino acid sequences of L chains of additional Type I cryoglobulins.

Other intrinsic characteristics

In addition to the protein moiety, carbohydrate content also plays an important role in determining the solubility of glycoproteins. Many sugar residues, e.g. hexoses, hexosamines and fucose, can effect the degree of surface hydration of a molecule, whereas sialic acid can directly contribute to the surface polarity via its negative electrostatic charge. The overall carbohydrate content of two IgM cryoglobulins has been found to be within the normal range [18, 29], but the amount of glucosamine was found to be smaller in an IgG monoclonal cryoglobulin when compared with other IgG myeloma proteins [5]. Removal of some sugar residues by means of glyco-sidases treatment decreased the solubility at 37 °C of one of the two IgM cryoglobulins [29] and caused the other to precipitate at a concentration lower than that needed for the native molecule to form cryoprecipitate [18]. However, removal of sialic acid by digestion with neuraminidase did not affect the cryoprecipitability of an IgM cryolgobulin [18].

Recently, Erickson et al. [30] compared the V_H-region amino acid se-quences of two monoclonal human cryoglobulins [31, 32] with each other and with the corresponding sequences of several non-cryoprecipitable mon-oclonal immunoglobulins. No common sequence that could differentiate cryoglobulin H chains from other H chains was found. However, compari-son of the data by metric analysis [30] showed that each of the two cryo-globulin H chains contains two unprecedented amino acid residues in the outer beta-sheet structure of the V-region. The analysis suggests that differ-ent monoclonal cryoglobulins may display cold-induced insolubility via dif-ferent perturbations of the outer surface of the V_H domain. This hypothesis can be examined by determination of V_H amino acid sequences of addition-al Type I cryoglobulins.

Examination of the amino acid information presented in Table I indicates that the contents of lysine, methionine and isoleucine are also lower whereas the amounts of leucine and threonine are higher in Ver kappa chain than in non-cryoglobulin kappa chains (Table III). The low content of lysine and methionine may be a subgroup-associated phenomenon because all V III proteins, cryo or non-cryo, have lower lysine and methionine content (Ta-bles I and IV). Since there is a preferential association between mixed cryo-gloublins and the V III subgroup [25, 28], a lower lysine and/or methionine content may be related to cold-enhanced antigen-binding activity or cold-induced precipitability of the mixed cryoglobulins. Lysine is probably the most exposed amino acid in globular proteins in aqueous solution [15]. It could conveivably exert more influence on the solubility of the protein molecule than most of the other amino acids. Examination of the V-region amino acid sequences [27] revealed that Ver has an arginine at position 107, whereas 34 out of 37 other human kappa chains have a lysine at this posi-tion. Two of the three remaining chains have a threonine and the other has an arginine at position 107. It appears worthwhile to examine if arginine, instead of lysine, also occurs at position 107 of other monoclonal cryo-Bence Jones proteins.

Another noticeable substitution in Ver is at position 44 where Ver has a leucine residue but all other human kappa chains sequenced to date have a proline residue [19, 27]. Since proline generally breaks the α-helix structure of the polypeptide chain, a proline to leucine substitution could also have a significant impact on the overall conformation and solubility of the pro-tein.

The hydrophobicity of amino acids contribute greatly to protein stability when a polypeptide chain is folded into a globular protein [15, 33]. An increase of hydrophobic amino acids in an IgG cryoglobulin was reported by Saha et al. [20] when comparison was made with non-cryoprecipitable IgG. On the other hand, using the amino acid hydrophobicity scale of Naza-

Table V. Comparison of human kappa chains by hydrophobicity. The mean solvent-accessible area (A) of amino acids (15) was used as the criterion for comparison. Calculation was based on the V-region amino acid content presented in Table I.

Kappa Chain	Cryo or Non-Cryo	Sub-group	Total Mean Solvent-Accessible Area (A)			Σ P.R.
			Σ P.R.*	Σ M.P.R.*	Σ H.R.*	Σ M.P.R.$+\Sigma$ H.R.
Ver	Monoclonal Cryo	$V_\kappa III$	2944	1316	765	1.414
Wol	Mixed Cryo	$V_\kappa III$	3109	1356	683	1.524
Sie	Mixed Cryo	$V_\kappa III$	3282	1266	654	1.709
Pom	Mixed Cryo	$V_\kappa III$	3206	1262	715	1.621
Lay	Mixed Cryo	$V_\kappa I$	3278	1230	710	1.690
Ti	Non-Cryo	$V_\kappa III$	3219	1253	713	1.638
Tew	Non-Cryo	$V_\kappa II$	3356	1105	872	1.697
Mil	Non-Cryo	$V_\kappa II$	3345	1067	843	1.752
Nim	Non-Cryo	$V_\kappa II$	3472	1069	870	1.791
Cum	Non-Cryo	$V_\kappa II$	3426	1277	844	1.615
Fr	Non-Cryo	$V_\kappa II$	3366	1254	844	1.604
Len	Non-Cryo	$V_\kappa IV$	3602	1291	745	1.770
Ou	Non-Cryo	$V_\kappa I$	3154	1369	655	1.558
Roy	Non-Cryo	$V_\kappa I$	3218	1183	788	1.632
Au	Non-Cryo	$V_\kappa I$	3282	1290	715	1.637
Rei	Non-Cryo	$V_\kappa I$	3199	1415	673	1.532
Hau	Non-Cryo	$V_\kappa I$	3250	1251	667	1.694
Gal	Non-Cryo	$V_\kappa I$	3559	1157	673	1.945
Scw	Non-Cryo	$V_\kappa I$	3260	1297	668	1.659
Wes	Non-Cryo	$V_\kappa I$	3056	1178	744	1.590
Eu	Non-Cryo	$V_\kappa I$	3341	1217	753	1.696
Den	Non-Cryo	$V_\kappa I$	3252	1291	697	1.636
Car	Non-Cryo	$V_\kappa I$	3265	1192	720	1.708
Bi	Non-Cryo	$V_\kappa I$	3458	1172	730	1.818
Ni	Non-Cryo	$V_\kappa I$	3416	1218	796	1.697
Ka	Non-Cryo	$V_\kappa I$	3209	1312	761	1.548
Kue	Non-Cryo	$V_\kappa I$	3425	1377	691	1.656

* Σ P.R. represents the summation of (A) of all polar residues; Σ M.P.R. represents the summation of (A) of all moderately polar residues; and Σ H.R. represents the summation of (A) of all hydrophobic residues.

Using the mean-fractional surface area loss (f) as the criterion for hydrophobicity, amino acids are classified into three groups: (a) polar, includes Lys, Gln, Glu, Asn, Asp, Arg, Pro and Ser; (b) moderately polar, includes Thr, Gly, Ala, Tyr, and His; and (c) hydrophobic, includes Leu, Met, Trp, Val, Ile, Phe, and Cys.

ki and Tanford [33] and of Jones [34] as the basis for measuring protein hydrophobicity, Meinke and Speilgelberg [26] found no significant increase in hydrophobic residues at the first 20 NH_2-terminal positions of three cryo-Bence Jones proteins. Indeed, using the Tanford-Nazaki-Jones scale [33, 34] as the basis for comparison, we also found the hydrophobicity of the monoclonal cryo-Bence Jones protein (Ver) as well as of the four mixed cryo-globulins to be within the range for non-cryoprecipitable immunoglobulins. The Tanford-Nazaki-Jones hydrophobicity scale is based on the free energy of transfer of amino acid side chains from water to organic solvents (e.g., ethanol or dioxane). This scale has been widely referred to but, nevertheless, not universally accepted [15, 35, 36]. Recently, Rose et al. [15] proposed a different scale for comparing hydrophobicity of amino acids and proteins. This new scale is based on the mean fractional surface area loss (f) of individual amino acids when a polypeptide chain is folded into a globular protein for defining degree of hydrophobicity. Table V presents the total solvent-accessible areas of polar, moderately polar, and hydrophobic residues calculated for V regions of the kappa chains listed in Table I. It is interesting to note that Ver appears to be more hydrophobic than any of the other kappa chains, since Ver has the lowest ratio of total solvent-accessible area of polar residues versus that of the hydrophobic plus moderately polar residues.

Concluding remarks

Comparison of V-region amino acid sequences reported in the literature indicates that the V region of a monoclonal (type I) cryo-Bence Jones protein (Ver) has a relatively lower amount of serine, lysine, methionine and isoleucine and higher amount of leucine and threonine than those of L chains of non-cryoprecipitable immunoglobulins. The low content of serine is particularly noteworthy, because a lesser amount of serine was also found in at least eight additional type I cryoglobulin kappa chains studied previously by others by means of gross amino acid composition determination. It is tempting to speculate that the absence of serine at certain key positions in the V region may be relevant to the cryoprecipitability of type I cryoglobulin kappa chains. This hypothesis can be critically evaluated by amino acid sequence determination of L chains of more type I cryoglobulins. The sequence information generated from such a study would also be helpful to ascertain whether unusual substitution involving other amino acids (e.g. the Leu/Pro exchange at position 44 or the Arg/Lys exchange at position 107) in the V region of protein Ver is characteristic of all type I cryoglobulin L chains.

The hydrophobicity of amino acids is a key factor to determine the manner in which a linear polypeptide chain is folded into a stable globular protein in physiological fluids. Attempts have been made to compare the hydrophobicity of Ver with those of non-cryoprecipitable immunoglobulins. The V-region of Ver kappa chain appears to have similar hydrophobicity as those of other human kappa chains when the Tanford-Nazaki-Jones hydrophobicity scale was employed. However, when the scale proposed by Rose and his colleagues was used for comparison, Ver seems to be more hydrophobic than any of the other chains. It appears that the interrelationship between hydrophobicity and cryoprecipibility merits further investigation.

Acknowledgements

This work was supported in part by National Science Foundation Research Grant PCM-82-01757 and South Carolina State Appropriation for Biomedical Research Grants CR-19 and CR-23.

References

1. Wintrobe MM and Buell MV: Hyperproteinemia associated with multiple myeloma. Bull Johns Hopkins Hosp 52:156–165, 1933.
2. Brouet JC, Clauvel JP, Danon F, Klein M and Seligmann M: Biological and clinical significance of cryoglobulins. Am J Med 57:775–788, 1974.
3. Winfield JB: Cryoglobulinemia. Hum Pathol 14:350–354, 1983.
4. Grey HM and Kohler PF: Cryoimmunoglobulins. Sem Hematol 10:87–112, 1973.
5. Saha A, Chowdhury P, Samburry S, Smart K and Rose B: Studies on cryoprecipitation. IV. Enzymatic fragments of a human cryoglobulin. J Biol Chem 245:2730–2736, 1970.
6. Nishimura Y and Nakamura H: Human monclonal cryoglobulins. I. Molecular properties of IgG3K (Jir protein) and the cryo-coprecipitability of its molecular fragment by papain. J Biochem 95:255–265, 1984.
7. Stone MJ and Fedak J: Studies on monoclonal antibodies. II. Immune complex (IgM-IgG) cryoglobulinemia: The mechanism of cryoprecipitation. J Immunol 113:1377–1385, 1974.
8. Pruzanski W, Jancelewicz Z and Underdown B: Immunological and physicochemical studies of IgA (μ) cryoglobulinemia. Clin Exp Immunol 15:181–191, 1973.
9. Zinneman HH: Cryoglobulins and pyroglobulins. In: 'Immunoglobulins', Litman GW and Good RA (eds), Plenum Pub, New York, pp 323–343, 1978.
10. Uki J, Young CA Suzuki T: A 22S cryoglobulin with antibody-like activity. I. Physicochemical characterization and modification of its cryoproperties. Immunochemistry 110:729–740, 1974.
11. Saluk PH and Clem W: Studies on the cryoprecipitation of a human IgG3 cryoglobulin: The effects of temperature-induced conformational changes on the primary interaction. Immunochemistry 12:29–37, 1975.
12. Feizi T: The monoclonal antibodies of cold agglutinin syndrome. Med Biol 58:123–127, 1980.
13. Weber RJ, Clem LW and Voss EW: The molecular mechanism of cryoimmunoglobulin precipitiation-II. Thermodynamic basis for self-association as determined by fluorescence polarization. Mol Immunol 21:61–67, 1984.

14. Middaugh CR, Litman GW: Effect of D20 on the temperature dependent solubility of cryoglobulin and noncryoglobulin IgM. FEBS Lett 79:200–202, 1977.
15. Rose GD, Geselowitz AR, Lesser GJ, Lee RH and Zehlus MH: Hydrophobicity of amino acid residues in globular proteins. Science 229:234–838, 1985.
16. Cummings, NA: Decreased tyrosine/tryptophan ratio in a 6.6S cryoglobulin, as determined by a spectrophotometric technique. Biochem Biophys Res Commun 33:165–171, 1968.
17. Zinneman HH, Fromke VL and Seal US: Some biochemical properties of a cryomacroglobulin. Clin Chim Acta 43:91–99, 1973.
18. Middaugh CR, Kehoe JM, Prystowsky MB, Gerber-Jenson B, Jenson JC and Litman GW: Molecular basis for the temperature-dependent insolubility of cryoglobulin — IV. Structural studies of the IgM monoclonal cryoglobulin McE. Immunochemistry 15:171–187, 1978.
19. Chersi A and Natali PG: Partial amino acid sequence of the V region of a K-type Bence Jones cryoglobulin. Immunochemistry 15:585–589, 1978.
20. Saha A, Edwards MA, Sargent AU and Rose B: Mechanism of cryo-precipitation. I. Characteristics of a human cryoglobulin. Immunochemistry 5:341–356, 1968.
21. Wang AC, Wells JV and Fudenberg HH: Chemical analysis of cryoglobulins. Immunochemistry 11:341–345, 1974.
22. Wang AC, Arnaud P, Fudenberg HH, Wang IY and Creyssel R: Biochemical study of a double paraprotein with cryoprecipitable component. In: 'Cryoglobulins', Chenais F (ed), INSERM Publ, Grenoble, France, pp 35–46, 1978.
23. Steinberg AG, Milstein CP, McLaughlin CL and Solomon A: Structural studies on Inv (1,2) kappa chain. Immunogenetics 1:108–117, 1974.
24. Meinke GC, Sigrist PH and Spiegelberg HL: The NH_2-terminal amino acid sequence of a κ and a λ Bence Jones cryoglobulin. Immunochemistry, 11:457–460, 1974.
25. Johnston SL, Abraham GN and Welch EH: Structural studies of monoclonal human cryoprecipitable immunoglobulins. Biochem Biophys res Comm 66:842–847, 1975.
26. Meinke GC and Spiegelberg HL: Amino acid sequence of the first hypervariable region of 2 κ and a λ Bence Jones cryoglobulin. Immunochemistry 13:915–919, 1976.
27. Kabat EA, Wu TT, Bilofsky H, Reid-Miller M and Perry H: 'Sequences of proteins of Immunological Interest'. National Inst. of Health Pub, Bethesda, MD pp 1–321, 1983.
28. Ledford DK, Goni F, Pizzolato M, Franklin EC, Solomon A and Frangione B: Preferential association of KIIIb light chains with monoclonal human IgM autoantibodies. J Immunol 131:1322–1325, 1983.
29. Andersen BR, Tesar JT, Schmid FR, Haisty WK and Hartz WH: Biological and physical properties of a human M-cryoglobulin and its monomer subunit. Clin Exp Immunol 9:795–807, 1971.
30. Erickson BW, Gerber-Jenson B, Wang AC and Litman GW: Molecular basis for the temperature-dependent insolubility of the heavy chain variable regions of the human cryoglobulins McE and Hil by metric analysis. Mol Immunol 19:357–365, 1982.
31. Chiu YYH, Lopez de Castro JA and Poljak RJ: Amino acid sequence of the V_H region of human myeloma cryoglobulin IgG Hil. Biochemistry 18:553–560, 1979.
32. Gerber-Jenson B, Kazin A, Kehoe M, Scheffel C, Erickson BW and Litman GW: Molecular basis for the temperature-dependent insolubility of cryoglobulins. X. The amino acid sequence of the heavy chain variable region of McE. J Immunol 126:1212–1216, 1981.
33. Nazaki Y and Tanford C: The solubility of amino acids and two glycine peptides in aqueous ethanol and dioxane solutions. J Biol Chem 246:2211–2217, 1971.
34. Jones DD: Amino acid properties and side-chain orientation in proteins: a cross correlation approach. J Theor Biol 50:167–183, 1975.
35. Wolfendent, R: Waterlogged molecules. Science 222:1087–1093, 1983.
36. Kyte J and Doolittle RF: A simple method for displaying the hydropathic character of a protein. J Mol Biol 157:105–132, 1982.

10. Cryoprecipitation as a consequence of globulin-antiglobulin interactions

G.N. ABRAHAM, S.L. JOHNSTON, C.G. HALL, C.D. SCOVILLE and D.N. PODELL

The causes of the cryoprecipitation of mixed IgM-IgG cryoglobulins have not been completely determined. However, investigations conducted in various laboratories have provided data partially clarifing the complex mechanisms involved. In order to understand this phenomenon, the role of the various components in the cryoprecipitation process, the characteristics of the IgM anti-IgG and of its interactions with IgG, and the biophysical processes which produce cryoprecipitation of a cryo-immunoglobulin complex will be discussed.

In mixed IgM:IgG cryoglobulins, while both immunogloublins are necessary, LoSpallutto et al. [1] and Meltzer et al. [2] have shown that the IgM anti-IgG is the *specific* component which mediates cryoprecipitation. In order to demonstrate this, these investigators separated the IgM and IgG fractions from mixed cryoglobulins and examined the ability of each to cryoprecipitate alone or when combined with other IgG or IgM obtained from normal serum. Their conclusions are schematized in Table I. As shown, neither the IgM anti-IgG or IgG purified from a patient's cryoglobulin (x) can cryoprecipitate by itself. However, IgM_x mixed with IgG purified from normal serum (NH) or the patient's serum (x), forms a cryopreci-

Table I.

	Cryoprecipitate formed
$(IgM_X - IgG_X)$	+
$IgM_X + IgG_{NH}$	+
$IgM_{NH} + IgG_X$	0
IgM_X	0
IgG_X	0

pitate. Thus, cryoprecipitation can occur after interaction of the patient's IgM anti-IgG with *any* normal IgG. The cryogloublin IgM anti-IgG has been shown by Stone and Metzger [3] and Chavin and Franklin [4] to combine with IgG through Fc-region antigenic determinants. Further, Stone and Metzger [3] provided excellent quantitative binding data for one IgM anti-IgG which strongly suggested that a single Fc-region antigenic determinant was involved in the IgM:IgG interaction.

Despite the fact that any human IgG may participate in cryoprecipitation, there still might be a common antigenic determinant shared by all IgG which reacts with an IgM cryoglobulin. Data published by Johnston and Abraham [5] show that this is not the case. The antigenic specificities of six monoclonal IgM anti-IgG cryoglobulins were determined using a panel of 20 IgG κ or λ myeloma proteins of the 4 gamma chain subclasses. As summarized in Table II, the IgM anti-IgG cryoglobulin of each patient showed a different reactivity pattern with the IgG myelomas. Thus, no IgM recognizes precisely the same antigen on the IgG Fc-region. Although not published, we have studied 6 other IgM anti-IgGs and all have different patterns of reactivity with this same panel of myeloma proteins. Thus, although there is a single Fc-region antigenic determinant on IgG which an IgM anti-IgG cryoglobulin identifies, there is no specific Fc-antigen which is selectively involved in or mediates, cryoprecipitation.

Since the cryoprecipitation process is clearly temperature related, perhaps lowering the temperature of the reaction causes an increase in the strength of binding of the IgM cryoglobulin to its IgG antigen. This does occur. Stone and Metzger [3], and Stone and Fedak [6] clearly demonstrated that the binding avidity of the IgM anti-IgG increases at lower temperatures. This is just the opposite effect of that which Drs. Clark, Vaughan and I [7] demonstrated for a monoclonal non-cryoprecipitable anti-IgG rheumatoid factor whose binding strength increased appreciably by increasing the temperature of the reaction from 4 °C to 37 °C.

However, while the cryoprecipitation process is temperature dependent, Stone and Fedak [6] clearly demonstrated that the small increases which

Table II.

IgM anti-IgG	γ-chain subclass specificity	
Teh	$IgG_1 = IgG_2 = IgG_4$	$IgG_3(-)$
Pla	$IgG_2 > IgG_1 > IgG_4$	$IgG_3(-)$
Gly	IgG_2	$IgG_1, IgG_3, IgG_4(-)$
Luc	$IgG_1 \geqslant IgG_2 = IgG_3$	$IgG_4(-)$
Jos	$IgG_3 \geqslant IgG_1 = IgG_2 = IgG_4$	
Cra	$IgG_1 > igG_2 = IgG_3 = IgG_4$	

occur in the binding constant of an IgM cryoglobulin at lower temperatures, are not sufficient in and of themselves to account for cryoprecipitation. It is also clear from their data that *minor* variations in the solvent ionic strength and pH *near neutrality,* do not appreciably change the strength of binding between the IgM and IgG, and also do not critically affect cryoprecipitation. Rather, they concluded that after the IgM:IgG interaction, the solubility of the *immune complexes* which are formed is significantly diminished over that of the individual components in the complex, and that precipitation of mixed cryoglobulins is due more to the size of the complexes and undefined interactions with the solvent which decrease their bulk solubility.

The types of mechanisms which affect the solubility of large immune complexes in solution and which cause cryoprecipitation have been most completely defined for the monoclonal IgG cryoglobulins. Scoville et al. [8, 9] demonstrated that for some cryoglobulins formation of an intermediate molecular nucleation center is necessary before cryoprecipitation can take place. Further, these intermolecular interactions occur at a very localized site on the cryoprotein molecules. In another instance, Hall and Abraham [9, 10] showed that self-association of IgG paraprotein molecules can proceed by a combination of weak nonionic and hydrophobic interactions. The polymerization of some IgG molecules and solubility of very large IgG:IgG complexes may be enhanced by an increase in the ionic strength of the solvent in which they are present. The net result of such a process clinically, is the development of a hyperviscosity syndrome in patients with this type of paraproteinemia, which is directly related to the presence of very large immunoglobulin polymers in a patient's blood. These two examples serve to demonstrate that various mechanisms may cause cryoprecipitation, and it may be difficult to precisely define the process responsible unless rather complex biophysical studies are performed. Regardless of the biophysical process involved, the most consistent parameter which affects cryoprecipitation is the solution concentration of a cryoprotein. Thus as would be expected, reduction of the cryoprotein level in blood is of paramount clinical importance.

Remarkably, regardless of how cryoprecipitation occurs all cryoglobulins assume three morphologic forms [12]: amorphous, crystalline, and gelatinous cryoprecipitates. The determination of the form may be ascertained by gross visual and light microscopic examination and may relate to the clinical signs. In general, the more rapid forming crystalline and amorphous cryoprecipitates produce more flagrant disease than gelatinous cryoglobulins.

In summary, cryoprecipitation is a complex process which is dependent upon interaction of the cryoglobulin IgM anti-IgG with an IgG antigen. Both immunoglobulins are necessary for cryoprecipitation, but the only specific component is the IgM anti-IgG. The determinant on the IgG with which the IgM reacts and the antigenic specificity of the IgM for Fc-region antigens seemingly have nothing to do with cryoprecipitation. While the process is enhanced by decreased temperature as evidenced by an increase in binding avidity of the IgM, this increase in avidity is not a major contributor to precipitation. Rather, cryoprecipitation occurs after diverse interactions between the IgM-IgG immune complexes which are formed. The solubility of these immune complexes is most-likely influenced by the solvent environment and changes in the interactions of these macromolecular complexes with this environment which may be influenced by temperature and ionic strength. Finally, regardless of the process involved, all cryoglobulins can be classified into three morphologic forms which are readily distinguished by visual and light microscopic examination.

Acknowledgement

Supported by U.S.P.H.S. research grant AI-19658, program project grant PO1-AI21288, and the James P. Wilmot Foundation.

References

1. LoSpalutto J, Dorward B, Miller W and Ziff M: Cryoglobulinemia based on interaction between a gamma macroglobulin and 7S gamma Globulin. Am J Med 32:142, 1962.
2. Meltzer M, Franklin EC, Elias K, McCluskey RT and Cooper N: Cryoglobulinemia — A clinical and laboratory study. Am J Med 40:837, 1966.
3. Stone MJ and Metzger HM: Binding Properties of a Waldenstrom macroglobulin antibody. J Biol Chem 243:5049, 1968.
4. Chavin SI and Franklin EC: Studies on antigen-binding activity of macroglobulin antibody subunits and their enzymatic fragments. J Biol Chem 244:1345, 1969.
5. Johnston SL and Abraham GN: Studies of human IgM anti-IgG cryoglobulins. I. Patterns of reactivity with autologous and isologous human IgG and its subunits. Immunology 36:671, 1979.
6. Stone MJ and Fedak JE: Studies on monoclonal antibodies. II. Immune complex (IgM-IgG) cryoglobulinemia: The mechanisms of cryoprecipitation. J Immunol 113:1377, 1974.
7. Abraham GN, Clark RA and Vaughan JH: Characterization of an IgA rheumatoid factor. Binding properties and reactivity with the subclasses of human gamma-G globulin. *Immunochemistry* 9:301, 1972.
8. Scoville CD, Abraham GN and Turner DG: Spectroscopic and kinetic analysis of a monoclonal IgG cryoglobulin. Effect of mild reduction on cryoprecipitation. Biochem 12:2610, 1979.
9. Scoville CD, Turner DH, Lippert JL and Abraham GN: Study of the kinetic and structural properties of a monoclonal Immunoglobulin G cryoglobulin. J Biol Chem 255:5847, 1980.
10. Hall CG and Abraham GN: Reversible self-association of a human myeloma protein. Thermodynamics and relevance to viscosity effects and solubility. Biochem 23:5123, 1984.

11. Hall CG and Abraham GN: Size, shape, and hydration of a self-associating human IgG myeloma protein: Axial asymmetry as a contributing factor in serum hyperviscosity. Arch Biochem Biophys 233:330, 1984.
12. Abraham GN, Packman CH and Podell DN: Morphologic properties of monoclonal IgG cryoglobulins. A light, and scanning and transmission electron microscopic study. Submitted for publication.

11. Fibronectin is a regular component of single-type and mixed cryoglobulins

FRANCO DAMMACCO and GIUSEPPE GALLO

Cryoglobulins are cold-insoluble immunoglobulins which reversibly precipitate at temperatures below 37 °C, giving rise to high molecular weight aggregates. On the basis of their immunochemical characteristics cryoglobulins can be classified into Type I, which are composed of isolated monoclonal immunoglobulins; Type II, which are accounted for by mixed cryoglobulins with a monoclonal component (usually a monoclonal IgM rheumatoid factor and polyclonal IgG); and Type III, consisting of mixed polyclonal cryoglobulins [3, 7].

While IgM cryoglobulins are the commonest and IgG cryoglobulins are the second most frequent of the Type I variety, IgA and Bence Jones cryoglobulins are of much rarer occurrence. In addition, single cryoproteins are usually found in patients with immunoproliferative diseases such as Waldenström's macroglobulinemia (WM) and multiple myeloma (MM). On the other hand, Type II and Type III cryoglobulins may be associated with several disease conditions, namely autoimmune disorders, acute and chronic infections, and liver dysfunctions. However, in the majority of instances no other diseases can be detected and the clinical picture consists of a purpura-weakness-arthralgia syndrome [8, 11, 15]: such patients are commonly defined as having essential mixed cryoglobulinemia (EMC).

All mixed cryoglobulins, and possibly also a minor number of the apparently single forms, are considered as immunoglobulin/anti-immunoglobulin complexes, but sometimes include other proteins such as C1q, β-lipoprotein, or DNA [6, 8]. Following the report by Anderson et al. [1] on the occurrence of fibronectin (FN) in the large majority of a group of cryoprecipitates isolated from patients with connective tissue and autoimmune diseases, a few papers have addressed the problem of the actual frequency with which this glycoprotein can be detected in cryoglobulins [2, 5, 12]. We now show that FN is a regular component of immunochemically different cryoglobulins and plays a significant role in cold-induced immunoglobulin precipitation.

Materials and methods

Specimens Studied

A total number of 29 cryoglobulins were included in this study and were grouped into three different categories. Group I consisted of 10 patients with histologically confirmed liver cirrhosis (LC), who have been the object of a previous report [5]. Alcoholism was consistently excluded in these cases by both an accurate history and morphologic criteria. Group II was accounted for by 13 patients with EMC who had been followed-up for periods ranging from 6 months to 9 years. Finally, 6 patients with a lymphoproliferative disease were gathered in group III: 4 of them had WM and 2 had MM.

Isolation and Purification of Cryoglobulins

Blood sample collection, isolation and purification as well as immunochemical characterization of cryoglobulins were carried out as described elsewere [7]. Separation of cryoglobulin components was achieved by gel filtration chromatography of the purified cryoprecipitates on Sephadex G-200 columns, using a Na-acetate buffer 0.2 M, pH 4.0.

Fibronectin Detection

FN was identified in both plasma samples and isolated cryoproteins by Ouchterlony double diffusion analysis and electroimmunoassay, using a strictly specific rabbit antibody to human FN (Behring Institute, Scoppito, Italy). For reference purposes as well as for the preparation of standard solutions, human plasma FN was isolated [19] by one-stop chromatographic separation on Gelatin-Sepharose 4B (Pharmacia Fine Chemicals, Uppsala, Sweden). The results of this separation procedure were checked by sodium dodecyl sulfate (SDS)-polyacrylamide slab gels, using a discontinuous buffer system.

Fibronectin Measurement

Quantitation of FN was accomplished by a turbidimetric assay, using a commercially available kit (Boehringer Mannheim GmbH, Milan, Italy), which is based on the kinetic turbidimetric measurement of the antigen-antibody reaction according to the 'fixed time' method. The procedure allows a measuring range of approximately 0–1,000 µg FN/ml plasma. A standard curve was drawn using known amounts of isolated FN.

Effect of FN Depletion and Reconstitution on Cryoprecipitation

In order to evaluate the role of FN in both the formation and amount of a cryoprecipitate, aliquots of each serum sample were selectively depleted of FN using the same affinity chromatography approach on Gelatin-Sepharose 4B columns already described for the isolation of FN. The same samples applied to simple Sepharose columns in the absence of gelatin were used as controls. Cryoprecipitation was then comparatively verified in each case before and after removal of the FN. Conversely, increasing quantities of FN were added to the system and the effects on the amount of cryoprecipitates were recorded.

Anti-FN Activity of Cryoprecipitates

Anti-FN activity of cryoproteins and/or their isolated constituents was looked for by an indirect solid-phase radioimmunoassay [2]. Plate wells were coated with FN, washed with buffered saline, filled with 1 % bovine serum albumin, and then washed again with buffered saline. Afterwards, solubilized whole cryoglobulins and their fractions were added and incubated overnight. Following a further washing, a ^{125}I-labelled goat antiserum to human IgG was added to the system and incubated for 18 h at room temperature. Controls included a rabbit antibody to human FN, followed by a ^{125}I-labelled goat antiserum to rabbit IgG. The sensitivity threshold of this assay was calculated to be approximately 40 ng/ml of the affinity-purified rabbit antibody to human FN.

Additional Tests

Total protein levels were determined by the Folin-Lowry method using human albumin as a standard. Fibrinogen concentrations were measured by single radial immunodiffusion and fibrinogen degradation products were detected by a latex agglutination test.

Results

The immunochemical typing of the 29 isolated cryoglobulins included in this study is reported in Table I. With the exception of the 4 Waldenström-type IgM and the 2 myeloma IgG cryoproteins, the remaining 23 cryoprecipitates were of the mixed IgM-IgG type, cryoglobulins with a monoclonal

Table I. Summary of clinical and laboratory features of patients studied.

| Patient No. | Age years | Sex | Diagnosis | Serum cryoglobulin | | FN | Fibrinogen anti FDP |
				Concen-tration (MG/ML)	Immuno-chemical analysis		
1	52	F	LC	3,7	IgMk-IgG	+	−
2	56	M	LC	5,0	IgM-IgG	−	−
3	47	F	LC	4,2	IgM-IgG	+	−
4	45	F	LC	3,3	IgMk-IgG	+	+
5	63	M	LC	3,0	IgMk-IgG	+	−
6	42	F	LC	2,8	IgM-IgG	+	−
7	57	M	LC	3,5	IgM-IgG	−	−
8	60	F	LC	3,5	IgM-IgG	+	−
9	64	F	LC	4,0	IgM-IgG	+	−
10	49	M	LC	4,2	IgM-IgG	+	−
11	61	F	EMC	8,0	IgM-IgG	+	−
12	40	M	EMC	5,4	IgMk-IgG	+	−
13	38	F	EMC	9,2	IgMk-IgG	+	−
14	45	M	EMC	5,0	IgMk-IgG	+	−
15	31	F	EMC	5,5	IgM-IgG	+	−
16	40	F	EMC	4,6	IgMk-IgG	+	−
17	38	F	EMC	3,8	IgM-IgG	+	+
18	35	F	EMC	10,0	IgM-IgG	+	−
19	52	M	EMC	4,2	IgMk-IgG	+	−
20	37	M	EMC	4,0	IgMk-IgG	+	−
21	41	F	EMC	7,5	IgM-IgG	+	−
22	63	F	EMC	6,4	IgMk-IgG	−	−
23	47	F	EMC	6,1	IgMk-IgG	+	+
24	67	F	WM	13,4	IgMk	+	−
25	59	M	WM	21,3	IgMk	+	+
26	62	M	WM	18,9	IgMk	+	−
27	60	F	WM	31,3	IgMk	+	−
28	60	F	MM	33,7	IgGk	+	−
29	72	M	MM	35,3	IgGk	+	−

component being more numerous in the EMC group and mixed polyclonal-type cryoglobulins in the LC group. In addition, the amount of the cryoprecipitable protein exceeded 5 mg/ml in all single-type as well as in over half of the mixed cryoglobulins with a monoclonal component, but in none of the mixed polyclonal cryoproteins. It should also be emphasized that the monoclonal components mounted kappa light chains in all cases and that the IgM fractions of mixed cryoglobulins consistently exhibited antihuman gamma-globulin (rheumatoid factor) activity. On the contrary, no such activity could be shown in any of the IgM or IgG Type I cryoglobulins.

With the exception of 2 instances of LC and 1 of EMC, FN as detected by both Ouchterlony double diffusion analysis and electroimmunoassay in all

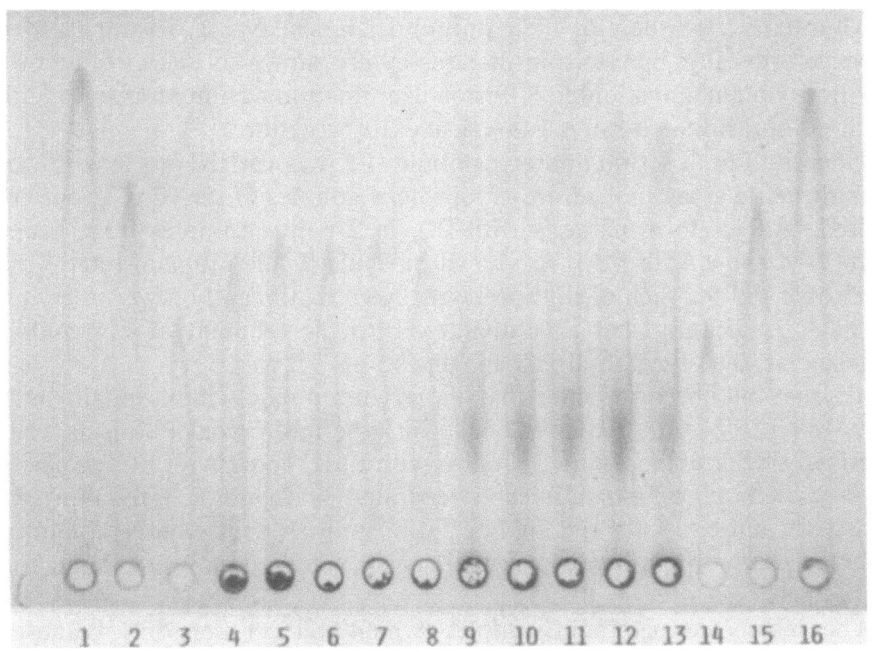

Figure 1. Laurell's electroimmunoassay in 1% agarose gel containing a rabbit antiserum to human FN. Ten different purified cryoglobulins (3 mg/ml) were placed in wells 1–10, whereas wells 1–3 and 14–16 were filled with standard FN solutions (1,000; 750, and 500 µg/ml, respectively). Despite poor solubility of cryoproteins, a 'rocket' is clearly visible with all samples from cryoglobulinemic patients.

Table II. Total Protein (TP) and FN concentration in sera and cryoprecipitates.

Patient No.	Diagnosis	TP/FN, MG/100 ML		Enrichment factor (ratio 1:2)
		Serum (1)	Cryoprecipitates (2)	
1	LC	6,900/28	370/24	16
4	LC	6,600/17	330/21	25
5	LC	7,000/22	300/44	47
8	LC	5,800/12	265/21	38
10	LC	5,700/23	61/15	62
13	EMC	7,400/19	920/32	13
15	EMC	7,000/12	550/36	38
16	EMC	8,200/32	460/19	10
20	EMC	7,800/29	400/28	19
25	WM	8,900/45	1,300/43	6
27	WM	7,300/49	2,650/33	2
28	MM	8,100/55	2,340/191	12

cryoproteins, regardless of their immunochemical typing. Examples of FN 'rockets' revealed by electroimmunoassay are shown in Fig. 1. In addition, FN lines obtained by double diffusion examination of human plasma and of each cryoprecipitate always gave an identity reaction.

Quantitation of serum and cryoglobulin FN was carried out by an *in vitro* turbidimetric assay in 4 serum-cryoprotein samples of the EMC group, in 5 paired samples from patients with LC, in 2 paired samples from patients with WM and 1 with MM. As shown in Table II, the ratios of total protein (TP) over FN for each of the specimens were significantly lower in cryoprecipitates, indicating that a comparatively higher content of FN could be detected in the cryoglobulins belonging to all 3 Types.

To rule out the possibility that the cryoimmunoglobulins might indeed possess anti-FN activity, 2 Waldenström-type IgM cryoglobulins as well as 4 mixed cryoproteins (from 2 patients with EMC and 2 with LC, respectively) and their chromatographically separated IgM and IgG fractions were tested for antibody activity to FN by an indirect solid-phase radioimmunoassay. Both whole cryoproteins and isolated fractions were found to be consistently negative in this assay.

The same 6 cryoglobulin samples (which were chosen only because of their larger availability) were employed to assess the effects of FN removal and reconstitution upon cryoprecipitation. After serum FN had been selectively removed by affinity chromatography on Gelatin-Sepharose columns, cryoprecipitate formation appeared to be significantly impaired, though to a variable extent from case to case. Conversely, cryoprecipitation was again recovered following stepwise addition of human purified FN to each sample.

Finally, it seems worth emphasizing that, with 4 exceptions, neither fibrinogen nor fibrinogen degradation products were detected in the cryoprecipitates (Table I) indicating that the occurrence of FN in the cryoprecipitates is not likely to result from FN-fibrinogen interactions.

Discussion

The pathogenetic significance of circulating cold precipitable proteins in patients with EMC [3, 7, 8, 11] and LC [5, 12] is to be found in their immune complex nature. This is obviously true for all mixed cryoglobulins of the gammaglobulin/anti-gammaglobulin type. Systemic vasculitis and renal damage, which may be frequently observed in these patients, are indeed typical features of an immune complex disease. In addition, it seems likely that even a certain number of seemingly Type I IgG cryoglobulin usually associated with lymphoproliferative disorders should indeed be considered of the IgG/anti-IgG type [6].

Whatever the exact nature of these cryoproteins in the different situations, the actual reasons for their cold insolubility still remain largely controversial. Attempts to disclose structural abnormalities of cryoglobulins in terms of aminoacid sequence, molecular conformation, carbohydrate moieties, and so on have so far remained inconclusive.

Recently, FN has been detected as a regular component of serum cryoglobulins from patients with connective tissue diseases [1, 2], acute viral hepatitis [12], EMC [2, 5] and chronic active hepatitis [12], as well as of synovial fluid cryoprecipitates from patients with rheumatic disease [4, 13], our results confirm and extend such findings, in that plasma FN has been demonstrated in all but 3 samples of Types I, II and III serum cryoproteins from patients with lymphoproliferative disorders, EMC and LC. Whether failure of FN detection in 3 cryoglobulins might be related to the relatively low cryocrit of both patients, or to the actual lack of this glycoprotein, remains to be ascertained.

That FN was not conceivably entrapped into cryoprecipitates in a passive way was clearly shown by comparative FN measurements in both sera and corresponding cryoglobulins, indicating a relative enrichment of FN in the cryoproteins. In addition, FN involvement in the formation of antigen-antibody complexes was also excluded because of the consistent lack of anti-FN activity by whole cryoglobulins as well as by their chromatographically isolated components. Although FN interactions with the fibrinogen-fibrin system has been suspected to be involved in the formation of cryoprecipitates in the synovial fluid of patients with rheumatic diseases [4, 13], such interactions do not seem to account for the occurrence of serum cryoglobulins in that fibrin-fibrinogen products could not be shown in the large majority of the cryoprecipitates.

FN appears to be involved in a number of seemingly different processes [14, 16], including cell to cell and cell to substratum adhesion, malignant transformation, reticuloendothelial function and removal of colloids by liver cells and macrophages [14, 18]. Confirming the findings of Beaulieu et al. [2], our own experiments of FN removal and reconstitution also indicate that this glycoprotein is essential for cryoprecipitation.

In the course of inflammatory processes, large normal serum proteins acting as acute-phase reactants may significantly increase making intermolecular attractive forces prominent, especially in the cold. Larger and less soluble molecular aggregates might then interact with FN and/or immune complexes, resulting in the formation of cryoprecipitates [9]. It seems, therefore, reasonable to suggest that the role of FN in cryoprecipitation is twofold [9, 10]: indeed, it may favor cold precipitation of IgM-IgG immune complexes (such as in Types II and III mixed cryoglobulins) or of a greatly expanded monoclonal immunoglobulin (as it occurs in Type I cryoglobulin [17]). On the other hand, it can also enhance the removal of cryoprecipitable immune complexes by the clearance system [12].

126

Summary

A total number of 29 cryoglobulins from 10 patients with LC, 13 with EMC and 6 with lymphophoproliferative diseases (LPD) were tested for the presence of plasma FN. This glycoprotein was identified in all EMC and LPD cryoglobulins, and in 8 out of 10 LC cryoprecipitates. In addition, quantitation studies showed a relative enrichment of FN in the cryoproteins as compared with the corresponding serum samples. No anti-FN activity could be demonstrated in 2 Waldenström-type IgM cryoproteins as well as in the isolated IgM or IgG fractions from 4 different cryoglobulins. Interactions fo FN with fibrin-fibrinogen products could also be excluded. FN depletion and reconstitution experiments showed a remarkable, though variable effect on cryoprecitation. It is suggested that FN may enhance both precipitation and removal of monoclonal proteins and/or cryoprecipitable immune complexes by the reticuloendothelial system.

Acknowledgement

Supported in part by a Grant from the Italian Ministry of Education.

References

1. Anderson B, Rucker M, Entwistle R, Schmid FR, Wood GW: Plasma fibronectin is a component of cryoglobulins from patients with connective tissue and other diseases. Ann rheum Dis 40:50-54, 1981.
2. Beaulieu AD, Valet JP, Strevey J: The influence of fibronectin on cryoprecipitate formation in rheumatoid arthritis and systemic lupus erythematosus. Arthritis Rheum 24:1383–1388, 1981.
3. Brouet J-C, Clauvel J-P, Danon F, Klein M, Seligmann M: Biologic and clinical significance of cryoglobulins. A report of 86 cases. Am J Med 57:775–788, 1974.
4. Carson S, Lavietes BB, Diamond HS, Kiney SG: The immunoreactivity, ligand, and cell binding characteristics of rheumatoid synovial fluid fibronectin. Arthritis Rheum 28:601–612, 1985.
5. Dammacco F, Carandente F, Vacca A, Campobasso N, Bonomo L: The occurrence of plasma fibronectin in mixed cryoglobulins from patients with liver cirrhosis. Front gastrointest Res 8:135–145, 1984.
6. Dammacco F, Gnisci G, Silvestris F, Bonomo L: New clinical and immunological trends in cryoglobulinemia. Ricerca Clin Lab 10:51–57, 1980.
7. Dammacco F, Lucivero G, Miglietta A, Antonaci S, Bonomo L: Cryoglobulinemia: a model of immune complexes disease. Immunochemical and structural studies. Ricerca Clin Lab 4:569–590, 1974.
8. Gorevic PD Kassab HJ, Levo Y, Kohn R, Meltzer M, Prose P, Franklin EC: Mixed cryoglobulinemia: clinical aspects and long-term follow-up of 40 patients. Am J Med 69:287–308, 1980).

9. Hardin JA: Cryoprecipitation from normal serum: mechanism for cryoprecipitation of immune complexes. Proc natl Acad Sci USA 78:4562–4565, 1981.

10. Hautanen A, Keski-Dja J: Affinity of myeloma IgG proteins for fibronectin. Clin Exp Immunol 53:233–238 1983.

11. Invernizzi F, Pioltelli P, Cattaneo R, Gavazzeni V, Borzini P, Monti G, Zanussi C: A long-term follow-up study in essential cryoglobulinemia. Acta haemat 61:93–99, 1979.

12. Levo Y: Presence of fibronectin in cold precipitates of patients with cryoimmunoglobulinemia. Int Archs Allergy appl Immun 68:179–181, 1982.

13. Lu-steffes M, Iammartino AJ, Schmid FR, Castor CW, Davis L, Entwistle R, Anderson B: Fibronectin in rheumatoid and non-rheumatoid arthritic synovial fluids and in synovial fluid cryoproteins. Ann clin Lab Sci 12:178–185. 1982.

14. McDonagh J: Fibronectin, a molecular glue. Archs Path Lab Med 105:393–396, 1981.

15. Meltzer M, Franklin EC: Cryoglobulinemia. A clinical and laboratory study. II. Cryoglobulins with rheumatoid factor activity. Am J Med 40:837–856, 1966.

16. Ruoslahti E, Engvall E, Hayman EG: Fibronectin: current concepts of its structure and functions. Collagen Res 1:95–128, 1981.

17. Strevey J, Beaulieu AD, Ménard C, Valet JP, Latulippe L, Hébert J: The role of fibronectin in the cryoprecipitation of monoclonal cryoglobulins. Clin exp Immunol 55:340–246, 1984.

18. Tsukamoto Y, Helsel WE, Wahl SM: Macrophage production of fibronectin, a chemoattractant for fibroblasts. J Immun 127:673–678, 1981.

19. Zardi L, Carnemolla B, Siri A, Santi L, Accolla RS: Somatic cell hybrids producing antibodies specific to human fibronectin. Int J Cancer 25:325–329, 1980.

Discussion Part III

CORDONNIER: Dr. Invernizzi, we looked to cryoglobulins since '71 and we have seen about 600 patients with more than 80 mcg/ml of cryoglobulins in the serum. I agree completely with your new classification which seems to be closer to the clinical situations. The second point concerns the prognosis of essential mixed cryoglobulinemia: I agree with you in that type II is more severe in the long and in the short term than type III; in that renal involvement is twice more frequent in type II than in type III; in that type II presents severe membranoproliferative GN whereas only proliferative GN in type III is usually seen. Moreover, in my opinion hepatic involvement is not identical in these two subgroups.

D'AMICO: I am not perfectly convinced about your classification in which you consider 'secondary' also type II cryoglobulinemia found in patients with liver disease, implying that cryoglobulin production, in this case, is a consequence of the hepatic disorder. I think type II cryoglobulinemia is something pathogenetically different from type III, being possibly due to the presence of an abnormal clone of monoclonal IgM-producing cells, a sort of 'paraneoplastic' disease. When we find a type II cryo and a concomitant liver disease we must consider the possibility that we are dealing with a primary essential mixed cryoglobulinemia complicated by secondary liver involvement.

INVERNIZZI: I don't think that type II cryoglobulinemia is a paraneoplastic disease, I think it is the best example of the continuum existing between the autoimmune diseases and the neoplastic proliferation. Other examples are the Sjögren syndrome and, in the experimental pathology, the autoimmune disease of the NZB mice. In our series we have a small number of cases of EMC type II (5 out of 70) who developed a malignancy after a period of 5–10 years. In patients with established liver cirrhosis we observed a type II cryoglobulinemia which clinically appeared secondary to the liver disease. Perhaps the hepatic failure might determine a continuous antigenic stimulation and trigger the production of a monoclonal IgM.

MIHATSCH: Can you explain why EMC is so frequent in Italy and so rare outside of Italy?

INVERNIZZI: I have no explanation for that.

DAMMACCO: Why do you say it is so rare elsewhere? There have been a lot of reports dealing with EMC in the USA and in Holland.

MIHATSCH: We are looking for mixed cryoglobulins in Switzerland since ten years and we found only one case.

CARSON: Dr. Wang, you didn't talk at all about carbohydrate composition of cryos. I wonder whether there is somebody, who knowns the new techniques for sequencing specific carbohydrates.

WANG: I don't know too much about carbohydrates. I don't think that carbohydrate involvement is a major factor, because many of the mono-clonal cryoglobulins are Bence Jones proteins and they generally do not have any carbohydrate. I should make one comment: if I gave the impression that I know the reason of cryoprecipitability, I apologize, I certainly do not know.

AGNELLO: Dr. Wang, have you done hydrophobic measurements with the monoclonals after binding to IgG?

WANG: No, we didn't do that kind of measurements. What we did is just a comparison based on the sequence analysis of informations available.

AGNELLO: What would you expect if you took a monoclonal antibody and added one molecule of IgG at a time to it? What it would happen to the hydrophobic measurement of that molecule?

WANG: I don't know if anybody has done that.

GLASSOCK: Dr Lalazeri has recently described the inhibition of cryopre-cipitation by long chain carboxylic acids. How does this inhibition work in terms of protein and carbohydrate content of the cryoimmunoglobulin?

WANG: I don't know.

GELTNER (Israel): Dr. Abraham, to the unexperienced eye, like mine, the organization of the cryoglobulin fibrils you have just shown us resembled the amyloid fibrils. Isn't that in support of the idea that both diseases, what we used to call primary amyloidosis and mixed cryoglobulinemia, could both be two sides of the spectrum of the same disease, namely plasma-cell dyscrasia?

ABRAHAM: I think there is probably a fundamental difference between of what amyloid proteins are in terms of structure and final morphologic form and the cryos. The amyloid fibrils are really different in the fact that they are composed of immunoglobulins, but there is no reason why, for example a longstanding cryo, if it is a lymphoproliferative disorder, could not ulti-mately wind up in an amyloid or as an amyloid protein. I would like to ask what is the experience of amyloid in mixed cryoglobulinemia.

DAMMACCO: The incidence of amyloid in cryoglobulinemia is low, prob-ably not higher than 8–10%. On the other hand, you know that to mimic amyloidosis it should have a Beta-pleated-sheet structure, which I don't think it has.

ABRAHAM: No, it hasn't.

CORDONNIER: Dr. Abraham, the picture you demonstrated concerned only experimental data *in vitro*, or were they from patients' sera? In IgM-IgG type II cryoglobulinemias do you regularly find the same picture?

ABRAHAM: I just called mixed IgG-IgM type II or IgG type I cryoglobu-lins according to the usual classification, but I can't get the interaction over it.

CORDONNIER: A systematic search for ultrastructural aspects of cryopre-cipitates conducted us to observe that we had to be fortunate to find these aspects which seem to be related to some ratio between IgM and IgG (for instance if you have 1:1 ratio, you have tha aspect, if you have 9:1 ratio, you do not see it.

ABRAHAM: You can actually change the form of the cryoglobulins simply by concentrations or by juggling antigen to antibody. But we usually just take as it comes out from the patients' serum. I don't bother to adjust the antigen-antibody concentrations.

PETERS: Dr. Abraham, how much of these conformational changes that, for example, lead to crystalization do you think are required for immunopathological consequences?

ABRAHAM: There is no real conformational change in the crystal protein. However our few patients with the pure monoclonal type I IgG cryoglobulins had a clinical course which seem to follow the type of cryoglobulin precipitation, the more indolent course seems to follow the formation of the cryo-gel, the more malignant and rapidly progressive course seems to follow the formation of the crystal protein. Looking at it simply on a biophysical basis, you can assume that the crystal falls out and is able to self-associate much more rapidly and at lower concentrations and can also form a smaller nucleus; on the other hand the cryogels take a much longer time to form, have to polymerize and you can tolerate much larger polymers in the serum before the protein actually falls out. Moreover in the cryo-gel forms symptoms of hyperviscosity are greater than in the cryocrystalling forms as the protein concentration goes up.

CORDONNIER: I will emphasize the fact that we can find such an ultrastructural aspect in the kidney, in the liver and in many circulating cells, for example monocytes or leukocytes.

DONINI (Bologna): Dr. Abraham, I have observed patient with Waldenstrom's disease and a type I IgM cryo, in whom the cryoprecipitate disappeared after washing in PBS. It was possible to get this cryoprecipitate only washing it with distilled water. So it seemed that the cryoprecipitation was really salt concentration-dependent. Did you ever observe this phenomenon? In this respect did you observe differences between type I, type II or type III cryoglobulinemia?

ABRAHAM: We have published two papers, recently, for monoclonal IgG cryoglobulins: one is in the Journal of Biochemistry and Biophysics and the other one is in Bicohemistry. We showed exactly what you showed: shielding charges, which maybe are on the surface of molecules, enhance the solubilization of cryoproteins or, indeed, of some immunocomplexes. Because of the ions in the solution you shield the interactions between the molecules. As you lower the concentration of the salt, you get a typical euglobulin effect in the cryoprotein, as complexes begin to self-associate, and they fall spontaneously out of solution.

MAGGIORE: Dr Dammacco, did you find any relationship between the plasma fibronectin level, the cryoglobulins level and the disease activity?

DAMMACCO: There was no relationship between the amount of fibronectin which we could quantitate in the whole serum and the amount which we could find in the isolated cryoprecipitates. And that's why in most cases there seemed to be a higher concentration in the cryoprecipitates as compared with the whole serum, suggesting that an enrichment factor could be calculated in the cryoprecipitate and that probably fibronectin was not passively entrapped in the cryoprecipitate but it was an active phenomenon. As regards a comparison with the clinical activity of disease, no relationship was present.

AGNELLO: I have one more question for Dr. Abraham. In the mixing experiments if you mix cryoprecipitable RF with Fc of normal IgG do you get cryoprecipitation?

ABRAHAM: We haven't actually done those studies, all we have done is to inhibit the cryoprecipitation with Fc fragments that regenerated after various periods of digestion.

DAMMACCO: In some experiments you can apparently get the same amount of cryoprecipitation whether you use the normal IgG or the Fc fragment.

ABRAHAM: I am surprised nobody asked if we found any fibronectin in our cryoprecipitates and whether they were responsible for that. The answer to the question is: we actually were not able to find any fibronectin in monoclonal IgG cryoglobulins nor in the mixed cryoglobulins in the serum or in purified cryoglobulins or equally in cryoprecipitates.

AGNELLO: What do you think the discrepancy is here?

ABRAHAM: I don't think there is any, which probably means that you can have fibronectin in some cryoprecipitates and it may contribute to it, while it may not be present in others.

DAMMACCO: We have tested 8 type I cryoglobulins, all of them from patients with Waldeström's macroglobulinemia and in none of them could we detect fibronectin in the cryoprecipitate, so it's not a rule which is always valid, of course. Even in two of ten cryoprecipitates from patients with liver cirrhosis we were not able to detect fibronectin.

AGNELLO: Was there fibronectin in the renal lesion in mixed cryoglobulinemia?

DAMMACCO: We haven't look for fibronectin in the kidney. Moreover, I would say that fibronectin is an ubiquitous glycoprotein which is synthesized by many cells, including kidney cells.

GLASSOCK: Is there any necessary relationship between C1q content of mixed cryo and fibronectin binding?

DAMMACCO: There is not a strict relationship: however, since we knew that fibronectin can bind C1q, we looked for C1q and we found it in two cases of essential mixed cryoglobulin.

Part IV. Immunological aspects of essential mixed cryoglobulinemia

12. Complement activation in patients with mixed cryoglobulinemia (cryoglobulins and complement)

IRMA GIGLI

Cryoglobulins are an abnormal group of serum proteins which share the common property of reversible precipitation at low tempartures [1]. It is now accepted that the majority of cryoglobulins are either intact monoclonal immunoglobulins (Igs) [2], or more often, Ig complexes in which one component, usually IgM, exhibits antibody activity to the Fc and F(ab')2 portions of IgG [3–5]. These latter complexes have been termed mixed cryoglobulins.

As a syndrome, cryoimmunoglobulinemia has been associated with a variety of hematopoietic malignancies, acute and chronic bacterial infections, and collagen-vascular diseases. Recently, it has been recognized that viral infections, most commonly the one of hepatitis B virus, appear to be involved in the pathogenesis of the essential form [6–8].

The most common clinical features of this syndrome are purpura, which is present in most patients, arthralgias, weakness, and renal involvement that can be rapidly progressive [5]. Histologic examination of the affected tissues shows involvement of the vessels compatible with leukocytoclastic vasculitis. Although these vascular lesions are most frequently seen in the skin, they are also found to a lesser extent in other organs such as the kidneys, heart, brain, and pancreas [9]. The cause of this vasculitis is unknown. However, it has been suggested that mixed cryoglobulins may function as immunecomplexes, and that their deposition in tissues may cause subsequent vascular inflammation. The demonstration of IgG, IgM, and deposits of components of complement at involved sites, lends support to this hypothesis [5, 10, 11].

Determinations of complement-component levels in the sera of patients with essential mixed cryoglobulinemia, have generally revealed low levels of C1, C4, and C2, with no effect on C3 levels in most cases [12–14]. There are, however, rare reports of low levels of C3 and CH_{50} [15, 16]. It has been hypothesized, that the lack of C3 activation in spite of markedly decreased levels of C4 and C2, is due to hyposynthesis of these early complement components, rather than a consequence of complement activation [13, 17]. Here we present evidence that the lack of effect upon C3, may be due to a previously undescribed regulatory mechanism of the classical pathway C3 convertase (C4b, 2a), mediated by two proteins, normally present in serum, the C4 binding protein (C4-bp) and the C3b/C4b inactivator (I) [18].

Materials and methods

Buffers

Veronal-buffered saline 0.15 M, pH 7.5, containing 0.1% gelatin (GVB$^=$), 0.15 mM CaCL$_2$ and 0.5 mM MgCl$_2$ (GVB^{++}); dextrose-veronal-buffered saline 0.075 M (D-GVB^{++}) and 0.04 M disodium ethylenediaminetetracetate (EDTA) buffer in GVB$^=$ (EDTA GVB$^=$) were prepared as previously described [19].

Purified Complement Components, Cellular Intermediates and Assays

Guinea pig [19] and human C$\bar{\text{l}}$ [20], human C4 [21], C2 [22], C3 [23], C4-bp [24], and C3b/C4b inactivator (I) [25, 26] were purified by previously published techniques. C4 was radiolabeled with ^{125}I by the lactoperoxidase method [27], the specific activity was $\cong 3 \times 10^5$ cpm/ug protein. EA and EAC$\bar{\text{l}}$ cells were prepared from sheep erythrocytes as previously described, and were converted to EAC4b,2a cells using highly purified C4 at a concentration of 6 ug/1 $\times$ 10^8 cells [28]. Measurements of C4, C2, and C3 were performed by hemolytic titrations [29]. Rat serum, diluted 1/20 in EDTA GVB$^=$, was used as a source of C3-C9. The C5, C6, C7, C8 and C9 used in C3 titrations were purcheased from Cordis Laboratories (Miami, FL).

Depletion of C4-bp from Normal Human Serum

Rabbit anti-C4-bp was prepared by injecting rabbits with purified C4-bp incorporated in complete Freund's adjuvant. By cross immunoelectrophoresis the antiserum reacted against a single protein in human serum and against purified C4-bp. The IgG fraction of this antiserum, obtained by DEAE-cellulose chromatography, was coupled to CNBr-activated Sepharose 4B (Pharmacia Fine Chemicals, Piscataway, NJ) following directions from the manufacturer.

Serum depleted of C4-bp was obtained by passage of 2 ml of fresh normal human serum containing 0.02 M EDTA through an anti-C4-bp immunoabsorbent column equilibrated with EDTA GVB$^=$. The effluent was concentrated to the original serum volume by ultrafiltration.

Structural Analysis of Bound ^{125}I-C4

Polyacrylamide slab gel electrophoresis (SDS-PAGE) was performed as described by Laemmli [30]. Cryoglobulins carrying ^{125}I-C4 were solubilized in a buffer containing 0.0625 M Tris-HCl pH 6.8, 2% SDS, 10% glycerol, and 0.1 M DTT. The samples were heated for 3 minutes in boiling water, applied to 7.5% SDS-PAGE gels, and subjected to electrophoresis. The gels were then stained, dried, and autoradiographs were made.

Cryoglobulin-Containing Serum and Purification of Cryoglobulins

Blood was obtained from ten patients with mixed cryoglobulinemia, who were previously found to have hepatitis B virus antigen, antibody, or both in their sera [8]. The clinical presentation of these patients was characterized by purpuric lesions on their lower extremities, weakness, and/or renal disease. Hepatomegaly, or evidence of hepatic dysfunction by laboratory examination, but with adequate clinical liver function, was also found in them [8]. The purpuric lesions were diagnosed as cutaneous vasculitis histologically.

Serum and EDTA plasma were separated at 37 °C, and either used immediately or stored at −70 °C. Cryoprecipitates were isolated from plasma samples by storing a 25 ml sample in a glass test-tube at 4 °C for 24 hours. The samples were than centrifuged at 2,000 g for 20 minutes at 4 °C, and the supernatant fraction was discarded. The precipitates were washed three times with ice-cold sterile saline and were then resuspended in saline at 37 °C for 20 minutes. The undissolved contaminants were removed by centrifugation, and the cryoproteins in the supernatant fraction were reprecipitated by storage at 4 °C. The concentration of the cryoglobulins was determined by measuring their optical density at E/280 nm while they were in a solubilized form. The redissolved cryoprecipitates were analyzed by Ouchterlony immunodiffusion using monospecific antisera, and were found to contain IgG and IgM. One cryoprecipitate contained trace amounts of IgA as well. No C1q, C3, or C4 were detected.

Results

Complement-Component Levels in the Sera of Patients with Cryoglobulinemia

Levels of C4, C2, and C3 were determined by quantitative hemolytic assays in the sera of ten patients with mixed cryoglobulinemia. Three patterns of complement activation were noted. The first pattern showed elevated or normal levels of C4, C2, and C3 in two patients who had purpura, skin ulcers, peripheral neuropathy, and mild renal disease. The second and most common pattern showed markedly decreased levels of C4, and moderately decreased or normal levels of C2, and C3. This was seen in six patients who had purpura, peripheral neuropathy, and laboratory evidence of abnormal liver function. The thid pattern showed markedly depressed levels of C4, C2, and C3 in two patients who had purpura and severe renal disease.

Activation of Complement in Normal Human Serum by Purified Human Cryoglobulins

The patient's cryoglobulins consisted of IgG and IgM, and as such, one might expect them to activate serum complement *in vitro*. In order to compare their relative complement-fixing abilities, 0.5 ml samples of purified human cryoglobulin, at a final concentration of 1 mg/ml, were incubated with 0.5 ml of normal human serum at 37 °C for 60 minutes. The cryoglobulins were then precipitated by incubation at 0 °C for 30 minutes, and the supernatants removed by centrifugation (2,000 g) at 4 °C for 20 minutes. The C4, C2, and C3 levels were measured in the serum supernatant as well as in a control sample of the same serum incubated without cryoglobulins.

Table I. Utilization of C4, C2 and C3 in normal human serum following incubation with purified human cryoglobulins.

Cryoglobulin Patient	% Uitlization [a]		
	C4	C2	C3
1	86	25	0
2	26	27	0
3 [b]	63	55	57
4	20	0	0

[a] Values áre expressed in terms of % utilization reflecting the difference between those values obtained when normal human serum was incubated either with or without cryoglobulins.

[b] This patient presented with severe renal disease.

The results (Table I) demonstrate that with only one exception (patient 4), each of the cryoglobulins tested was able to activate C4 and C2 to a variable degree as evidenced by the reduced levels of hemolytic activity of C4 and C2. However the cryoglobulins failed to activate C3 in every patient except one (patient 3), who had severe renal disease.

In order to determine whether the lack of C3 utilization by these cryoglobulins, was due to poor formation of the enzyme responsible for cleavage of the C3 molecule known as the classical pathway C3 convertase, C4b,2a, an attempt was made to generate this C3b,2a enzyme complex with purified human cryoglobulin. One-half milliliter of cryoglobulin solubilized in GVB^{++} at a concentration of 1 mg/ml, was incubated with 0.02 ml of highly purified Cl (6,600 units) at 30 °C for 15 minutes, and then 0 °C for 15 minutes. The cryoprecipitate was centrifuged, the supernatant saved for measurement of Cl, and the cryoprecipitate then washed twice in D-GVB^{++} to prevent C̄l̄ dissociation. Finally, the solubilized cryoglobulins were incubated with 0.1 ml of purified C4 (100,000 units), under the same conditions described above. Following precipitation and removal of the supernatant for measurement of C4, the cryoprecipitate was incubated at 37 °C for 15 minutes with a mixture of C2 and C3 (100 units each), and the supernatant of this reaction mixture was assessed for residual C2 and C3 activity. As shown in Table 2, the cryoglobulins consumed 65 % of the Cl, 100 % of the C4, 85 % of the C2, and 86 % of the C3. Thus, it may be concluded, that the failure of the cryoglobulins to activate C3 in whole serum was not due to an impaired formation of the classical pathway C3 convertase.

Modulation of the Cryoglobulin-Induced C̄1̄4̄2̄ Enzyme by C4-bp

As previously reported, C4b, the cleavage product of C̄l̄ action on C4, is degraded in the fluid phase by the serum enzyme C3b/C4b inactivator (I), only in the presence of a recently recognized serum protein, C4 binding protein, C4-bp [31, 32]. In addition, C4-bp accelerates the natural decay of the thermolabile enzyme, C4b,2a, thus serving as an important control mechanism of the function of this enzyme [18]. Based on these observations, it seemed of interest to investigate the role that C4-bp might have as a control protein in the activatin of complement by cryoglobulins.

Cryoprecipitates carrying C̄l̄ and C4b, (cryo-C4b,2a) were prepared as in the previous experiment. The cryoprecipitates were divided into two 0.5 ml samples each containing cryoglobulin at a final concentration of 1 mg/ml. After redissolving the cryoprecipitates by warming them at 37 °C, one sample was mixed with C2 and C3 (100 units each), and the other with C2 (100 units), C3 (100 units) and C4-bp (0.16 mg). After 15 minutes of incubation at 30 °C, the samples were centrifuged, and the residual C3 and C2 activities

140

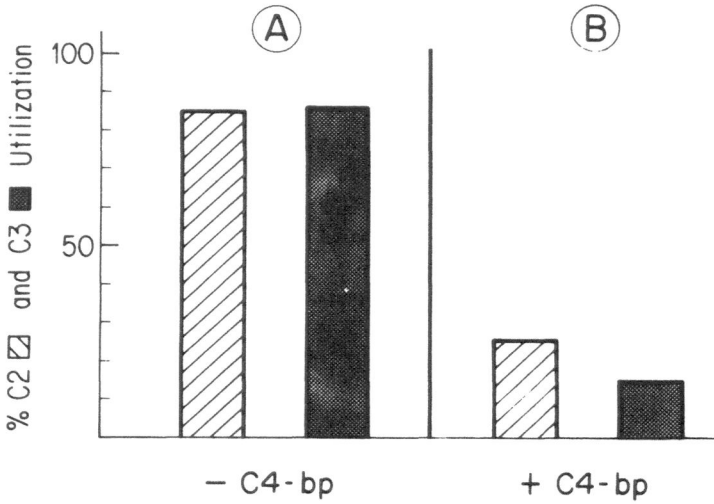

Figure 1. Modulation of Cryoglobulin-Induced C142 Enzyme by C4-bp. Cryoglobulins carrying C1 and C4b were incubated with C2 and C3 diluted either in buffer alone (panel A), or in buffer containing C4-bp (panel B). C2 and C3 activities were measured in these samples and compared with the same complement components incubated in the absence of cryoglobulins.

were measured in the supernatants. As shown in Fig. 1, the C4b,2a enzyme formed in the presence of C4-bp, utilized only 15% of the C3 added whereas in the absence of C4-bp, 86% of the C3 was utilized. Similarly, only 26% of the C2 added was utilized in the presence of C4-bp as compared to 85% utilization of C2 in its absence.

Control of Complement Activation by Cryoglobulins in Normal Human Serum by C4-bp

The previous experiments clearly demonstrated that purified cryoglobulins were capable of initiating the formation of the classical pathway C3 convertase when mixed with purified complement components. They also showed that C4-bp controlled the assembly and function of this convertase. However, the question remained as to whether the function of C4-bp in normal human serum was similar. This was studied in the following experiment. Duplicate 0.5 ml samples of normal human sera were depleted of their C4-bp by passage through a specific immunoabsorbent column. One of these samples was incubated with 0.5 ml of D-GVB^{++}, and the other with 0.5 ml of solubilized cryoglobulin (final concentration 1 mg/ml). As controls, samples of the same normal human sera were passed through a column which did not contain the anti-C4-bp antibody, and these samples were then incu-

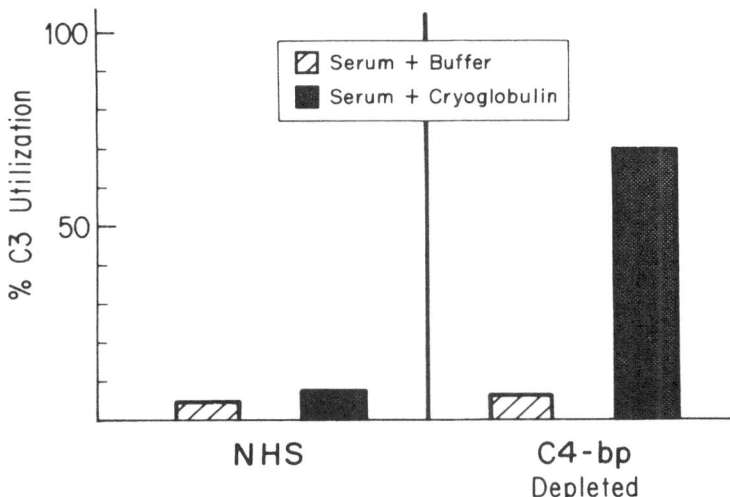

Figure 2. Control of Complement Activation by Cryoglobulins in Normal Human Serum by C4-bp. In the left panel, cryoglobulins incubated with normal human serum (containing C4-bp) were unable to utilize C3. When incubated with normal human serum depleted of C4-bp, as depicted in the right panel, cryoglobulins were able to utilize 71% of the C3 present. No C3 consumption was observed in serum incubated with buffer alone.

bated with either D-GVB^{++} or solubilized cryoglobulin as before. The cryoprecipitates were removed by centrifugation and the serum supernatants analyzed for residual C3 activity. As shown in Fig. 2, cryoglobulins incubated with normal serum failed to utilize C3 whereas those incubated with serum depleted of C4-bp utilized 71% of the C3 present.

Cleavage of C4b Bound to Cryoglobulins by C4-bp and I

These last experiments demonstrated that C4-bp controls the formation of the C4b,2a enzyme and thus the utilization of C3. C4-bp also functions as a co-factor in the proteolysis of C4b, when in the presence of another serum enzyme, the C3b inactivator (I) [31]. In the next experiment, we examined whether C4-bp and C3bINA could change the structure of C4b bound to purified cryoglobulins. Cryoglobulin-C$\overline{1}$ was prepared as in the previous experiment. It was incubated with ^{125}I-C4, centrifuged, and washed with D-GVB^{++} until no counts were found in the supernatant. The cryo ^{125}I-C4b was resuspended in 0.5 ml of buffer and divided into four 0.1 ml samples. Each sample was incubated for 60 minutes at 37 °C with 0.15 ml of either D-GVB^{++}, C4-bp (0.08 mg), I (30 units), or both C4-bp and I. After washing, the solubilized cryoprecipitates were subjected to slab gel electrophore-

142

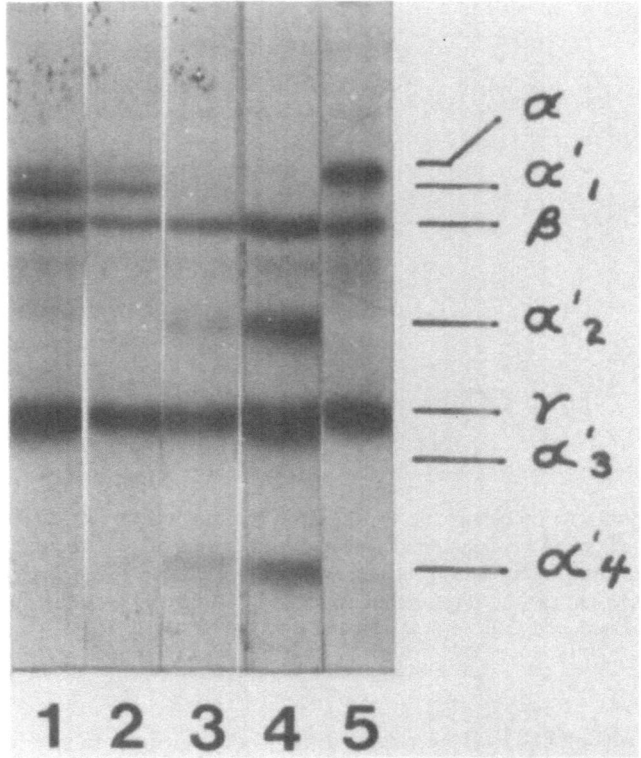

Figure 3. Cleavage of C4b Bound to Cryoglobulins by C4-bp and C3bINA. Autoradiography was performed after SDS-PAGE of samples of cryoglobulin-C14 prepared with ^{125}I-C4 and incubated with either D-GVB^{++} (track 1), C4-bp (track 2), I (track 3), or I and C4-bp (track 5). ^{125}I-C4 (track 5), was used as the reference standard. Track 5 shows the a, β and λ chains of native C4. Tracks 1 and 2 show the a', β, and γ chains which characterize C4b. Tracks 3 and 4 show, in addition to the β and γ chains of C4b, the fragments of cleavage of the a' chain, as evidenced by the appearance of the additional bands $a'2$ (C4d) and $a'4$. The $a'3$ fragment is not seen in this preparation as it contains the least amount of radioactive label, but its relative position has been indicated in the figure.

sis and then an autoradiograph was made (Fig. 3). Gel samples 1 and 2, in which the cryo ^{125}I-C4b was incubated with either buffer, or C4bp, showed three chains, a', β and γ which characterize activated C4 (C4b). Samples 3 and 4, those in which the cryo ^{125}I-C4b was incubated with either I or I and C4bp together, showed further cleavage of the a' chains of C4b as evidenced by the appearance of the $a'2$ (c4d), $a'3$ and $a'4$ fragments derived from a'. These fragments correspond to those previously described as the cleavage products of the two control proteins [31]. In addition, I alone, can cleave C4b [18].

Discussion

Analysis of complement components in the sera of patients with mixed cryoglobulinemia have shown activation of the classical pathway [33–35]. The pattern of complement activation that has been found is unusual in that the early complement components C1, C4, and C2, show variable degrees of utilization, but C3 levels are normal, except in patients with severe renal disease. Studies by Ruddy et al. [17], of complement component synthesis and catabolism in the sera of three patients with essential cryoglobulinemia, suggested that the lowered levels of early complement components and, C4 in particular, was due to their hyposynthesis and hypercatabolism. Tarantino et al. [13], studied serum complement patterns in twenty-six patients with essential mixed cryoglobulinemia and found marked depression of C1q, and C4 levels, in the presence of normal C3 levels. These authors also hypothesized that the main mechanism responsible for these characteristic complement profile was hyposynthesis of the early complement components.

The findings of our studies on complement-component levels in the sera of ten patients with mixed cryoblogulinemia are in agreement with other reports [33–35]. Most of our patients showed markedly decreased levels of C4, moderately decreased or normal levels of C2, and normal levels of C3. The same pattern of serum complement-component utilization was observed when cryoglobulins obtained from sera were purified, and then incubated with normal human serum (Table I). This suggested that a mechanism other than complement hyposynthesis could be involved. The possibility that cryoglobulins were unable to initiate the formation of the C4b,2a enzyme, thereby preventing activation of C3, was investigated by incubating purified cryoglobulins with purified complement components, in an attempt to form the C4b,2a enzyme. The resultant comsunption of C3 in this experiment (Table II), showed that cryoglobulins were in fact capable of initiating the formation of the C4b,2a enzyme. Thus, it was concluded, that some other mechanism was responsible for the lack of C3 activation in normal serum.

Table II. Formation of the C4b, 2a enzyme using purified cryoglobulins and purified complement components

No. of units	C1	C4	C2	C3
Input	6,600	26,500	100	72
Residual	2,300	0	15	10
% Utilization	65%	100%	85%	86%

Recently, Gigli et al. [18] described in normal human serum, a previously unrecognized control protein of the C$\overline{42}$ enzyme, the C4-bp. This protein serves as a modulator of the C4b,2a enzyme by accelerating its decay. In addition, C4-bp acts as an accelerator of I, an enzyme which cleaves bound C4b to form fragments (C4c, C4d) which can no longer participate in the regeneration of the classical pathway convertase.

In view of the properties of these newly described serum proteins, several experiments were carried out to determine whether C4-bp might be responsible for the characteristic pattern of complement component utilization seen in our patients with mixed cryoglobulinemia.

The addition of C4-bp to the purified complement components used in formation of the C3 converting enzyme C4b,2a, was shown to control the degree of C3 activation, as evidenced by the decreased consumption of C3 (Fig. 1). C4-bp was also shown to control the degree of C3 activation in normal human serum incubated with purified human cryoglobulins, in that removal of the C4-bp from normal human serum prior to its incubation with purified human cryoglobulin, resulted in the consumption of all complement components tested, including C3 (Fig. 2).

However, C4-bp was not the only control protein involved. As shown by experiments in which both C4-bp and I were incubated with C4b bound to cryoglobulins, I alone, could cleave C4b, to form C4c and C4d (Fig. 3). Yet, maximal cleavage of C4b required the presence of both I and C4-bp.

In conclusion, although the characteristic serum complement-component abnormalities seen in patients with mixed cryoglobulinemia may be related to complement hyposynthesis, our findings offer an alternative explanation. The consumption of the early serum complement-components C1, C4, and C2 with the characteristic sparing of C3, can be attributed to the action of a recently described control mechanism of the classical pathway C3 convertase.

It is of interest to speculate whether there are differences in the chemical composition of cryoglobulins, that allow for a greater accessibility of C4b or C4b,2a to these control proteins.

Acknowledgement

This work was supported by National Institutes of Health Grant AI20476.

Abbreviations

C4-bp — C4 binding protein

I — C3b/C4b inactivator
C4b,2a — classical pathway convertase
D-GVB^{++} — half-isotonic veronal buffered saline, 0.1% gelatin, 0.5 mM
    magnesium, 0.15 mM calcium, and 2.5% dextrose
DTT — DL-dithiothreitol
EDTA — disodium ethylenediaminetetracetate
SDS — sodium dodecyl sulfate

References

1. Lerner AB and Watson CJ: Studies of cryoglobulins: Unusual purpura associated with the presence of a high concentration of cryoglobulins (cold precipitable serum globulin). Am J Med Sci 214:410–415, 1947.
2. Lo Spalluto J, Dorward B, Miller W Jr and Ziff M: Cryoglobulinemia based on interaction between a gamma macroglobulin and 7S gamma globulin. Am J Med 32:142–147, 1962.
3. Metzger H: Characterization of a human macroglobulin V. A Waldenström macroglobulin with antibody activity. Proc Natl Acad Sci 57:1490–1497, 1967.
4. Geltner D, Franklin E and Frangione B: Anti-idiotypic activity in the IgM fractions of mixed cryoglobulins. J Immunol 125:1530–1535, 1980.
5. Goldman M, Renversez JD and Lambert PH: Pathological expression of idiotypic interactions, immune complex and cryoglobulins. Springer Semin Immunopathol 6:33–90, 1983.
6. Steinhard MJ and Fisher GS: Essential cryoglobulinemia. Ann Intern Med 43:848–858, 1955.
7. Inernizzi F, Galli M, Serirro G et al.: Secondary and essential cryoglobulinemias. Acta Haematol 70:73–82, 1983.
8. Levo Y, Gorevic PD, Kassab HJ, Zucker-Franklin D and Franklin EC: Association between hepatitis B virus and essential mixed cryoglobulinemia. N Engl J Med 296:1501–1504, 1977.
9. Reza MJ, Roth BE, Pops ME and Goldberg LS: Intestinal vasculitis in essential mixed cryoglobulinemia. Ann Intern Med 81:632–634, 1974.
10. Golde D, Epstein W: Mixed cryoglobulins and glomerulonephritis. Ann Intern Med 69:1221–1227, 1968.
11. Meltzer M, Franklin EC, Elias K, McCluskey RB and Cooper N: Cryoglobulinemia — a clinical and laboratory study. II. Cryoglobulins with rheumatoid factor activity. Am J Med 40:837–856, 1966.
12. Zimmerman SW, Dreher WH, Burkholder PM, Goldfarb S and Weinstein AB: Nephropathy and mixed cryoglobulinemia: Evidence for an immune complex pathogenesis. Nephron 16:103–115, 1976.
13. Tarantino A., Anelli A, Costantino A, DeVecchi A, Monti G and Massaro L: Serum complement patterns in essential mixed cryoglobulinaemia. Clin Exp Immunol 32:77–85, 1978.
14. Soter NA, Austen KF and Gigli I: The complement system in necrotizing angiitis of the skin. Analysis of complement component activities in serum of patients with concomitant collagen-vascular diseases. J Invest Dermatol 63:219–226, 1974.
15. Klein F, van Rood JJ, van Furth R and Radema H: IgM-IgG cryoglobulinaemia with IgM paraprotein component. Clin Exp Immunol 3:703–716, 1968.
16. Cream JJ: Clinical and immunological aspects of cutaneous vasculitis. Q J Med 45:255–276, 1976.

17. Ruddy S, Carpenter CB, Chin KW, Knostman JN, Soter NA, Gotze O, Muller-Eberhard HJ and Austen KF: Human complement metabolism: An analysis of 144 studies. Medicine (Baltimore) 54:165-178, 1975.

18. Gigli I, Fujita T and Nussenzweig V: Modulation of the classical pathway C3 convertase by plasma proteins C4-binding protein and C3b inactivator. Proc Natl Acad Sci USA 76:6596-6600, 1979.

19. Nelson RA, Jensen J, Gigli I and Tamura N: Methods for the separation, purification and measurement of nine components of hemolytic complement in guinea pig serum. Immunochem 3:111-135, 1966.

20. Gigli I, Porter RR and Sim RB: The unactivated form of the first component of human complement, Cl. Biochem J 157:541-548, 1976.

21. Gigli I, von Zabern I and Porter RR: The isolation and structure of C4, the fourth component of human complement. Biochem J 165:439-446, 1977.

22. Kerr MA and Porter RR: The purification and properties of the second component of human complement. Biochem J 171:99-107, 1978.

23. Tack BF and Prahl JW: Third component of human complement: Purification from plasma and physicochemical characterization. Biochemistry 15:4513-4519, 1976.

24. Scharfstein J, Ferreira A, Gigli I and Nussenzweig V: Human C4-binding protein. 1. Isolation and characterization. J Exp Med 148:207-222, 1978.

25. Whaley K and Ruddy S: Modultion of the alternative complement pathway by β1H globulin. J Exp Med 144:1147-1163, 1976.

26. Fearon DT and Austen FK: Activation of the alternative complement pathway due to resistance of zymosanbound amplification convertase to endogenous regulatory mechanisms. Proc Natl Acad Sci USA 74:1683-1683-1687, 1977.

27. David GS and Reisfeld RA: Protein iodination with solid state lactoperoxidase. Biochem 13:1014-1021, 1974.

28. Ferreira A., Nussenzweig V and Gigli I: Structural and functional differences between the H-2 controlled Ss and Slp proteins. J Exp Med 148:1186-1197, 1978.

29. Rapp JH and Borsos T: Molecular Basis of Complement Action. Appleton-Century-Crofts, Meredith Corporation, New York, pp 75-111, 1970.

30. Laemmli UK: Cleavage of structural proteins during the assembly of the head of basteriophage T4. Nature (London) 227:680-685, 1970.

31. Fujita T, Gigli i and Nussenzweig V: Human C4-binding protein 11. Role in proteolysis of C4b by C3b-inactivator. J Exp Med 148:1044-1051, 1978.

32. Shiraishi S and Stroud RM: Cleavage products of C4b produced by enzymes in human serum. Immunochem 12:935-939, 1975.

33. Ruddy S., Gigli I and Austen KF: The complement system of man. N Engl J Med 287:642-646, 1972.

34. Potter BJ, Truenan AM and Jones EA: Serum complement in chronic liver disease. Gut 14:451-456, 1973.

35. Perrin LH, Lambert PH and Miescher PA: Complement breakdown products in plasma from patients with systemic lupus erythematosus and patients with membranoproliferative orother glomerulonephritis. J Clin Invest 56:165-176, 1975.

13. Human type II mixed cryoglobulins as a model of idiotypic interactions

J.C. RENVERSEZ, S. ROUSSEL, M.J. VALLE and
P.H. LAMBERT

Introduction

Among the autoimmune diseases those associated with the production of antibodies directed against immunoglobulins (Ig), for example diseases with rheumatoïd factor (RF) may be anticipated in the disturbance of the regulation of the immune response [1]. The most common of these anti-immunoglobulin auto-antibodies, such as RF, are directed against antigenic determinants localized on the Fc fragment of Ig G [2]. Other anti-immunoglobulin auto-antibodies react with determinants on the constant regions of immunoglobulins [3] but a particular attention has been recently given to antibodies reacting with the variable region of immunoglobulin molecules (anti-idiotypes) [4–5]. An internal network of idiotypes and anti-idiotypes has been hypothesized to modulate antibody production against exogenous antigens [6]. It seems possible that a similar mechanism may play some role in controlling the synthesis of RF autoantibodies [7].

A disease associated with a high incidence of anti-immunoglobulin antibodies is cryoglobulinemia in which a monoclonal Ig M possesses an antibody reactivity against a polyclonal Ig G (mixed type II cryoglobulins) [8]. The question of whether the Ig M cryo-antiglobulins select certain subspecies of Ig G from the seric heterogeneous Ig G pool has been postulated in the reactivities of some monoclonal or mixed cryoglobulins [9, 10].

The purpose of this study was to investigate the nature of immunoglobulin interactions involved in a series of 18 type II mixed cryoglobulinemia and to evaluate the possible role of idiotypic interactions in the formation of those cryoglobulins. First, the spectrotypes of the cryoprecipitating Ig G were analyzed to determine whether the formation of the Ig M-Ig G complex would involve a selection of Ig G molecules produced by particular B cell clones. Secondly, the cross-reactivities of each of the 18 cryoprecipitating Ig G with each of the cryoprecipitating Ig M were studied in solid phase assays. These specificities were then better defined using absorption or inhibition experiments and fragmented cryo-components.

Materials and methods

Patients selection

Eighteen patients with mixed cryoglobulinemia unassociated with any underlying disease were choosen. Most of them had renal biopsy proven membrano-proliferative glomerulonephritis.

As controls monoclonal Ig G or Ig M were obtained from myeloma or Waldentröm macroglobulinemia patients.

Mixed cryoglobulins

Cryoglobulins were isolated from 50 ml blood stored at 4 °C for 7 days, followed by a series of centrifugations and sterile washes to separate the cryoprecipitates from the remaining serum [11].

Separation of Ig G and Ig M from cryoglobulins

Separation of the cryocomponents was done by ultracentrifugation in linear sucrose density gradients [12].

The two Ig G and Ig M fractions were then concentrated and quantified by radial immunodiffusion (Hoechst Behring, Marburg, Germany). Further identifications were carried out using agar gel immunoelectrophoresis with the specific gamma, mu, kappa, lambda and whole human serum antisera (Organon, Tecknika b.v., Oss, Holland). Some Ig G containing traces of albumin were thereafter passed through a DEAE ion-exchange chromatography column. Pure Ig G were eluted in 0,015 M Na Cl. Purity of the two fractions was assessed by electrophoresis on polyacrylamide gradient slab gels containing sodium dodecyl sulfate (SDS) with a discontinuous buffer system [13]. Ig G subclasses were determined using specific antisera (Organon) by agar gel double diffusion. Ig G heavy and light chains V region subgroups were revealed also with the same technique using monospecific antisera kindly provided from the Blood Transfusion Center in Rouen (France).

Digestion of the Ig G and Ig M fractions

To prepare Fab and Fc fragments from the cryo Ig G fractions, papaïn (Worthington Biochemical Corp., Freehold, USA) was added to Ig G [14]. Proteolytic fragments were separated from undigested Ig G immediately by gel filtration on a Sephadex G-100 column (Pharmacia Fine Chemicals, Uppsala, Sweden). Fab and Fc fragments were isolated with the same ion exchange chromatography as described above; Fab was desorbed in 0,025 M Na Cl and Fc in 0,300 M Na Cl. To prepare $(Fab')_2$ fragments from the cryo Ig M fractions, TPCK-trypsin (Worthington) was added to Ig M with mild reduction ways [15]. Fragments were separated by Sephadex G200 gel filtration. All fragments were finally purified from residual impurities by affinity chromatography performed with anti gamma and anti mu chains immunosorbents (Dako antiserums-Dakopatts ab., Hägersterl, Sweden) prepared by insolubilization [16].

Fv fragments of some Ig M and Ig G were prepared by treatment of the Ig with thiocyanobenzoïc acid (NTCB SIGMA Chem. Comp., St-Louis, USA). Fragments were separated from other products by gel chromatography with Sephadex G 200 in 6 M guanidine-HCl buffer containing 10 mM sodium phosphate, pH 7 and immediately passed through a Sephadex G 25 column to eliminate guanidine [17].

Purity of the fragments was controlled by immunoelectrophoresis and ELISA with specific antisera. SDS slab gel electrophoresis was used to verify the molecular weight of the fragments.

Control immunoglobulins

7 Monoclonal Ig G were isolated from serum samples by ion exchange chromatography. 3 Monoclonal Ig M and a polyclonal R.F. positive Ig M were purified by gel filtration on Biogel A 1,5 m (Biorad Laboratories, Richmond, USA) followed by affinity chromatography performed with an anti-Ig M immunosorbent (Dako antiserum).

Isoelectric focusing procedure

The isolated cryo Ig M fractions were focused on agarose slab gels containing sorbitol [18]. An ampholine mixture of 2 % final concentration was used corresponding to a pH gradient ranging from 3,5 to 11. The isolated cryo Ig G fractions were isoelectro focused on 5 % polyacrylamide slab gels [19]. After fixing the proteins all gels were stained using a silver staining [20]. Normal polyclonal Ig G or Ig M and pI calibration markers (Pharmacia) were run in parallel.

Solid phase RF ELISA test

A solid phase RF enzyme linked immunosorbent assay (ELISA) was used first to determine the total reactivity of the separated cryo Ig M fractions against pooled human Ig G. The same test was also done to analyze the activity of each cryo Ig M against monoclonal Ig G, each cryo Ig G fraction and proteolytic Ig G fragments. Controls included 7 monoclonal Ig G, an RF positive polyclonal Ig M and 3 monoclonal Ig M. The test was performed in flat bottom microtiter plates specially treated for the ELISA (Titerteck-Flow Laboratories, Richmond, USA) and was done in duplicate. Intact Ig G or Ig G fragments were usually used to coat the microplates for 16 hours at 37 °C. Pooled human Ig G were checked at 1 or 10 microgr/ml concentrations; monoclonal Ig G, cryo Ig G and Ig G fragments were tested at 1,5 and 10 microgr/ml concentrations, always diluted in phosphate buffer saline (PBS). After coating, plates were rinced 3 times in PBS and the wells were filled with 1% bovine serum albumin (BSA) during 2 hours. After removal of the BSA the various cryo or control Ig M and cryo Ig M (Fab')$_2$ were added at the same concentrations in the wells. After incubation 1 h 30 at 37 °C plates were washed and an alkaline phosphatase conjugated mu-chain antiserum was added in each well and allowed to incubate for 2 hours. After washing a nitro-phenyl-phosphate (NPP) substrate (1 mg/ml) was added and after 15 min incubation the optical densities in the wells were read with an automatic spectrophotometer (Multiscan-Titertek) at 405 nm.

Absorption experiments

Anti-immunoglobulin reactivities and cross-reactivities of the cryo Ig M were tested in absorption experiments using the same ELISA test. Plates were coated with polyclonal or cryo Ig G Fab and Fc fragments. After incubation of control or cryo Ig M in the wells, these samples were transferred in a second series of plates coated with the same Ig G Fab or Fc fragments to test their residual reactivities. The percentage of residual binding was calculated from the optical densities obtained with or without absorption.

Fluid phase inhibition experiments were done by incubating cryo Ig M (Fab')$_2$ (10 microg) with cryo Ig G Fab and Fc fragments (1 to 20 microg/ml) in glass tubes. After 2 hours incubation and centrifugation the fluid phase was transferred in plates coated with the same cryo Ig G fragments (5 microg/ml) and the residual reactivities measured by ELISA. Control non absorbed cryo Ig M were tested in the same way. Analysis of the cross-reactivities between the different cryo-Ig M was done by the same ELISA absorption experiments. Cryo Ig M (Fab')$_2$ (5 microg/ml) were subsequently absorbed on different cryo Ig G Fv fragments (5 microg/ml) before testing their residual reactivities against the same and other cryo Ig G Fv fragments. Results of the cross-absorptions were compared in optical densities by reference to non absorbed cryo Ig M (Fab')$_2$ studied in the same conditions.

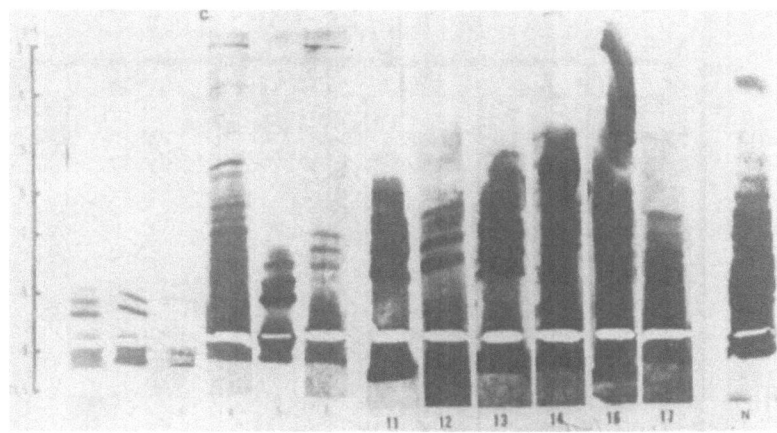

Figure 1. Isoelectrofocusing spectrotypes of some cryo IgG (–17) and of normal human IgG (N) compared to the reference pH gradient scale.

Results

General characteristics of the studied cryoglobulins

All 18 cryoglobulins show proper immunochemical characteristics.

The Ig M components contained only one type of light chains, either kappa (15 cases) or lambda (3 cases), one type of VH and VL subgroups with a particular frequency of VH I (12 cases) and VL K I (9 cases). In all cases the Ig G fractions contained both kappa and lambda chains. The Ig G3 subclass was present in all Ig G fractions; it was associated with traces of Ig G 1 in 4 cases or Ig G 2 in 1 case, but Ig G 3 was the only detected subclass in 13 cases. In 9 cases, only the Ig G VH subgroup I was detected. In those patients, the cryoprecipitated Ig M was also of the VH I subgroup. Such a restriction was not observed for VL subgroups.

Isoelectric focusing analysis of the Ig M and Ig G fractions of the cryoglobulins

The spectrotypes of the 18 Ig M fractions analyzed by isoelectrofocusing confirmed their homogeneity. Only one major band was observed in 14 samples, while some additional minor bands were also seen in 4 samples.

The spectrotypes of the 18 Ig G fractions separated by polyacrylamide gel isoelectric focusing were quite different from each others (Fig. 1). In marked contrast to the large heterogeneity of the pooled normal human Ig G used as control the majority of the Ig G from cryoglobulins presented a restricted

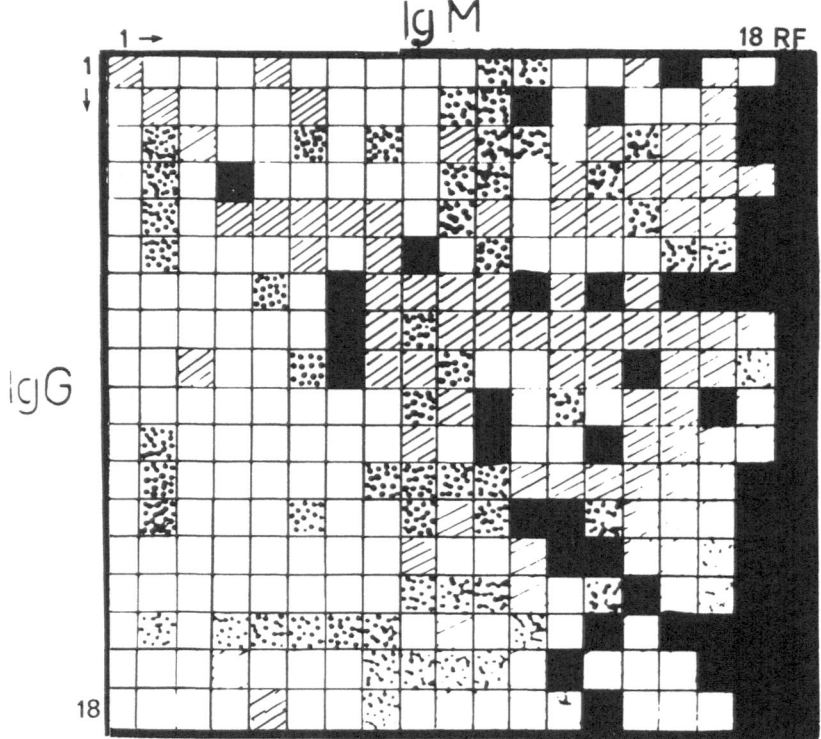

Figure 2. Interactions of each Cryo IgM fraction and of one RF IgM with each cryo IgG fraction. Dark areas represent strongly positive reactions (OD over 600); hatched areas represent positive reactions (OD over 400); pointed areas represent slight positive reactions (OD over 200).

profile with a very limited number of bands. Indeed in 10 cryo Ig G only 2 to 6 bands, often on the cathodic side of the gel, were seen. The other 8 Ig G fractions were more heterogeneous.

Interaction of Ig M fractions with intact Ig G molecules

The interaction of the 18 Ig M fractions was studied with each one of the 18 Ig G fractions obtained from the precipitates. The results, summarized in Fig. 2, indicate that there is often a high degree of restriction in the Ig M-Ig G interactions, probably reflecting marked differences in avidity. In general most Ig M fractions reacted very well with a significant binding (O.D. > 200) with the Ig G fraction isolated from the same cryoprecipitate. In addition some of the Ig M fractions (n° 1-2-3-4-5-6) reacted only with one to three Ig G fractions from other cryoprecipitates. Others Ig M fractions (n° 7-8-9-10-11-12) reacted with four to eight Ig G fractions from other

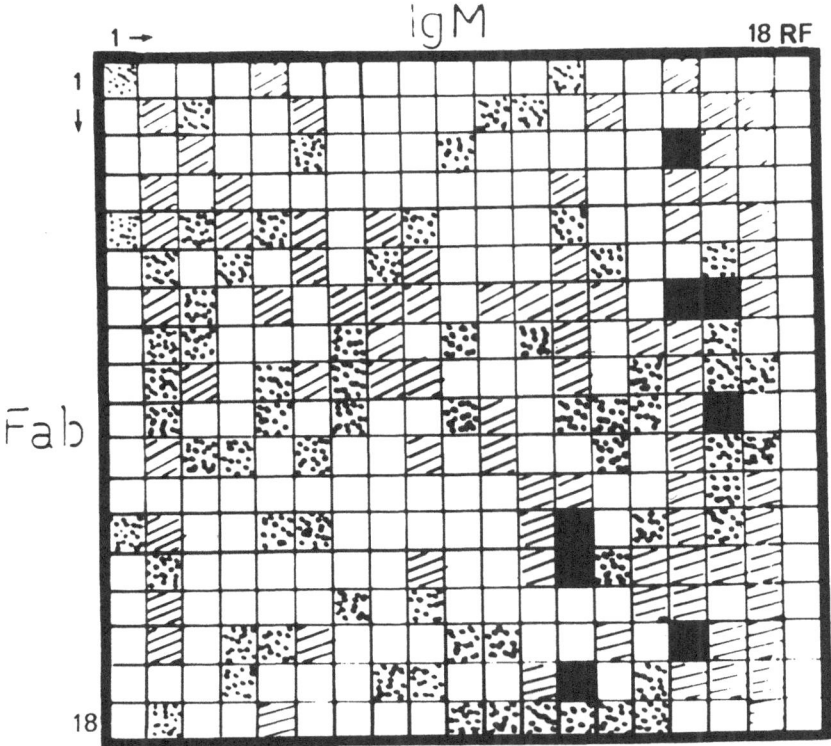

Figure 3. Interactions of each cryo IgM fractions and of one RF IgM with Fab fragments frome each cryo IgG fractions. Representation similar to figure 2.

cryoprecipitates. Only six Ig M fractions (n° 13-14-15-16-17-18) reacted with more than eight Ig G fractions. In similar experiments, there was no binding of monoclonal Waldenström Ig M to any of the solid phase cryo Ig G.

Interactions of Ig M fractions with Ig G fragments

The reactivity of the 18 Ig M fractions was then studied with the Fab and Fc fragments obtained from the 18 cryo Ig G fractions. Each Ig M fraction from cryoglobulins were tested with each of these 18 Fab or Fc preparations. Most positive reactions previously observed with solid phase Ig G fractions were also seen using Fab coated plates with a similar restricted profile (Fig. 3). The binding of Ig M to Fab fragments was usually lower than to intact Ig G fractions. Most of the Ig M to Fab fragments was usually lower than to intact Ig G fractions. Most of the Ig M fractions exhibited a maximal binding to Fab fragments obtained from the same cryoprecipitate. The control

154

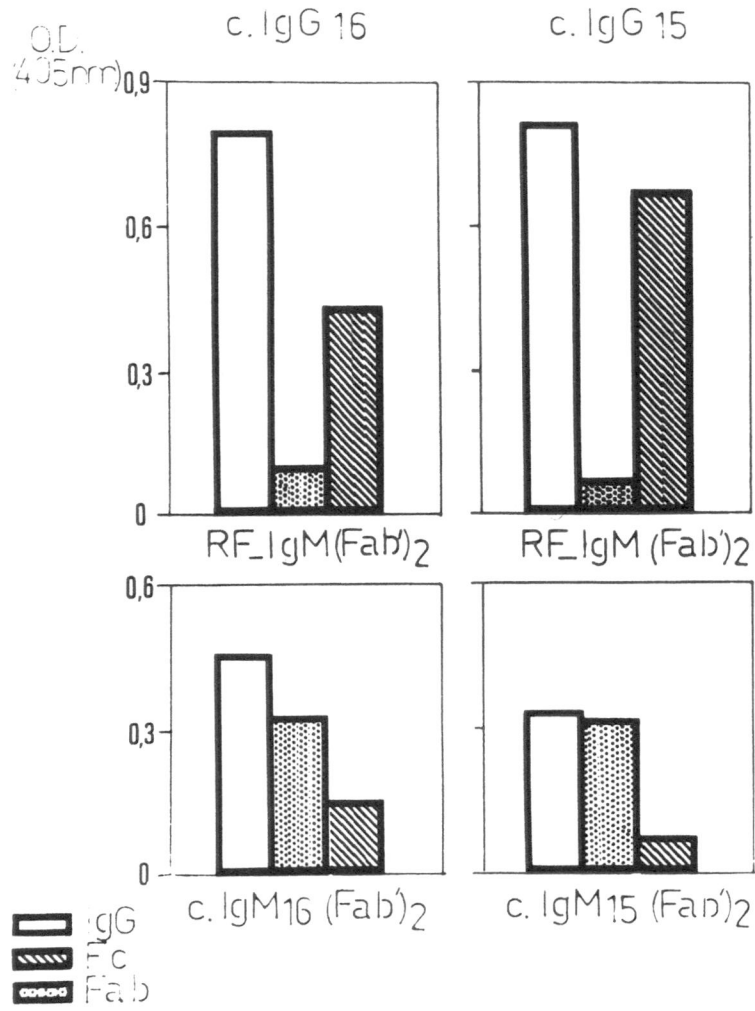

Figure 4. Interactions of 2 cryo IgM (Fab')$_2$ fragments and one RF IgM (Fab')$_2$ with 2 intact autologous cryo IgG fractions or their Fab and Fc fragments.

polyclonal RF did not react with any of the Fab fractions tested. When Fc fractions were used for coating plates instead of Fab fractions, the pattern of reactivity was different from that obtained with intact Ig G fractions. This binding was always rather low as compared to that of the RF Ig M used as control.

The same types of interactions were obtained by replacing in the ELISA the total cryo Ig M by their (Fab')$_2$ fragments (Fig. 4).

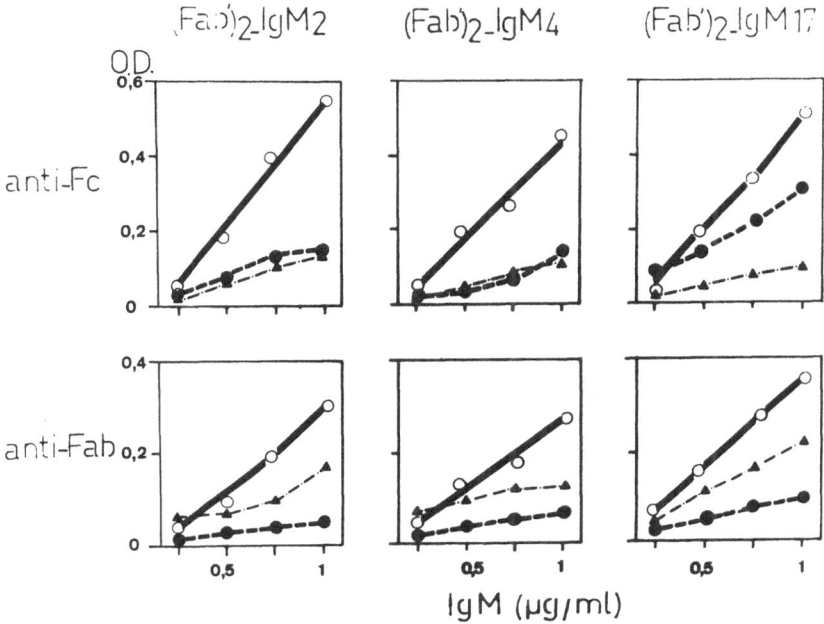

Figure 5. Absorption of 3 cryo IgM (Fab')₂ anti-immunoglobulin activities on solid-phase IgG Fc (▲), or Fab (●) or on uncoated tubes (○). The absorption was done at various IgM (Fab')₂ concentrations and the residual anti-IgG Fc or Fab activities were measured in a second time by the ELISA, using corresponding cryo IgG fragments.

Absorption of anti immunoglobulin activities with Fab or Fc fragments

In a first series of experiments, Fc from normal pooled Ig G was used as a solid phase absorbant for the 18 Ig M samples. These ones were then tested for their reactivity with Fc from polyclonal Ig G or from the corresponding cryo Ig G as well as with Fab from the corresponding cryo Ig G. For all Ig M, there was an extensive absorption of the anti-Fc activity; a similar decrease was observed for a polyclonal RF Ig M after absorption on Fc from polyclonal Ig G. There was also a significant decrease (more than 50%) of the binding of 10/18 Ig M to the corresponding cryo Ig G Fab.

In a second series of experiments, Fab fragments from each cryo Ig G were used to absorb the corresponding Ig M fraction and the results were compared with the absorption with polyclonal Fab from normal pooled Ig G. With all Ig M fractions, there was an extensive decrease of the reactivity with Fab after the incubation with the corresponding solid phase Fab (4 to 18% of residual activity). This absorption with Fab also led to a variable but often very significant decrease of the anti Fc activity of the Ig M fractions (less than 50% residual activity) in 10/18 Ig M. A similar absorption of a polyclonal RF Ig M on Fab from polyclonal Ig G did not lead to any decrease of the anti-Fc activity.

These results were confirmed using 3 cryo Ig M (Fab')$_2$ at various concentrations (Fig. 5). Quantitative absorption experiments confirmed a more efficient depletion of the reactivity with Ig G Fab after absorption on solid phase Ig G Fab, than on solid phase Ig G Fc. Inversely the reactivity with Fc is better absorbed on solid phase Fc. So it was not possible to separate two types of Ig M each showing a proper specificity against Ig G Fab or Fc fragments.

These fluid phase experiments were repeated with cryo Ig M (Fab')$_2$ replacing cryo Ig G Fab by cryo Ig G Fc. Absorptions identified different proper cross-reactivities shared by many of the Ig M (Fab')$_2$, separating it in different groups, as presented in 3 cases on Table I*.

Table I. Fluid phase inhibition assays showing cross-reactivities shared by 3 cryo Ig M (Fab')$_2$ interacting with different cryo Ig G Fv fragments. Siginificant O.D. values are underlined.

	no abs.		abs. on Fv_1		abs. on Fv_4	
	reaction with		reaction with		reaction with	
(Fab')$_2$	Fv_1	Fv_4	Fv_1	Fv_4	Fv_1	Fv_4
Ig M$_1$	238	102	21	92	203	109
Ig M$_4$	36	359	17	302	36	19
	Fv_1	Fv_5	Fv_1	Fv_5	Fv_1	Fv_5
Ig M$_1$	272	242	39	35	41	28
Ig M$_5$	403	327	52	26	57	39
	Fv_4	Fv_5	Fv_4	Fv_5	Fv_4	Fv_5
Ig M$_4$	326	402	15	103	78	102
Ig M$_5$	101	359	57	237	71	39

Ig M → Ig M$_1$ = WH II, K I; Ig M$_4$ = VH I, K I; Ig M$_5$ = VH I, K III

Ig G → 1 = VH I, III; K I, III; L II, III
4 = VH I, III; K III; L II, III
5 = VH I; K III; L II

* First there was no significant cross-reactivity between cryo Ig M$_1$ and Ig M$_5$. Secondly there was an extensive cross-reactivity between IG M$_1$ and IgM$_5$. Thirdly there was a limited cross-reactivity between Ig M$_4$ and Ig M$_5$: Ig M$_4$ and Ig M$_5$ were binding to Fv$_5$ but only Ig M$_4$ was binding to Fv$_4$.

Discussion

The aim of this work is the demonstration of a frequent restriction in the clonotypes of the Ig G molecules involved in the formation of cryoprecipitates with monoclonal Ig M from type II mixed cryoglobulinemia. It also suggest the possibility of idiotypic interactions in many of these cryoprecipitates.

By definition the Ig M component of mixed type II cryoglobulins is a monoclonal immunoglobulin. In the present study, each Ig M fraction was found homogeneous by immunoelectrophoresis and by isoelectrofocusing. Furthermore, there was a prevalence of VH I and VK I variable region subgroups, which suggests that some physicochemical characteristics may be common to some of these Ig M, although they differed from those analyzed by other authors who found a prevalence of VK III in their series of monoclonal RF Ig M [21–23]. Monoclonal Ig M antiglobulins have also been studied with respect to their idiotypes and cross-idiotypic reactions. Cross-idiotypic specificities were clearly demonstrated among a group of monoclonal Ig M antiglobulins, using antisera prepared against single monoclonal Ig M [24].

Our analysis of the Ig G component of mixed type II cryoglobulins indicated a particular selection of Ig G molecules during cryoprecipitation. All these fractions contained mostly Ig G 3 subclass molecules. Although both kappa and lambda light chains were represented, there was a very restricted charge heterogeneity in the Ig G and a very homogeneous profile was seen for some of them. So clonally restricted anti-Ig G antibodies have been recently described with the same alcaline pI [25]. VH I subgroup was predominant since it was found alone in 9/18 Ig G and in association with VH II and/or VH III in 6 other Ig G fractions. There was no such restriction for the light chain V subgroup. These results support the hypothesis of a selection of certain subspecies of Ig G from the heterogeneous Ig G pool during cryoprecipitation and are consistant with a restricted reactivity between the two components in the Ig G-Ig M cryoglobulins. Similarly a restricted reactivity profile was exhibited for cryo Ig M with antiglobulin activity against autologous or isologous human Ig G or their subunits [26]. In a population of 11 monoclonal Ig M from type II cryoglobulins, multiple antiglobulin specificities were shown [10]: Some of the Ig M were reactive with Fc fragments; some others reacted with Ig G (Fab')$_2$ fragments. Other authors suggested that the Ig M anti-Fab may react as anti-idiotypic antibodies with Ig G [27, 28].

In our investigations, we have confirmed that all of the 18 cryo Ig M studied reacted with autologous and isologous cryo Ig G. However this reaction was often of relatively low avidity since, for most of the cryo Ig M, it was only demonstrated when at least 10 microgrìml of Ig G were used for

158

coating in the solid phase assay. The pattern observed suggests a preferential reactivity of the cryo Ig M for some Ig G preparations. The fact that most of the cryo Ig M react with both Fab and Fc fragments of the autologous Ig G suggests two types of interactions between cryo Ig M and cryo Ig G. Indeed, we can exclude the possibility that the reactivity of cryo Ig M with Fab would be due to contaminating Fc since (a) many cryo Ig M react more with Fab than with Fc, (b) each cryo Ig M exhibits a proper pattern of reactivity with the Fab fragments from the 18 cryo Ig G and (c) polyclonal RF did not react with any of the Fab preparations used. The reaction between cryo Ig M and Ig G Fab is specific and involves Ig M (Fab')$_2$. No (Fab')$_2$ of other monoclonal Ig M from patients with Waldenström macroglobulinemia share those specificities. One should note that if the absorption of cryo Ig M on solid phase Fc did lead to a decrease of their binding to Fc there was not a parallel decrease of their binding to Fab fragments from the corresponding Ig G. Inversely, although the absorption of cryo Ig M with Fab from the corresponding cryo Ig G did inhibit completely the binding of all cryo Ig M to Fab, there was only a partial parallel depletion of the anti-Fc activity. These absorption data suggest the existence of a certain heterogeneity in the monoclonal Ig M molecules and confirm the involvement of 2 different sites of reaction. Some cryo Ig G Fv appear to interact with cryo Ig M (Fab')$_2$ similarly to anti-idiotypic antibodies directed against the paratope of the Ig M RF, as epibodies [29], but subsequent analysis should be necessary to point out and subgroup the different cross-idiotypes detected in most of these cryocomponents.

Thus, all these data are consistant, with the idea that in about two thirds of the studied cryoglobulins, the Ig M RF would preferentially interact with anti-idiotypic Ig G Fv. Some of these anti-idiotypes are probably directed against determinants outside the paratope, but in some cases, they would react with the anti-Fc paratope. The coexistence of two reactions, anti-Fc Ig M with Ig G-Fc and anti-idiotype Ig G Fv with Ig M (Fab')$_2$ idiotypes or vice versa, should confer a higher stability to cryoprecipitable Ig M-Ig G complexes. One may wonder whether these cross-reactive idiotypes will be involved in the disturbance of the immune network concerning the pathogenesis of the disease [30].

Summary

Interactions between immunoglobulin molecules within cryoglobulins has been carried out from 18 type II mixed cryoglobulinemia. In this series, there was a prevalence of VH I and VK I variable regions subgroups in the monoclonal Ig M component, a prevalence of Ig G 3 and of the VH I subgroup and a very restricted spectrotype of the isoelectrofocusing pattern in two thirds of the Ig G components. These results suggested a selective reactivity between cryo-Ig M and Ig G fractions and were confirmed by an analysis of the cross-reactions between each Ig G and each Ig M from all cryoprecipitates. All Ig M reacted with intact Ig G or Fc fragments but another reaction was observed between cryo-Ig M and Fab fragments from a limited number of cryo-Ig G. Results of the absorption of each cryo-Ig M $(Fab')_2$ on Fc, Fab or Fv from the corresponding cryo-Ig G also suggested the existence of a reaction between Ig M $(Fab')_2$ and Ig G Fv in addition to that involving Ig M $(Fab')_2$ and Ig G Fc with a pattern suggestive of idiotypic specificities. The coexistence of these two reactions should confer a higher stability to the cryoprecipitating complexes.

Acknowledgements

We are grateful to Mrs N. COLLET for her secretarial help.

References

1. Zubler RE, Nydegger U, Perrin LH, Fehr K, Vormick J.Mc, Lambert PH, Miescher PA: Circulating immune complexes in patients with rheumatoïd arthritis. J Clin Invest 57:1308, 1976.
2. Schrohenloher RE, Kunkel HG, Tomasi TB: Acticity of dissociated and reassociated 19 S anti-gammaglobulins. J Exp Med 120:1215, 1964.
3. Kunkel HF, Mannik M, Williams RC: Individual antigenic specificity of isolated antibodies. Science 140:1218, 1963.
4. Kunkel HG, Agnello V, Joslin FG, Winchester RJ, Capra JD: Coss idiotypic specificity among monoclonal IgM proteins with anti-gammaglobulin activity. J Exp Med 137:331, 1973.
5. Bona CA, Finley S, Waters S, Kunkel HG: Anti-immunoglobulin antibodies. III. Properties of sequential antiidiotypic antibodies to heterologous anti-gammaglobulins. Detection of reactivity of antiidiotype antibodies with epitopes of Fc fragments and with epitopes and idiotypes. J Exp Med 156:986, 1982.
6. Jerne NK: Towards a network theory of the immune system. Ann Immunol (Inst Pasteur) 125:373, 1974.
7. Fong S., Gilbertson TA, Carson D: The internal image of IgG in cross-reactive anti-idiotypic antibodies against human rheumatoïd factors. J Immunol 131:719, 1983.
8. Franklin EC: Cryoglobulinemia. Am J Med Sci 262:50, 1971.
9. Abraham GN, Podell DN, Welch EH, Johnston SL: Idiotypic relatedness of human monoclonal IgG cryoglobulins. Immunology 48:315, 1983.
10. Geltner D, Franklin EC, Frangione B: Antiidiotypic activity in the IgM fractions of mixed cryoglobulins. J Immunol 125:1530, 1980.
11. Renversez JC, Vialtel P, Seigneurin JM, Cordonnier D: Cryoglobulins as immune complexes: an immunochemical study of 376 cryoprecipitates. In: 'Protids of the Biological Fluids', Peters H, Editor, p 391, Pergamon Press, Oxford, 1979.
12. Renversez JC, Groslambert P, Vialtel P, Cordonnier D, Groulade J: Analyse des cryoglobulines par ultracentrifugation en gradient de densité stabilisé suivie d'immunodiffusion. Ann Biol Clin 37:163, 1979.

13. Laemmli UK: Cleavage of structural proteins during the assembly of the head of bacterio-phage T4. Nature (Lond) 227:680, 1970.
14. Nisonoff A, Markus G, Wissler FC: Separation of univalent fragments of rabbit antibody by reduction of a single labile disulfide bond. Nature (Lond) 4761:293, 1961.
15. Plaut AG, Tomasi TB: Immunoglobulin M: Pentameric Fcµ fragments released by trypsin at higher temperatures. Proc Natl Acad Sci , USA 65:no 2, 318, 1970.
16. Avrameas S, Ternynck T: Coupling of enzyme to proteins with glutaraldehyde. Use of the conjugates for the detection of antigens and antibodies. Immunochem 6:43, 1969.
17. Rodnell JD, Karush F: A general method for the isolation of the VH domain from IgM and other immunoglobulins. J Immunol 121:no 4, 1528, 1978.
18. Rosen A, Ek K, Amn P: Agarose isoelectric focusing of native human immunoglobulin M and alpha 2 macroglobulin. J Immunol Methods 28:1, 1979.
19. Brendel S, Mulder J, Verhaar MA: Heterogeneity of monoclonal immunoglobulin G pro-teins studied by isoelectric focusing. Clin Chim Acta 54:243, 1974.
20. Oakley BR, Kirsch DR, Morris NR: A simplified ultrasensitive silver stain for detecting proteins in polyacrylamide gels. Analyt Biochem 105:361, 1980.
21. Kunkel HG, Winchester J, Joslin FC, Capra JD: Similarities in the light chains of anti-gammaglobulins showing cross-reactive specificities. J Exp Med 149:128, 1974.
22. Andrews DW, Capra JD: Complete aminoacid sequence of variable domains from two monoclonal human antigammaglobulins of the Wa cross-idiotypic group. Suggestion that the J segments are involved in the structural correlate of the idiotype. Proc Natl Acad Sci USA 78:no 6, 3799, 1981.
23. Pons-Estel B, Goni F, Solomon A, Frangione B: Sequence similarities among KIII b chains of monoclonal human IgM K autoantibodies. J Exp Med 160:893, 1984.
24. Forre OT, Dobloug JH, Michaelsen TE, Natvig JB: Evidence of similar idiotypic determi-nants on different rheumatoïd factor populations. Scand J Immunol 9:281, 1979.
25. Persselin JE, Lovie JS, Stevens RH: Clonally restricted anti-IgG antibodies in rheumatoïd arthritis. Arthr Rheumat 27:no 12, 1378, 1984.
26. Johnston SL, Abraham GN: Studies of human IgM anti-IgG cryoglobulins. I. Patterns of reactivity with autologous and isologous human IgG and its subunits. Immunology 36:671, 1979.
27. Greenstein JL, Solomon A, Abraham GN: Monoclonal antibodies reactive with idiotypic and variable region specific determinants on human immunoglobulins. Immunology 51:17, 1984.
28. Chen PP, Goni F, Fong S, Jirik F, Vaughan JH, Frangione B, Carson DA: The majority of human monoclonal IgM rheumatoïd factor express a primary structure dependant cross-reactive idiotype. J Immunol 134:no 5, 3281, 1985.
29. Chen PP, Fong S, Houghten RA, Carson DA: Characterization of an epibody. An antiidio-type that reacts with both the idiotype of rheumatoïd factors (RF) and the antigen recog-nized by RF. J Exp Med 161:323, 1985.
30. Geha RS: Idiotypic-antiidiotypic interactions in man. Ric Clin Lab 15:1, 1985.

14. Monoclonal antibodies to idiotypic determinants on monoclonal rheumatoid factors – application to patients with type II cryoglobulinaemia

M. ONO, C.G. WINEARLS, D. GRENNAN, D.K. PETERS and J.G.P. SISSONS

1. Introduction

Type II (mixed essential) cryoglobulinaemia (MEC) presents many unanswered questions. Clearly the major obvious abnormality in these patients is their production of monoclonal rheumatoid factor (MRF). However the factors involved in the initiation and maintenance of MRF production are obscure: for instance is this a primary clonal proliferative disorder, or does a distinct antigen lead to immune complex formation and production of MRF as a secondary consequence as some form of abnormal immunoregulation? Patients with MRC may remain stable for many years without developing clinical or morphological evidence of the B cell clone producing MRF – what is the size and location of this clone? What are the mechanisms involved in the pathogenesis of the disease – the physical basis for cryoprecipitation, mechanism of complement activation, and reasons for the variable clinical pattern of disease? Finally, what is the most appropriate therapy? Many of these questions are addressed by others in this volume. Our own interest has been in developing reagents to facilitate the recognition and enumeration of MRF producing cells, for possible use in the monitoring and clinical investigation of patients with MEC.

In view of the drawbacks of using aggregated IgG to detect RF producing cells we elected to produce a series of monoclonal antibodies to MRF idiotypes and apply these to the clinical investigation of our patients. The existence of a common cross reactive idiotype on MRFs (the Wa idiotype) was first reported by Kunkel and colleagues [1], and the same authors also reported that restricted idiotypes existed on individual MRFs. More recently the molecular structure of some of these idiotypic determinants has been established [2], and anti idiotypic circuits involving MRF described as examples of the network theory [3].

2. Patients and methods

2.1. Patients

This study involved 5 patients with *Type II MEC*. All had monoclonal IgM kappa rheumatoid factors and variable organ involvement. MRFs from four of these patients were purified from their cryoglobulins and used for the production of monoclonal antibodies. One of these patients (patient F) also had acquired hypogammaglobulinaemia as discussed later.

2.2. Methods

MRFs were purified from cryoglobulins by gel filtration on Sepharose 6B, and used to immunise mice. Hybridomas were prepared from the immunised mice by standard techniques and supernatants were screened by solid phase RIA against normal IgM and MRF. Hybrids producing antibody against MRF but not normal IgM were selected, and cloned three times. *The ability of the MAb to inhibit the binding of MRFs to solid phase IgG was tested in a RF assay as previously described* [4].

Pokeweed mitogen (PWM) induced Ig synthesis was studied as described [5]. *Cytospin preparations of* PWM induced blasts and bone marrow were stained immuno-histochemically with monoclonal antibodies and horseradish peroxidase coupled anti-mouse Ig.

Table I. Monoclonal antibodies to monoclonal RFs.

mAb	subclass	donor of MRF
Against cross reactive idiotypes		
* C82G11	IgG1	Co
* F9B8	IgG1	Fr
Against restricted idiotypes		
C8G9	IgG1	Co
* C8E3	IgG1	Co
F8D3	IgM	Fr
* F3EBG	IgG2a	Fr
* K7D10	IgM	Ka
K4C38	IgM	Ka
L8B10	IgG1	La
* L8C3	IgM	La

* Indicates those monoclonal antibodies discussed in this paper.

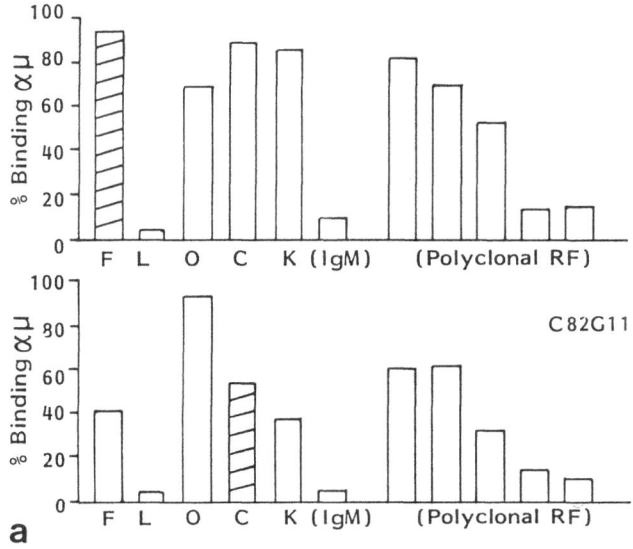

Figure 1a. The binding of two cross-reactive MAbs F9B8 and C82G11 to the MRFs, IgM or polyclonal Rfs (× axis) is represented on the y axis as a % of the binding obtained with a mouse monoclonal anti-u chain antibody (Dako). The cross hatched bar represents the immunizing MRF.

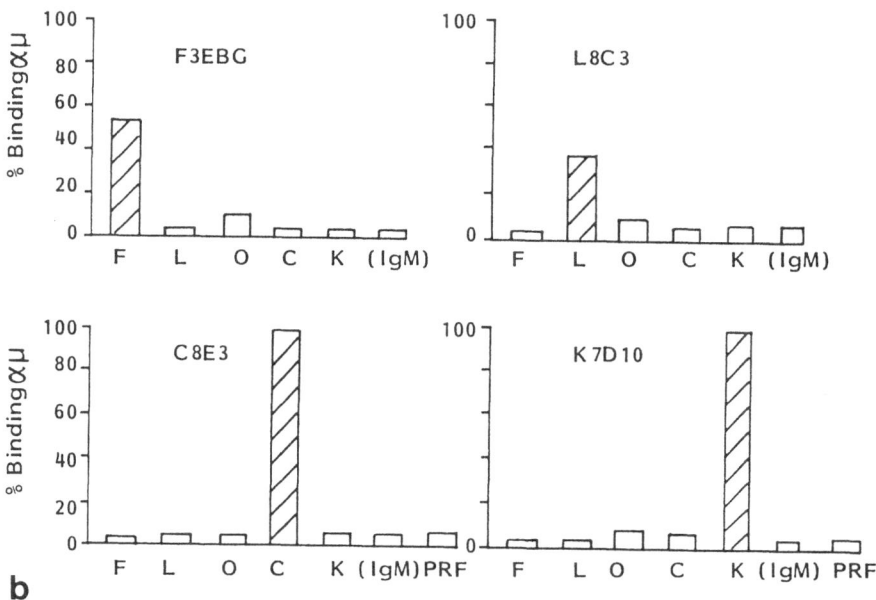

Figure 1b. The binding of four restricted MAbs to the MRFs, IgM or polyclonal RFs (× Axis) is represented on the y axis as a % of the binding obtained with a mouse monoclonal anti-u chain antibody (Dako). The cross hatched bar represents the immunizing MRF.

164

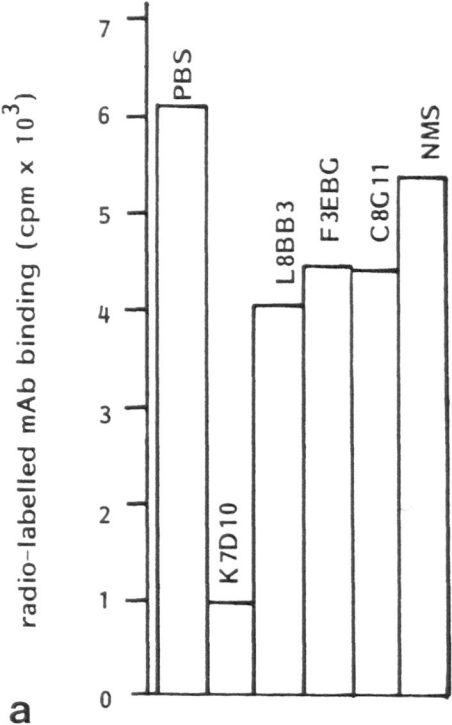

Figure 2a. Inhibition of the binding of I[125] labelled MAB K7D10 to its immunising MRF (K) by unlabelled antibody and not by other MAbs. MAbs L8B3 and F3EGB did not bind to MRF (K) but the cross-reactive MAB C8G11 did.

3.   Results

3.1. Binding specificity of MAbs

A number of MAb which showed specific binding to MRFs were selected for further study. The nomenclature of these MAbs is shown in Table I. Two MAb bound to most of the MRFs studied whereas a number of others bound only to the MRF used for immunisation (Fig. 1a and 1b). The MAb which bound to only a single MRF were subjected to further study. As shown in Fig. 2 when one of these MAb was directly radiolabelled its binding to the autologous MRF could not be inhibited by other cold MAbs recognising a single MRF or an MAb recognising multiple MRFs. Similarly, only the autologous MRF would competitively inhibit the binding of individual MAbs to solid phase MRF. From these characteristics we concluded that the MAbs recognising a single MRF were directed against restricted idiotypes on these MRFs. The two MAb which bound to most of the MRFs

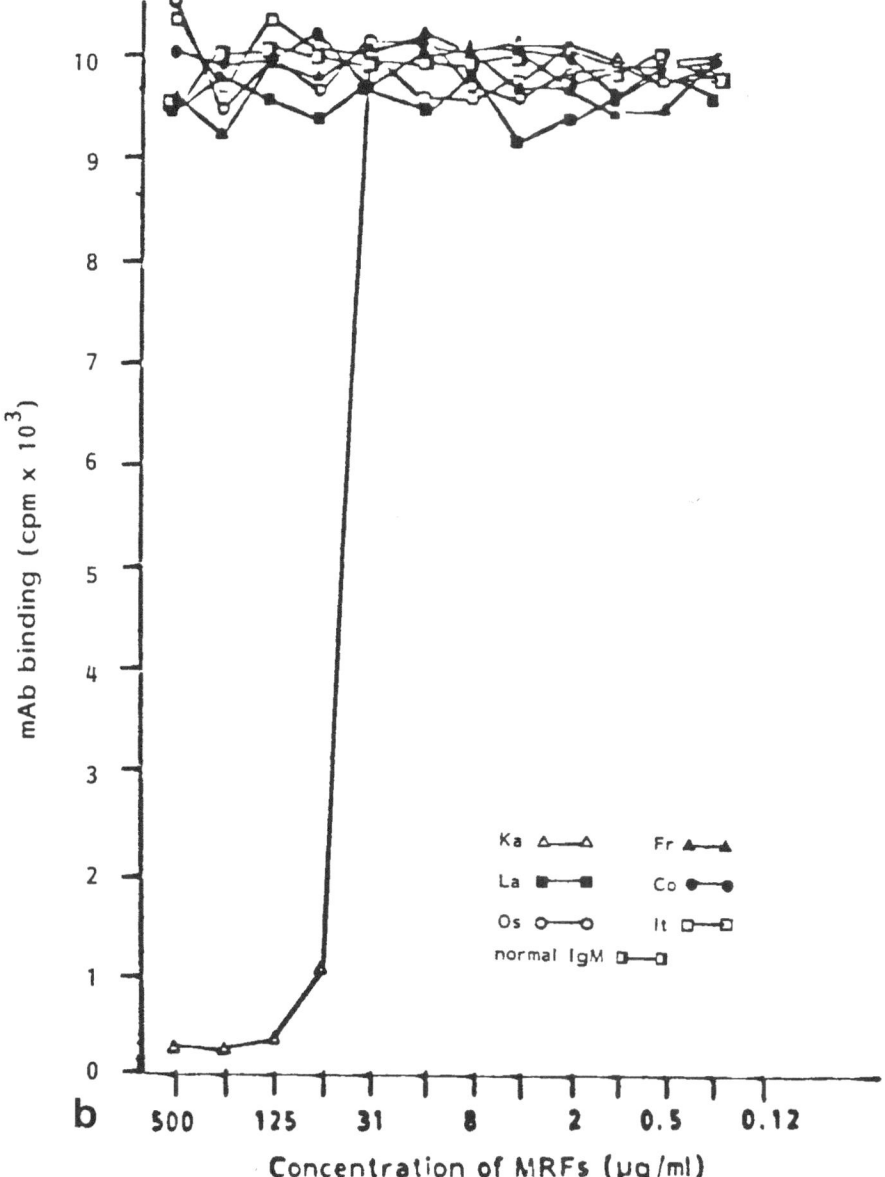

Figure 2b. This figure illustrates that the binding of MAb K7D10 to its solid phase immunising MRF(k) could only be inhibited by MRF(K) and not by five other MRF or IgM.

studied, but of course not to normal human IgM, were presumed to be directed against cross reactive idiotypes – these two MAb also bound to polyclonal RFs when tested in solid phase RIA, indicating that this cross reactive idiotype is shared between MRFs and many polyclonal RFs (as indeed previously described for the Wa idiotype).

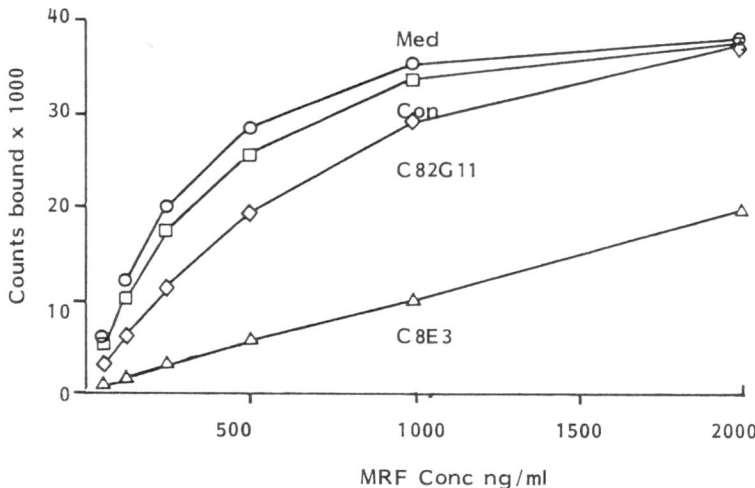

Figure 3. This figure illustrates the inhibition of the binding of the MRF (C) to solid phase IgG by the MAb against a restricted idiotype (C8E3) and to a lesser extent the MAb against the cross-reactive idiotype (C82G11) but not by a control MAb (Con) which did not bind to MRF (C). With this control antibody binding was similar to that obtained in medium alone (Med).

When the MAb recognising a restricted idiotype on MRFs were tested against a panel of polyclonal RFs they showed binding to occasional individual RFs. This would be consistent with these clonally restricted idiotypes being present within some populations of polyclonal RF. (It would be of interest to determine whether these restricted idiotypes can be recognised by the MAb in relatives of the patients, as normal subjects have the capacity to produce RF and the idiotype could be heritable).

Table II. Inhibition of TF activity by MAb.

X reactive Id	Inhibition of autologous MRF	Inhibition of other MRFs
C82G11	+	+
F9B8	+	+
Restricted Id		
K7D10	+	−
C8E3	+	−
F3EBG	−	−
L8C3	+	−

3.2. Inhibition of RF activity by MAb

The ability of selected MAb to inhibit RF activity was assayed using a solid phase assay for RF activity. The results are shown in Fig. 3 and Table II where it can be seen that all except one of the MAb to restricted idiotypes inhibited the RF activity of the MRF to which they bound. This suggests that they are directed against idiotypic determinants associated with the combining site of the MRF molecule. The two MAbs recognising a cross-reactive idiotype also produced some inhibition of RF activity.

3.3. Potential applications of monoclonal anti-idiotypes to patients with MEC

These monoclonal anti-idiotypic antibodies to MRFs can obviously be used to explore the basic mechanisms of idiotypy, as has already been done by others. However, our main intention was to apply these to the clinical investigation of patients with type II MEC. They could be used in a number of ways: for identifying MRF producing B cells in patients, as reagents to detect small amounts of MRF, to examine the regulation of MRF production *in vitro* and its possible modulation by anti-idiotypic antibody. Thus far our preliminary studies have been limited to attempting to identify and enumerate idiotype positive cells in these patients.

3.4. Clinical investigation of patients with type II MEC using monoclonal anti-idiotypes

We have begun to use these monoclonal antibodies to determine the number of idiotype positive cells in the peripheral blood and bone marrow of patients with MEC. The results are shown in Table III. There is little information in the literature on the frequency of MRF producing cells in various compartments. In their study (principally investigating the cellular localization of idiotypes in patients with rheumatoid arthritis), Bonagura et al. [6] found that a high proportion of PWM induced blasts from the peripheral blood of 2 patients with Type II MEC stained with polyclonal antibody to a cross reactive RF idiotype. We have not detected significant numbers of cells bearing RF idiotypes on their surface by direct flow cytometric analysis of peripheral blood mononuclear cells using our monoclonal anti-idiotypes. We therefore studied PWM induced blasts from peripheral blood.

As expected, PWM blasts from control subjects gave a very small number of cells expressing the cross reactive idiotype, confirming that normal subjects have cells capable of producing RF. However no cells from normals

Table III. Expression of monoclonal RF idiotypes in pokeweed mitogen induced blasts (PWMB) and bone marrow (BM) cells of patients with type II cryoglobulinaemia.

Patient	Ctrl. PWMB	F PWMB	F BM	O PWMB	O BM	K PWMB
Ig+	10%	—	10%	8%	5%	—
u+	4%	2%	6%	4%	4%	13%
Kappa	8%	1%	7%	—	3%	
Lambda	3%	1%	1%	—	1%	
MRF+ (X reactive Id)	0.1%	2% (F9B8)	7%	3% (C82G11)	3%	2% (C82G11)
MRF+ (Restricted Id)	0	0 (F3EBG)	6%	—	—	1.5% (K7D10)
MRF+ * (C8E3 Control)	0	0	0	0	0	0

* This MAb was used as a specificity control and recognises a restricted idiotype on a different MRF.

stained with the MAb to restricted RF idiotypes, emphasising the highly restricted specificity of these reagents. It can be seen that in three patients the number of idiotype positive cells in PWM induced blasts ranged from 15–100% of the number of u positive cells. It may be significant that the lowest number of idiotype positive blasts were seen in the patient (K) with the least severe clinical symptoms. Bone marrow from the other two (more severely affected) patients was available for study – here the number of idiotype positive cells was 75% and 100% the number of u+ cells.

3.5. Conjunction of type II cryoglobulinaemia and acquired hypogammaglobulinaemia

Patient F deserves further mention in that he has acquired hypogammaglobulinaemia in addition to type II MEC. His serum IgG concentration is consistently below 2 g/l. At first it seemed possible that this was a result of accelerated catabolism of IgG consequent on its complexing with MRF. However turnover studies (previously reported [7] clearly showed *decreased* catabolism of both normal homologous IgG and the autologous IgG isolated from his cryoprecipitate. In addition this patient had increased numbers of T8+ and Leu 7+ cells in peripheral blood. Studies of the *in vitro* synthesis of IgG in response to PWM suggested his peripheral blood (E−) T cells suppressed IgG synthesis by normal B cells (Table IV). The T8+/Leu7+ population in normal subjects has been reported to be capable of suppressing Ig

Table IV. Mechanism of hypogammaglobulinaemia in Patient F with Type II MEC and acquired hypogammaglobulinaemia.

- IgG turnover

	^{125}I normal IgG	^{131}I Cryo IgG	NR
FCR %/day	3.3	2.8	4.3–9.8
T1/2 days	31	25	14–28
Synthesis mg/kg/day	1.0		
% IgG incorporated in cryo.	42	51	

- PWM Induced Ig synthesis in vitro

E^+ cells	E^- cells	Ig synthesis (ng/ml/10^{-6} E^- cells)	
		IgM	IgG
Normal	Normal	2000	300
Pt. F	Pt. F	350	~20
Pt. F	Normal	350	~20
Normal	Pt. F	1500	800

synthesis *in vitro* [8]. Although not definitively established in this patient the data suggest there may be active suppression of Ig synthesis *in vivo* by the abnormal Leu7$^+$ population. The conjunction of these two conditions seems unlikely to be coincidence, and raises the possibility that the suppressor mechanism may be a secondary response to the type II MEC, and possibly an attempt at its regulation.

4. Discussion

The development of this panel of monoclonal antibodies should facilitate the clinical investigation of these patients, as well as confirming the existence of common and restricted idiotypic determinants on MRFs. *We have not addressed the question of the molecular identity of the idiotypes recognised by our monoclonal antibodies. The cross reactive MAb seem unlikely to be the "internal image" type of anti-idiotype – if they were conformationally similar to the IgG epitope recognised by RFs, then they might be expected to bind to all RFs (which they did not). Experiments to determine whether they bind to isolated kappa or u heavy chain are in progress.*

Obviously our results on their use in identifying idiotype positive cells in patients with type II MEC are preliminary. However, they do suggest that the ability to identify cells of the MRF producing clone might be of use in the serial monitoring of disease activity and severity in these patients. They may be especially useful in determining the effect of therapy aimed at reducing the size of the abnormal clone. The amount of cryoglobulin has, (from previous studies by others) been found not to correlate well with *clinical* evidence of disease, strengthening the case for using an alternative method for assessing the size and extent of the MRF producing clone.

The question arises of whether the MAB themselves could be of any therapeutic use. This seems unlikely at present, although anti-idiotypic MAb have already been used to treat B cell lymphomas [9]. In type II MEC the high concentration of the secreted product (the MRF) would presumably mitigate against the MAb ever reaching the target cell – on which there may anyway be relatively little surface idiotype.

Nevertheless by applying these reagents to our patients with MEC we anticipate being able to approach their management and treatment on a more rational and informed basis.

Acknowledgement

This work was supported by the Medical Research Council.

References

1. Kunkel HG, Agnello V, Joslin FG, Winchester FJ, Capra JD: Cross-idiotypic specificity among monoclonal IgM proteins with anti-globulin activity. J Exp Med 137:331–342, 1973.
2. Chen PP, Fong S, Houghten RA, Carson DA: Characterization of an Epibody — An anti-idiotype that reacts with both the idiotype of Rheumatoid Factors (RF) and the Antigen Recognized by RF. J Exp Med 161:323–331, 1985.
3. Bona CA, Finley S, Waters S, Kunkel HG: Anti-immunoglobulin antibodies. III. Properties of sequential anti-idiotypic antibodies to heterologous anti-gamma globulins. Detection of reactivity of anti-idiotype antibodies with epitopes of Fc fragments. J Exp Med 156:986–993, 1982.
4. Elkon KB, Caeiro K, Gharavi AE, Patel BM, Ferjencik PP and Hughes GRV: Radioimmunoassay profile of antiglobulins in connective tissue diseases: elevated levels of IgA antiglobulin in systemic sicca syndrome. Clin exp Immunol 46:547, 1981.
5. De La Concha EG, Oldham G, Webster ADB, Asherson GL, Platts-Mills TAE: Quantitative measurements of T and B cell function in 'variable' primary hypogammaglobulinaemia: evidence for a consistent B cell defect. Clin Exp Immunol 27:208–215, 1977.
6. Bonagura VR, Kunkel HG, Pernis B: Cellular localisation of rheumatoid factor idiotypes. J Clin Invest 69:1346–1365, 1982.
7. Schifferli JA, Amos N, Pusey CD, Sissons JGP, Peters DK: Metabolism of IgG in type II mixed essential cryoglobulinaemia — autologous cryoprecipitated and normal homologous IgG are incorporated into complexes and metabolized in vivo at similar rates. Clin exp Immunol 51:305–315, 1983.
8. Landay L, Gartlend GL, Clement LT: Characterization of a phenotypically distinct subpopulation of Leu^{-2+} cells that suppresses T cell proliferative responses. J Immunol 131:2757–2761, 1983.
9. Levy R, Miller RA: Tumour therapy with monoclonal antibodies. Fed Proc 42:2650–2656, 1983.

Discussion Part IV

D'AMICO (Milano): When we treat acutely ill patients with type II essential cryoglobulinemia with plasma exchange and intravenous pulses of steroids plus cyclophosphamyde we frequently observe very good clinical results and regression of the histological lesions. What is really difficult to explain for us is the persistence of hypocomplementemia for C4 during remission unlike what happens in patients with systemic lupus. How can you explain this behaviour? Might we not be able anyway to remove enough circulating cryo to avoid activation of C4 bp even if we perform multiple plasma exchanges?

GIGLI: I agree, most probably we don't remove all the cryos. This is also our experience, with the patients of dr Franklin's group. This modality of therapy was stopped because we didn't see good clinical results, moreover in a very short time we saw the reappearance of all the serological manifestations present prior to therapy.

D'AMICO: Also in your experience did C4 levels remain low?

GIGLI: We did not make a very careful study, such as taking samples at one hour, at two hours, at 24 hours after plasmapheresis; therefore it is difficult for me to say at which point the C4 levels change, if they do change. Also one has to take into consideration that complement proteins are not a static series of proteins and there is a balance between activation and synthesis.

I think that you have certain situations in which C4 behaves as a reactive protein and very large amounts are being produced, however I don't know if that is the case in essential mixed cryoglobulins.

PETERS: If I understand you properly, dr Gigli you've shown C4 bp can account for the failure of the activation of C2 and C3 in some patients. On the other hand when you put cryoglobulins in normal human sera you observe C2 and C3 activation: do I understand you properly that this activation is not accountable for a difference in C4 bp but must relate to some other properties of the cryoglobulins?

GIGLI: It is correct. If we take the cryoglobulins from a patient and put it in a normal human serum we get basically the same pattern that we observe in the patient's serum. I had a question to ask on the biological functions of the mixed cryoglobulins, which have either RF exclusively or RF activity and anti-idiotype activity. Is this cryo biologically different from a cryo that has only one activity? If the exposure of the molecules is different, that may account for different types of binding, for complement activation and for the accessibility to the control protein: I believe that as biochemical techniques will be available, one will be able to answer these questions. The other point is that when you activate complement the amount of activated protein that goes into the target, being this target an immune complex or a cell, is really very small, in the order of 5 %. The rest is a fluid phase reaction and therefore when one looks at the events that take place in the circulation, one may be looking at the wrong place.

PETERS: Has anybody ever observed a patient with the typical complement profile of a low C1 and C4 but normal C3, change to the complement profile of complement consumption? I am talking particularly about patients who have monoclonal type II mixed essential cryoglobulinemia because that is bearing upon whether it is a characteristic of the IgM itself, that is the determinant of the complement profile, or whether it is some other consequence of the reaction which one could expect to respond.

GIGLI: I have not observed it and I think that this is an extremely important point. Unfortunately samples for complement studies stored for long periods are almost worthless, therefore long term studies we are very difficult to interpret. One also should point out that although we know a great deal about IgG interaction with complement proteins, we know very little of the interaction of IgM with complement proteins.

NAISH: Dr Gigli, presumably the cooperation between C4 bp and I in controlling the activation of C3 is absolutely crucial since C1 inhibitor seems to be contributing almost nothing to the control of the activation. Would you like to speculate about that?

GIGLI: There are very interesting studies bearing on that point that may be relevant to cryoglobulins. These studies have been done in patients with hereditary angioedema, particularly with the acquired type. It will appear that the C1 inhibitor is much more efficient in preventing C1 activations in the fluid phase, than when C1 is bound to a target. On the other hand activated C1 is very efficient as an enzyme, therefore the reactions are essential to kinetics analysed at this point. I am not aware of any laboratory that has taken this point especially and looked at the interaction of C1 with IgM in relation with the actions of the C1 inhibitor. I also think that there is an element here that has not been touched upon and it may have considerable bearing. When I presented the picture of the C4 bp I didn't make the point that this is another protein of the complement system that interacts with proteins of the clotting system. There is a portion in the C4 bp that binds to protein C. We know very little about protein C, but there must be a reason why C4 bp have two functional domains. If one brings also into the picture fibronectin and the interaction of fibronectin with C1q and the evidence coming from many laboratories that fibronectin has a very high affinity for C1q, one has a setting that tells us that we are really beginning to scratch to the surface of the problem of complement interaction with cryoglobulins.

AGNELLO: Dr Renversez, do some IgM monoclonal RF react better with the Fab than the Fc fragments of cryo-IgG?

RENVERSEZ: It depends of cases. In some cases Fab from cryo-IgG reacts with higher O.D. values than Fc fragments against cryo IgM fractions. In most other cases the reactivity is better recovered with Fc fragments similar to the reactivity of a polyclonal RF IgM. What is interesting is the fact that these two types of interactions are observed in the same time.

AGNELLO: What percentage of proteins react better with Fab?

RENVERSEZ: One third of the cryoglobulins studied.

CARSON: Dr. Renversez, is the IgM binding to the Fc and Fab region with the same combining site or do you think that there are two different combining sites? Second, how could you absorb a monoclonal IgM with a Fab fragment and still have reactivity with Fc fragment and viceversa, if it is monoclonal? Usually monoclonal proteins are absorbed all the way or are not, unless they have two combining sites or are not monoclonal.

RENVERSEZ: We have tried to absorb these two types of reactivities and to discriminate the type of IgM. But when we absorb in solid phase experiments, as in fluid phase experiments, the reactivity against Fc, we decrease also the Fab reactivity of more than 50%, and inversely with Fab fragments. So we are notable to separate two kinds of IgM molecules. The same IgM molecules interact both with Fab and Fc fragments. If IgM interact in a first time with IgG Fc fragments, we can hypothesize that in a second step another reaction will involve IgG Fv against the IgM anti-Fc combining site.

CARSON: I don't understand: is the IgG sometimes an anti-idiotype against the IgM or is always the IgM that's doing the binding?

RENVERSEZ: We cannot answer this question directly, because we have no results in favour of one hypothesis or in favour of the other one. It's possible that cryo IgG would react as anti-idiotypic antibodies because they react with IgG Fv fragments and will be directed against the anti-Fc paratope in some cases, but most of these antibodies can also be directed against determinants of the framework. We try to identify and separate all these cross reactivities to delimitate different populations in these cryo-monoclonal IgM.

AGNELLO: One problem may be the criteria we are using for assessing monoclonality. In fact, restriction of light chain may not be sufficient since on isoelectrofocusing multiple bands are frequently present which may have different specifities. This would explalin the absorption studies.

RENVERSEZ: In all cases IgM fractions were monoclonal. First, because only one type of light chain content was determined as kappa or lambda. Secondly, restricted VH and VL region subgroups were found in all these components. Third a very limited pattern of spectrotypes was revealed, including two or three bands with a definite isoelectric point. Monoclonal non cryoprecipitable IgM, that we have previously studied, also presented a very restricted isoelectric focusing pattern but we have never found in man only one band to account for monoclonality. When we use a very sensitive staining of the gels, as silver stain, we can appreciate much more bands than with classic stains, but it's always a very restricted number of bands very different from oligoclonal or polyclonal IgM.

CARSON: Since immunoglobulins were made up of domains, it seems to me reasonable that some antibodies, that would react with the Fc domain, could occasionally react with the Fab domain, particularly if the interactions led to an increased cryoprecipitation. Secondly, if the dual reactivity of some of these monoclonal anti-IgGs has been observed for a number of antigens, if any of them had any anti-idiotype activity against anyone of the IgG's, the interaction between that IgG and the monoclonal RF would be greatly favoured thermodynamically. These complexes would be sucked up out of the blood in such way to have like an affinity column for any possible cross-reaction between an anti-Fc and an anti-Fab idiotype and this could be quite interesting.

LAMBERT: A very critical observation is the fact that when you analyze the IgG's which cryprecipitated in your tubes with the IgM, you find that in a third of patients, you have a very restricted selection of the IgG which came down related to this RF activity. Therefore, independently of what mechanism will be involved for this selection, obviously you must have a selective mechanism to pick up only this limited number of clones IgG against the RF IgM. Reactivity with an anti-idiotype will obviously be the easiest way at this time to explain this type of selection.

MONTAGNINO: Dr. Sissons, I wonder whether you have tested whether your monoclonal anti-idiotypes inhibit the reaction of the IgM with the corresponding cryo IgG. This would be also interesting from a therapeutical point of view.

SISSONS: They inhibit the RF reactivity in ordinary solid phase with normal IgG, but we haven't looked at that with the corresponding cryo IgG.

DAMMACCO: Dr. Sissons, you mentioned that maybe one of the most interesting applications would be in the clinical situations, with the potential possibility of controlling the production of monoclonal RF. Wouldn't you expect some kind of antigenic modulation in this way?

SISSONS: I really mentioned that possibility only to dismiss it.

Even if you are a believer in the use of monoclonal antibodies, it doesn't seem to me to be a very practical possibility for *in vivo* use when you have got this enormous concentration of the secreted product. Where they have been used, as I understand it, for the treatment of surface idiotype positive B cell there has been no secreted product. We haven't studied the ability to modulate RF production *in vitro*.

ABRAHAM: What was the percentage of the idiotype positive cells that you were able to detect in the total peripheral blood lymphocyte pool when you did not stimulate with pokeweed mitogen?

SISSONS: We have only just begun these studies. We haven't looked, unfortunately, very critically at cytoplasmic percentages, cytoplasmic staining, idiotype-positive cells, stimulation, etc.

ABRAHAM: What about surface idiotype?

SISSONS: We have looked at the surface idiotype by fluorocytometric analysis: we've done it on fractionated peripheral blood mononuclear cells and it was vanishing (low to absent). We haven't actually done it on separated E-negative cells, to get a selected subpopulation and then see if we detect a very small percentage of surface idiotype positive cells, but at best they could only be very few.

ABRAHAM: We have done it in collaboration with dr Gorevic's laboratory trying to determine what the percentage of the idiotype positive cryoglobulin cells is in the peripheral blood and we just can't detect any. In addition, we even used some specific anti V region antibodies to be sure we were identifying minor subpopulations of cells also at low levels. The number of the idiotype positive B cells in the peripheral circulation of these patients, unless they have a lymphoproliferative disease, is incredibly low and we just can't detect them.

CARSON: I had only monoclonal anti-idiotype that reacts against RF. And this reacts with both the CDR and the La proteins, which are both completely sequenced, that have absolutely nothing in common and react with all of the RF. So it seems to be so analogous to your monoclonal in some way, and this monoclonal appears to be what we call 'internal image' and the Fab fragments of the monoclonal somehow are selected to look like an Fc fragment, so we are just using the anti-iditoype like an antigen. Another comment on this monoclonal is that it also reacts weakly with Fc receptors, and if you look in the blood you can see it in a number of even normal people who seemed to be standing with it and I don't think it is specific. Particularly one of the work-ups of the anti-idiotypes perhaps should include such an analysis of known primary sequence to try to see whether or not it does pick up the Wa group or the Po group because, if it is an internal image, then one is using a form of aggregated IgG in a way to pick up the RF producing cells. Aggregated IgG binds to many different things and so the anti-idiotype might also bind to many different things to the extent that it makes the IgG Fc region.

ABRAHAM: Dr. Sissons, could you tell us how did you perform the DEAE studies with the injection of the two IgG preparations? I just have trouble visualizing how you can get good fractional catabolic rates in individuals who have the ability to form immune complexes as well as tissue deposits.

SISSONS: These studies were done by Dr. Schifferli. There is one just doing conventional plasma disappearance curve and, as you implied the multiple mechanisms for clearance in these patients aside from the normal catabolic pathways. When you say FcR that's not actually imply one normal catabolic pathway, just the reflection of the disappearance rate. Most of the mechanisms could be operating. The interesting in that particular patient is that although a high proportion of the radio-labelled immunoglobulin was incorporate into the cryoprecipitate when you took his blood and form the cryoglobulin *in vitro* during the turnover studies, there in fact was low clearance: we were rather expecting an accelerated clearance due to the complex.

ABRAHAM: Are these really computed fractional catabolic rates during theoretical compartmentalization studies of the antigen that you inject or are just plasma disappearance percent?

SISSONS: They are computed fractional catabolic rates as done by the conventional method of computing fractional catabolic rates from the plasma curve, but obviously a number of factors could be contributing to that plasma curve such as normal catabolism, clearance as complex material, an abnormal pathway which would not operate in a normal person when you are measuring fractional catabolic rates.

ABRAHAM: The reason I am getting at it is because we have published studies on fractional catabolic rates in patients with cryoglobulins, and we had actually considered doing it in patients with mixed cryoglobulinemia, but we could not come to grip with what model to use. What was the size of the compartments when you actually applied the mathematical models? Because of these problems we were only able to study patients with monoclonal IgG cryoglobulins. We were also not able to come to grip with how to correct the data. But we actually plasmapheresed the patient way down, and then did a plasma disappearance. But we found that we were actually doing it in the face of a synthetic way, where the cryo was gradually increasing in the serum. We actually couldn't figure out how to compute the models.

SISSONS: In the latter case I don't think you can, because obviously all the methods of computation assume a steady state, and if you had someone recovering from a plasma exchange, you wouldn't have a steady state.

So the normal, circular method of calculating synthetic rate wouldn't apply. I'm not an expert on the various models of the number of compartments you use, but in practical terms, how big the difference would actually be?

AGNELLO: Dr. Sissons, you described an inhibition assay for detecting idiotypic determinants. Did you do direct screening with the labelled monoclonals on your panel of RFs?

SISSONS: We have not done that with all of them.

AGNELLO: The problem when you use the homologous protein is that you are going to pick up the private idiotype. If your monoclonal has cross idiotypic specificity, then you will not pick it up if you don't have heterologous protein.

SISSONS: That's true. During the selection they were screened on others as well. We were interested and really attempting to acquire a selection of different monoclonals.

Part V. Clinical and morphological findings in E.M.C.

15. Mixed Cryoglobulinemia: An Update of Recent Clinical Experience

PETER D. GOREVIC

Mixed cryoglobulins have been identified in the sera of patients with various disease states in which hyperglobulinemia or hyperimmunization may occur [1-3]. The term 'essential' mixed cryoglobulinemia has been used to designate a group of patients with a specific syndrome consisting of purpura, weakness, arthralgias and renal disease [4]. The exact incidence of this syndrome among patients found to have cryoglobulins in their blood has varied with the series, as well as with clinical and serological criteria utilized for inclusion, but has generally ranged 15–55% when either all types of cryoprecipitates or specifically IgM-IgG mixed cryoglobulins are sampled [1-3, 5]. Pathologic correlates of the clinical syndrome include cutaneous vasculitis and immune complex glomerulonephritis. A direct role for the cryoprotein constituents in the pathogenesis of these lesions is suggested by immunohistological studies showing specific immune reactants and antiglobulin activity to be present in kidney or skin [6, 7], as well as by *in vitro* [8] and *in vivo* [9] evidence for activation of complement.

A comprehensive review of the clinical, laboratory and pathologic features of 'essential' mixed cryoglobulinemia was first published by Meltzer et al. in 1966 [4]. Follow-up of some of the initial nine patients, as well details regarding 31 additional cases subsequently seen by referral from throughout the New York City area was reported in 1980 [2]. The purpose of this communication is to update this clinical experience to include an additional ten cases seen at New York University and at the State University of New York at Stony Brook over the period 1979-85.

Patient Population

Patients included in this series have been referred for conformation of diagnosis, clinical evaluation, therapy, or a specific research protocol. Additional cases of cryoglobulinemia found to have a lymphoproliferative disorder or defined collagen-vascular disorder have been excluded.

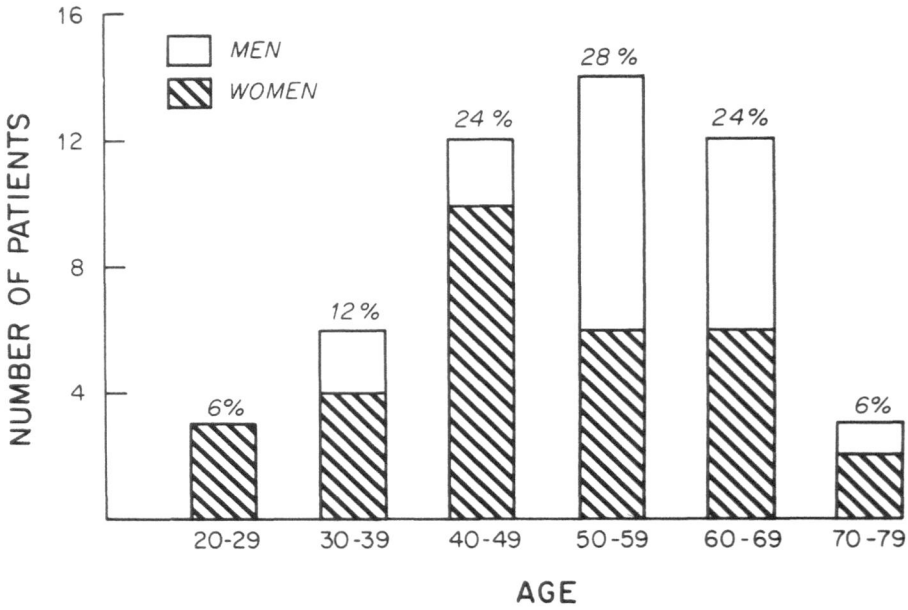

Figure 1. Age and sex distribution of 50 patients with mixed cryoglobulinemia.

Table I. Clinical features of mixed cryoglobulinemia.

	1960–79 (n = 40)	1979–85 (n = 10)	Total No.	Percent
Female	27	6	33	66
Purpura	40	10	50	100
Leg ulcers	12	3	15	30
Raynauds phenomenon	10	1	11	22
Arthralgias	29	6	35	70
Renal disease	22	4	26	54
Edema	20	3	23	46
Hypertension	18	4	22	44
Hepatic involvement	28	7	35	70
Abdominal pain	8	1	9	18
Lymphadenopathy	7	1	8	16
Sjogren's syndrome	6	1	7	14
Paresthesias	5	5	10	20
Foot drop	3	1	4	8
Thyroiditis	2	0	2	4
Herpes zoster	7	1	8	16
Bacterial pneumonia	8	3	11	22

Clinical Features

Mixed cryoglobulinemia remains predominantly a disease of women (Fig. 1), with onset in the fourth and fifth decades of life. We have seen no cases below age 20 and the oldest age of onset was at 72 years.

The fact that purpura is a universal clinical feature of our 50 patients probably reflects retrospective case acquisition and pattern of referral. In recent years, cutaneous vasculitis has been documented in all cases by skin biopsy. Routine histological stains have invariably showed a small vessel vasculitis, but the yield of positive results by direct fluorescence using antisera to immunoglobulin class-specific determinants and complement has been low (<10%).

Recent experience has not seen major changes in the incidence of leg ulcers, arthralgias, symptoms of Sjögren's syndrome, or hepatic involvement when compared to patients seen over the period 1960-79 (Table I). Raynaud's phenomenon, renal disease, and episodes of abdominal pain have been somewhat less common, and 5/10 patients seen since 1979 have had neurological involvement (paresthesias, motor neuropathy).

Renal Disease

Of the 10 patients seen since 1979, four have had clinical renal disease, a somewhat lower incidence than (but identical clinical presentation to), that

Table II. Clinical and laboratory findings in renal disease.

	1960–79 (n = 22)	1979–85 (n = 4)	Total No.	Percent
Clinical Data				
Hypertension	14	3	17	65.4
Edema	17	3	20	76.9
Hypertension and Edema	13	3	16	61.5
Hypertensive Retinopathy	8	1	9	34.6
Azotemia	10	3	13	50.0
Nephrotic Syndrome	5	1	6	23.1
Urinanalysis				
Hematuria	20	4	24	92.3
Pyuria	18	3	21	80.8
Proteinuria				
> 4 g/day	5	0		19.2
1–4 g/day	14	3	17	65.4
> 500 mg/day < 1 g/day	2	1	3	11.5

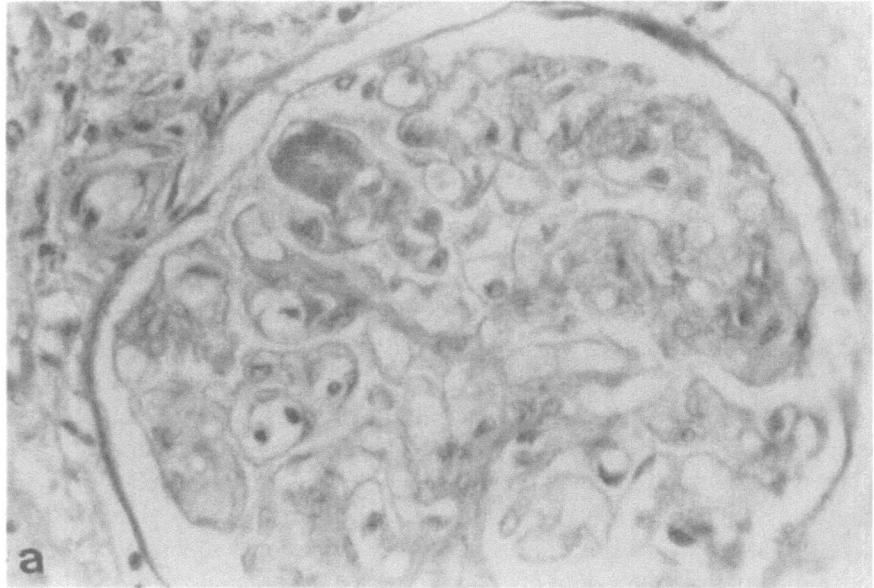

Figure 2a. Postmortem renal tissue from a patient with mixed cryoglobulinemia showing multiple PAS-positive intraluminal glomerular inclusions; hematoxylin and eosin, × 350.

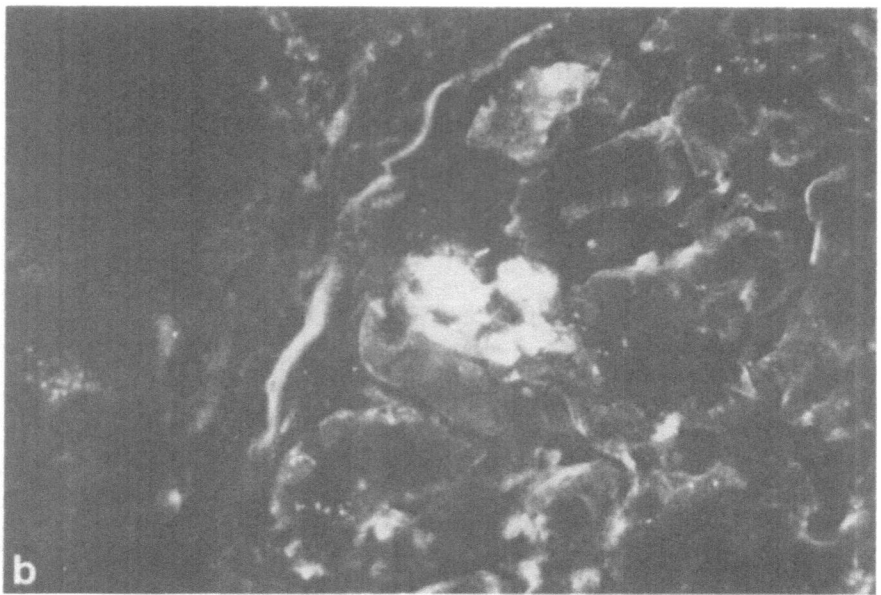

Figure 2b. Kidney tissue incubated with FITC-labelled anti-juman IgM, showing localization to glomerular inclusions, × 350.

seen previously. Of these four patients, pathologic confirmation is available for two, one obtained postmortem. Both had diffuse proliferative glomerulonephritis, with striking hyaline intraluminal glomerular deposits (Fig. 2a), staining positively for IgM and IgG by immunofluorescence (Fig. 2b) and immunoperoxidase (not shown) techniques. Of particular interest has been a 36 year old women who presented with purpura, hypertension, nephrotic syndrome, hematuria and red cell casts. An attempt at a renal biopsy was unsuccessful; a mixed cryoglobulin was appreciated and characterized shortly thereafter. Over the next few months, there was slow clearing of renal sediment, even though she was treated only with antihypertensive medications and never received corticosteroids or other immunosuppressives. Two years later, she still has occasional purpura and an easily detectable cryoglobulin, but has had no recurrence of symptoms or abnormal urinalaysis.

Hepatic Involvement

Previous publications have detailed the incidence of hepatic abnormalities [10], as well as serological evidence of prior hepatitis B virus infection [11], among our patients with 'essential' mixed cryoglobulinemia. It should be stressed that these are not persons who have established liver disease and that a history of hepatitis, if present (Table III), was self-limited

Table III. Clinical, laboratory and pathologic features of hepatic involvement.

	1960–79 (n = 28)	1979–85 (n = 7)	Total (n = 50) No.	Percent
↑ Serum alkaline phosphatase	26	7	33	66
↑ Transaminases	20	7	27	54
Serum (39 tested)				
HBsAg	3	2	5	12.8
HBsAb	12	2	14	35.9
Cryo (33 tested)				
HBsAg	6	2	8	24.2
HBsAb	11	2	13	39.4
History of hepatitis/jaundice	2	2	4	
Subsequent liver failure	2	0	2	
Pathology (21 patients)				
Normal	8	1	8	
Triaditis or focal inflammation	1	0	1	
Chronic hepatitis	7	2	9	
Cirrhosis	6	0	6	
Vasculitis	2	0	2	

184

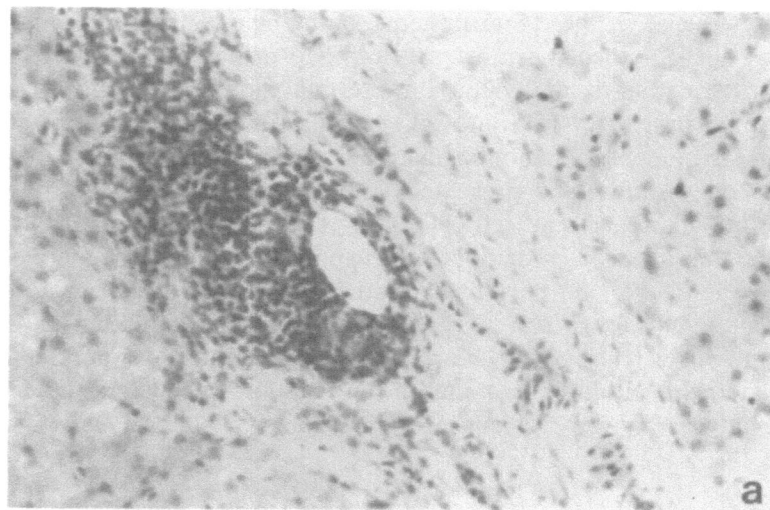

Figure 3a. Liver biopsy showing chronic hepatitis with a striking mononuclear cell infiltrate; hematoxylin and eosin, × 150.

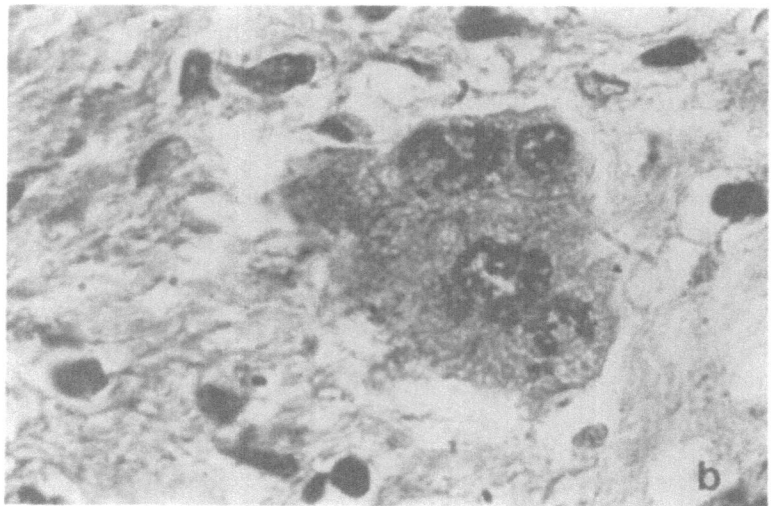

Figure 3b. Close-up of a hepatocyte from the liver biopsy of a patient (FC) reported by Meltzer et al. (4). Cytoplasmic staining is seen by the immunoperoxidase technique using a rabbit anti-serum (1:100 dilution) to hepatitis B surface antigen (kindly provided by Dr. David Gocke); hematoxylin and eosin, × 600.

and predated by many years the onset of purpura. More characteristically, mildly elevated liver function abnormalities have been noted soon after presentation and the patients are rarely symptomatic from liver involvement. In those cases in whom biopsy confirmation has been pursued, a characteristic histology consisting of chronic hepatitis, often with a striking mononuclear cell infiltrate (Fig. 3a), has been seen. In several instances, including a retrospective study of biopsy material from one of the cases reported in 1966, it has been possible to demonstrate the presence of hepatitis surface antigen (HBsAg) in a cytoplasmic distribution in hepatocytes by immunoperoxidase staining (Fig. 3b).

Laboratory Data

Characteristic features include serological evidence of IgM rheumatoid factor activity and high levels of immune complex-like material, assessed by C1q binding assay [12]. Both may be only partly removed by standard methods of cryoprecipitation; the latter is unaffected by reduction with $10^{-2}M$ mercaptoethanol and localizes to the IgG fraction of the mixed cryoglobulin [12]. Also characteristic, though not invariable, is a specific pattern of complement activation in serum, with selective depletion of early components of the classical pathway (i.e. C4) and normal factor B levels [9, 13]. *In vitro* studies with isolated dissociated and fractionated mixed

Table IV. Laboratory data.

	1960–79 (n = 40)	1979–85 (n = 10)	Total No.	Percent
Cryoglobulins				
Mixed "monoclonal"				
IgMK-IgG	12	6	18	36
IgAK-IgM-IgG	1	0	1	2
Mixed polyclonal				
IgM-IgG	23	4	27	54
IgA-IgM-IgG	4	0	4	8
Serumprotein electrophoresis				
Normal	12	7	19	38
Diffuse ↑ immunoglobulin	24	3	27	54
Hypoimmunoglobulin	2	0	2	4
Spike	2	0	2	4
Quantitative immunoglobulins				
↑ IgM	14	2	16	32
↑ IgA	11	0	11	22
↑ IgG	8	3	11	22
Serum latex fixation (48 recorded)				
> 1:650	17	8	25	50
> 1:160 < 1:640	9	1	10	20
< 1:160	12	1	11	22
Serum complement				
↓ C4	12/19	7/10	19	65.5
↓ C3	14/24	6/10	20	58.8

186

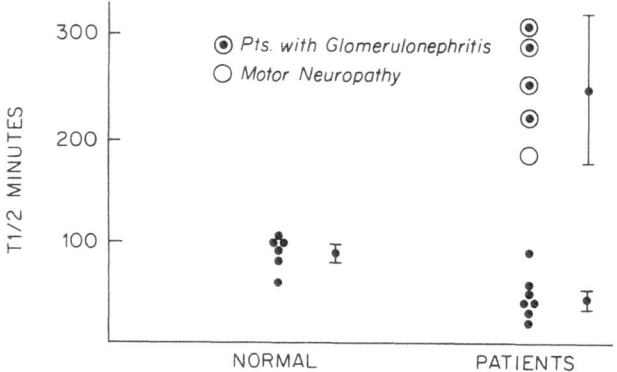

Figure 4. Fc receptor functional activity in the sera of normal volunteers and in 13 patients with mixed cryoglobulinemia. (Data updated from reference 13).

cryoglobulins have indicated that the IgM fraction contains most of the activity responsible for complement activation [14].

Previous studies in a small number of patients with this disorder have shown some to manifest a defect in the clearance of IgG-coated autologous erythrocytes [13]. Retarded clearance, indicative of abnormal Fc-receptor function, appears to be specific for mixed cryoglobulinemia patients who have renal involvement or progressive motor neuropathy (Fig. 4). By contrast, patients who are free of renal disease or neuropathy have normal or fast clearances compared to controls.

In recent experience, 6/10 isolated cryoproteins from patients with this symptom complex have had type II cryoglobulins, the IgM component invariably having kappa light chains. This restricted specificity has been even more apparent in amino acid sequence data that has resulted from the study of isolated IgM K IIIb light chains isolated from the cryoglobulins of several patients in this series [15]. The exclusively kappa light chains of the cryoglobulin IgM may not be apparent as a monoclonal arc on routine serum immunoelectrophoresis and may require isolation and fractionation of the mixed cryoglobulin for its demonstration. Whether this is due to the small quantities of cryo IgM circulating in blood or masking of light chain determinants, possibly secondary to complex formation, is unclear.

Clinical Course and Prognosis

Figure 5 updates the clinical course of 40 patients with and without renal disease reported in 1980. Average follow-up for the 22 patients with clinical renal disease is now 6.3 years vs 10.3 years for the 18 patients with no evidence of nephritis. The clinical course of patient VD, who was first

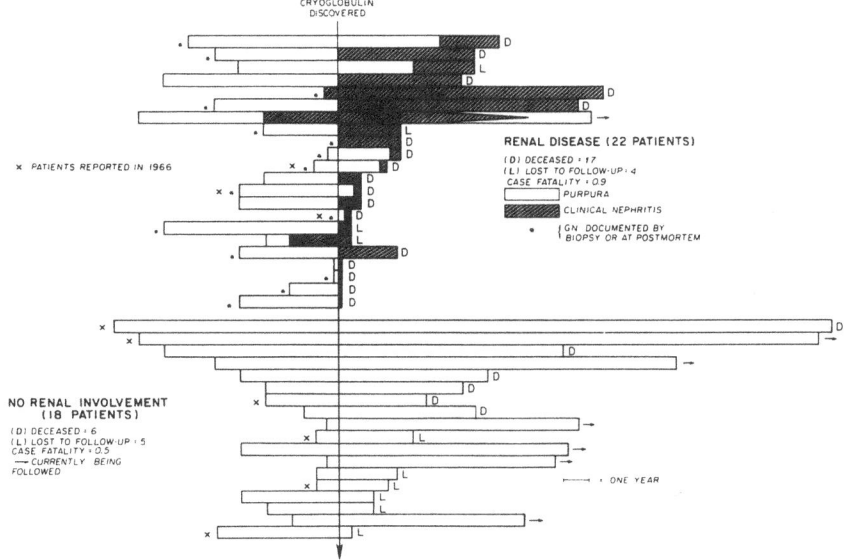

Figure 5. Updated clinical course of 40 patients reported in 1980.

reported in 1966 and whose clinical cryoglobulinemia dates back to 1955 is of particular interest. In recent years, purpura diminished considerably, though refractory leg ulcers continued to be a problem, requiring skin grafting and prolonged periods of bedrest. She developed increasing ascites and became progressively leukopenic. In late 1982, subcutaneous masses involving the left upper eyelid and right side of the nose were noted and removed surgically. Both bone marrow examination, and the subcutaneous nodules were found to be a poorly differentiated lymphoma. Chemotherapy was refused and was followed by a slow deterioration and death in hepatic coma two years later. In this patient with known cirrhosis a lymphoproliferative disorder developed following 30 years of known cryoglobulinemia.

Figure 6 updates the clinical course of patients 3 and 4 reported in 1980. The first patient (FO) was subsequently treated with high doses of corticosteroids, chlorambucil and plasmapheresis for deteriorating renal function, with good response, as detailed by Geltner et al. [16]. Immunosuppressive therapy was discontinued in early 1980, and he subsequently remained mildly azotemic with an active renal sediment and occasional purpura. In 1983 and 1984 he was hospitalized for heart failure and transient unexplained pulmonary infiltrates. Hypertension became increasingly refractory to treatment and he died suddenly at home, apparently of a cerebral hemorrhage. The second patient now has a 25 year follow-up, but is currently free of clinical disease and has had no detectable cryoglobulinemia since

188

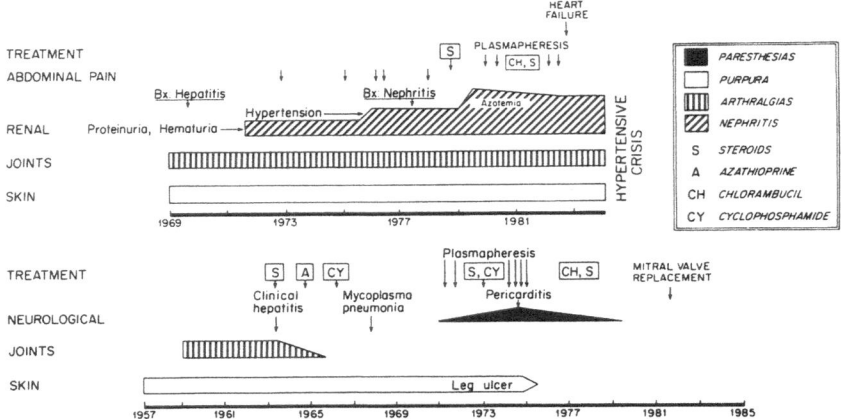

Figure 6. Clinical course of 2 patients reported in 1980 (reference 2, page 298, patients No. 3 and 4).

1976. Polyclonal hyperglobulinemia and a persistently positive IgM rheumatoid factor have been noted in follow-up blood testing.

Comments

Several clinical series [1–3, 17] have delineated the major features of 'essential' cryoglobulinemia occurring in individuals without lymphoproliferative, collagen-vascular or chronic infectious diseases, and provided some information as to the natural history [2, 18] of this disorder. The major cutaneous [19], articular [20], renal [21], hepatic [10, 22], pulmonary [23] and neurological [24] manifestations of this symptom complex have been reviewed. Long-term follow-up studies [2, 18] have made it clear that symptoms may remain static over long periods of time, may wax and wane spontaneously, and that a small percentage of patients may eventually be found to have a defined collagen disease, such as lupus erythematosus [25] or polyarteritis nodosa [26], or lymphoproliferative disorders [27], notably Waldenstrom's macroglobulinemia [18, 26].

The incidence of liver involvement and the strength of an association between hepatitis B virus infection and mixed cryoglobulinemia remain issues of some contention. This association was first noted by Realdi et al. [28] and has been confirmed in subsequent reports [11, 17, 22, 29]. Other series, however, have failed to show a significant incidence of HBV-related serological markers [30], noted comparable frequences in controls, or found a lower yield of positive serologies when isolated cryoprecipitates are analyzed [31]. These differences are partly nosological, resulting to some extent

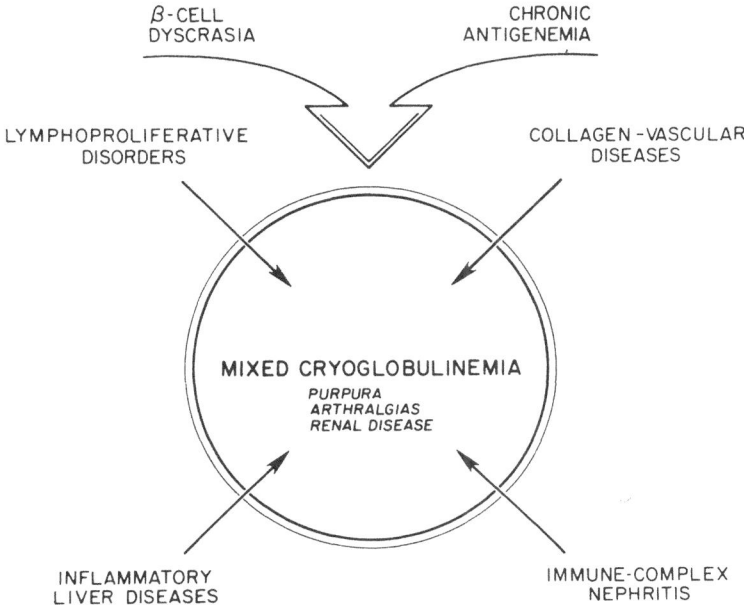

Figure 7. Schema.

from patient selection [3, 32]. They also reflect the fact that this symptom complex may result from multiple pathogenic mechanisms (Fig. 7) which is why the term 'essential' may be inappropriate, as it implies the existence of a unique disease. The exact role of the hepatitis virus in the genesis of tissue lesions also remains ill-defined. Serological evidence of both HBsAg and anti-HBs [11], as well as specific antiidiotypic antibody activity [33], in isolated mixed cryoglobulins has been presented. Nevertheless, the correlation between serological findings and clinical disease remains inexact. The incidence of inflammatory liver disease, often inapparent clinically, considerably exceeds the serological findings. Although HBsAg may be demonstrated in liver biopsies by immunohistological studies (Fig. 3b), in other 'typical' cases negative results are obtained. The specificity of immunohistological studies in skin and kidney has been questioned because of artefacts introduced by the concomitant presence of antiglobulin activity [7, 34]. Direct elution studies demonstrating virus-antibody complexes, ultrastructural definition of viral particles in tissue lesions, or immunohistological studies of vasculitic lesions with monospecific antisera to viral or idiotypic antigenic determinants, have not as yet been forthcoming.

Many patients with only cutaneous involvement can be managed symptomatically and do not require aggressive therapies. Major clinical problems are the identification of which patients will develop renal disease, as well as which of these individuals will have a progressive course. Possible factors include (a) a defect in Fc-specific reticuloendothelial system clearance function (Fig. 4) due to dysfunctional or blocked receptors, or an actual decrease in the number of receptors available for the clearance of immune complexes [13] (b) unknown factors, perhaps only operative in some patients, that lead to precipitation of complexes in glomeruli or blood vessels, giving rise in turn to characteristic hyaline inclusions [21, 35] (Figs. 2a and b) and corresponding crystalloid structures apparent by electron microscopy [36, 37] (c) a specific mononuclear cell response, as suggested by Tarantino et al. [21] (d) effector functions of circulating immune complexes, possibly mediated by complement split products or the secondary generation of vasoactive amines (e) other antibody activities in mixed cryoglobulins that may in turn be responsible for specific localization to kidney. It is also clear that renal disease is not always progressive, may remit, and can be managed conservatively in many cases. Clinical course is as much determined by adequate control of hypertension or attention to other indirect sequelae of disease as by therapy directed to an underlying disease process [21].

Studies of isolated cryoglobulins have provided evidence to suggest that the humoral immune response in many of these individuals is of restricted specificity. This has been apparent in serological [38] and structural studies [15] of the isolated IgM fraction, as well as in the demonstration of antiidiotypic antibody activity directed against autologous immunoglobulin [33, 39]. The potential thus exists for multiple circulating immune complexes, only some of which may be pathogenic or cryoprecipitable [12, 40]. These considerations, along with a further delineation of their clinical correlations, will need to be further clarified before a more rational approach to therapy becomes available.

Acknowledgements

The secretarial support of Mrs. Karen Abramowski is gratefully acknowledged. Work Supported in part by NIH Grant AM 26588.

References

1. Brouet JC, Clauvel JP, Danon F, Klein M, Seligmann M: Biological and clinical significance of cryoglobulinemia. Report of 86 cases. Amer J Med 57:775–788, 1974.
2. Gorevic PD, Kassab HJ, Levo Y, Kohn R, Meltzer M, Prose P, Franklin EC: Mixed cryoglobulinemia: clinical aspects and long-term follow-up of 40 patients. Amer J Med 69:287–308, 1980.
3. Invernizzi F, Galli M, Serino G, Monti G, Meroni PL, Granatieri C, Zanussi C: Secondary and essential cryoglobulinemias. Acta Haemat 70:73–82, 1983.

4. Meltzer M, Franklin EC, Elias K, McCluskey RT, Cooper NS: Cryoglobulinemia: a clinical and laboratory study II. Cryoglobulins with rheumatoid factor activity. Amer J Med 40:837–856, 1966.

5. Dammacco F, Guisci G, Silvestri F, Bonommo L: New Clinical and immunological trends in cryoglobulinemia Ricerca Clin Lab 10:51–57, 1980.

6. Miescher PA, Paronetto F, Koffler D: Immunofluorescent studies in human vasculitis, Fourth International Symposium on Immunopathology, Graber P, Mischer PA,eds. New York, Grune and Stratton, 1965.

7. Maggiore Q, Bartolomeo F, L'Abbate A, Misefari V, Martorano C, Caccamo A, Di Belgiojoso GB, Tarantino, A, Colasanti G: Glomerular localization of ciculating antiglobulin activity in essential mixed cryoglobulinemia with glomerulonephritis. Kidney Int 21:387–394, 1982.

8. Haydey RP, Pattaroyo DE, Rojas M, Gigli I: A newly described control mechanism of complement activation in patients with mixed cryoglobulinemia. J Invest Dermat 74:328–332, 1980.

9. Tarantino, A, Anelli A, Costantino A, DeVecchi A, Monti G, Massaro L: Serum complement pattern in essential mixed cryoglobulinemia. Clin Exp Immunol 32:77–85, 1978.

10. Levo Y, Gorevic PD, Kassab HJ, Tobias H, Franklin EC: Liver involvement in the syndrome of mixed cryoglobulinemia. Ann Int Med 87:287–292, 1977.

11. Levo Y, Gorevic PD, Kassab HJ, Zucker-Franklin D, Franklin EC: Association between hepatitis B virus and essential mixed cryoglobulinemia. New Engl J Med 296:1501–1504, 1977.

12. Lawley TJ, Gorevic PD, Hamburger MI, Franklin EC, Frank MM: Multiple types of immune complexes in patients with mixed cryoglobulinemia. J Invest Dermat 75:297–301, 1980.

13. Hamburger MI, Gorevic PD, Lawley TJ, Franklin EC, Frank MM: Mixed cryoglobulinemia. Association of glomerulonephritis with defective reticuloendothelial Fc receptor function. Trans Assoc Amer Phys 93:104–112, 1979.

14. Fox S, Ghebrehiwet B, Gorevic PD: Unpublished observations.

15. Pons-Estel B, Goni F, Solomon A, Frangione B: Sequence similarities among KIIIb chains of monoclonal human IgMK autoantibodies. J Exp Med 160:893–904, 1984.

16. Geltner D, Kohn RW, Gorevic P, Franklin EC: The effect of combination therapy (steroids, immunosuppressives and plasmapheresis) on 5 mixed cryoglobulinemia patients with renal, neurologic and vascular involvement. Arth Rheum 24:1121–1127, 1981.

17. Utsinger PD, Stimmel WH, Hicks JT: Essential mixed cryoglobulinemia (EMC): The syndrome of purpura, polyarthritis and nephritis. Arth Rheum 24:589 (Abstr), 1981.

18. Invernizzi F, Pioltelli P, Cattaneo R, Gavazzeni V, Borzini P, Monti G, Zanussi C: A long term follow-up study in essential cryoglobulinemia. Acta Haematol 61:93–99, 1979.

19. Cream JJ: Clinical and immunological aspects of cutaneous vasculitis. Quart J Med 178:255–276, 1976.

20. Weinberger A, Berliner S, Pinkhas J: Articular manifestations of essential cryoglobulinemia. Sem Arth Rheum 10:224–229, 1981.

21. Tarantino A, DeVecchi A, Montagnino G, Imbasciatti E, Mihatsch MJ, Zollinger HU, Barbiano G, Belgiojoso DI, Busnach DI, Ponticelli C: Renal disease in essential mixed cryoglobulinemia. Quart J Med: 197:1–30, 1981.

22. Bombardieri S, Ferri C, DiMunno O, Pasero G: Liver involvement in essential mixed cryoglobulinemia. Ric Clin Lab 9:361–368, 1979.

23. Bombardieri S, Paoeletti P, Ferri C, Dimunno O, Fornai F, Guntini C: Lung involvement in essential mixed cryoglobulinemia. Amer J Med 66:748–756, 1979.

24. Abramsky O, Slavin S: Neurologic manifestations in patients with mixed cryoglobulinemia. Neurology 24:245–249, 1974.

25. Perek J, Mittelman M, Eisbruch A, Djarletti M: Systemic lupus erythematosus preceded by long-term cryoglobulinemia. Ann Rheum Dis 43:339–34g43:339–340, 1984.
26. Mackecknie HL, Ogryzlo M, Pruzanski W: Heterogeneity of IgM IgG cryo-complexes. Immunological-clinical correlation. J Rheumat 2:225–240, 1975.
27. Kassab HJ, Prose P, Franklin EC, Gorevic PD: Mixed cryogloblinemia: follow-up 28 years later. Arch Dermat 117:65, 1981.
28. Realdi G, Alberti A, Rigoli A, Tremolada F: Immune complexes and Australia antigen in cryoglobulinemia sera. Immunforsch 147:114–126, 1974.
29. Garcia-Bragado F, Vilardell M, Fonollosa, V, Ruibal A, Gallart T, Cuxart A: Cryoglobulinemia mixte essentielle: relations avec le virus de L'hepatite B. Nouv. Presse Med 10:2955–2957, 1981.
30. Popp JWJ, Dienstag JL, Wands JR, Bloch KJ: Essential mixed cryoglobulinemia without evidence for hepatitis B virus infection. Ann Int Med 92:379–383, 1980.
31. Galli M, Invernizzi F: Hepatitis B virus and cryoglobulinemia. Ann Int Med 95:522, 1981.
32. Dienstag JL: Letter to the editor, New Eng J Med 312:187–188, 1985.
33. Geltner D, Franklin EC, Frangione B: Antiidiotypic activity of the IgM fraction of cryoglobulins. J Immunol 125:1530–1535, 1980.
34. Maggiore Q, Bartolomeo F, L'Abbate A, Misefari V: HBsAg glomerular deposits in glomerulonephritis: fact or artefact? Kidney Intl 19:579–586, 1981.
35. Verroust P, Morel-Maroger L, Preud'Homme JL: Renal lesions in dysproteinemias Springer Sem. Immunopathol 5:333–356, 1982.
36. Feiner H, Gallo G: Ultrastructure in glomerulonephrits associated with cryoglobulinemia. Amer J Pathol 88:145–162, 1977.
37. Feiner HD: Relationship of tissue deposits of cryoglobulin to clinical features of mixed cryoglobulinemia. Human Pathol 14:710–715, 1983.
38. Kunkel HG, Agnello V, Joslin, FG, Winchester RJ, Capra JD: Cross-idiotype specificity among monoclonal IgM proteins with anti gamma globulin activity. J Exp Med 137:331–342, 1973.
39. Goldman M, Renversez JC, Lambert PH: Pathologic expression of idiotypic interactions: immune complexes and cryoglobulins. Springer Semin Immunopathol 6:33–49, 1983.
40. Bombardieri S, Maggiore Q, L'Abbate A, Bartolomeo F, Ferri C: Plasma exchange in essential cryoglobulinemia. Plasma Therap 2:101–109, 1981

16. Histological and immunohistological features in essential mixed cryoglobulinemia glomerulonephritis

FRANCO FERRARIO, GIULIANO COLASANTI,
GIOVANNI BARBIANO DI BELGIOIOSO, GIOVANNI BANFI,
MARIA ROSARIA CAMPISE, ROBERTO CONFALONIEREI
and GIUSEPPE D'AMICO

Introduction

The glomerulonephritis (GN) of essential mixed cryoglobulinemia (EMC) shows some characteristic histological lesions which differentiate the renal involvement in this form from the glomerular lesions found in various types of idiopathic or systemic GN.

Four main lesions can be identified histologically in kidney biopsy specimens.

(1) *Intraluminal 'thrombi'*, variable both for size and diffusion, sometimes entirely filling the capillary lumen [1–4] (Fig. 1). They appear amorphous, eosinophilic, PAS positive and Congo red negative. No fibrin is pre-

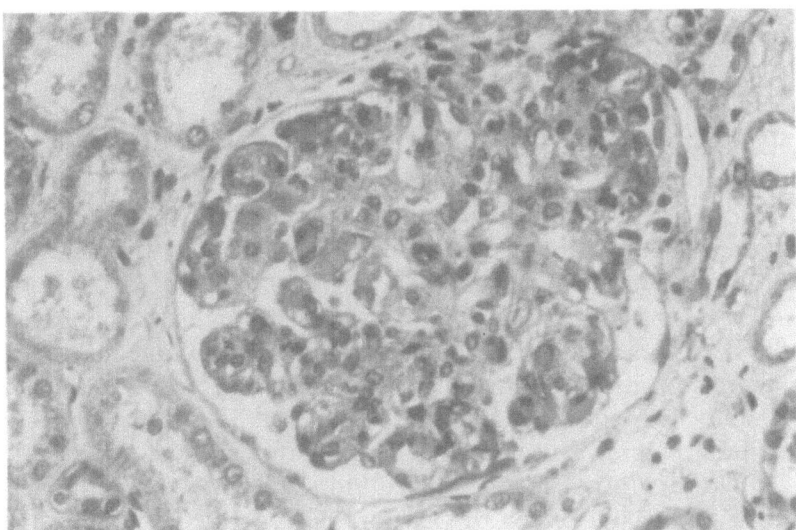

Figure 1. Membranoproliferative exudative GN with prevalent thrombi: diffuse amorphous intraluminal thrombi entirely filling the capillary lumina. (PAS × 250).

194

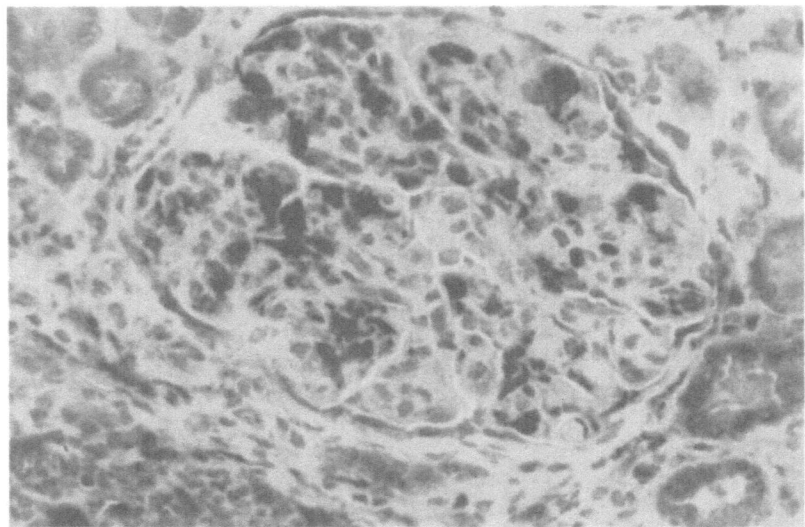

Figure 2. Membranoproliferative exudative GN: massive intracapillary infiltration of monocyte (dark cells). (Non-specific esterase × 250).

sent within 'thrombi, which are likely to be formed by precipitate cryoglobulins as suggested by their peculiar ultrastructural fibrillar and crystalloid appearance [5–7], by their immunoglobulin composition (IgG-IgM) [8] and finally by their antiglobulin activity [9].

(2) *Marked glomerular infiltration of monocytes* migrated from the bloodstream [10–13]. Staining with esterase method, which is rather specific for monocytes, shows that their infiltration may be massive in this disease (more than 60–70 cells per glomerulus) [10] (Fig. 2).

These cells show a close contact with endoluminal thrombi indicating a possible phagocitosing activity, as already suggested by electron microscopy finding of structured intracytoplasmic deposits in EMC-GB [12].

(3) *Thickening of the glomerular basement membrane* (GBM), with diffuse and conspicuous double-contoured appearance characterized by interposition of monocytes and their cytoplasms between the GBM and newly formed basement membrane-like material lying on its inner side [14, 15] (Fig. 3). Peripheral interposition of mesangial matrix and cells is not as prominent as in idiopathic mesangiocapillary GB [1, 10].

Subendothelial deposits may also be seen together with areas of translucent material possibly due to degradation of the deposits [2, 13].

(4) *Renal vasculitis* of small and medium-size vessels present in about 1/3 of patients and characterized by fibrinoid necrosis of the vessel walls, with infiltration of monocytes around the wall [1, 2, 14, 16] (Fig. 4). By immunofluorescence (IF), fibrin deposits are usually seen in the vessel walls. Peri-

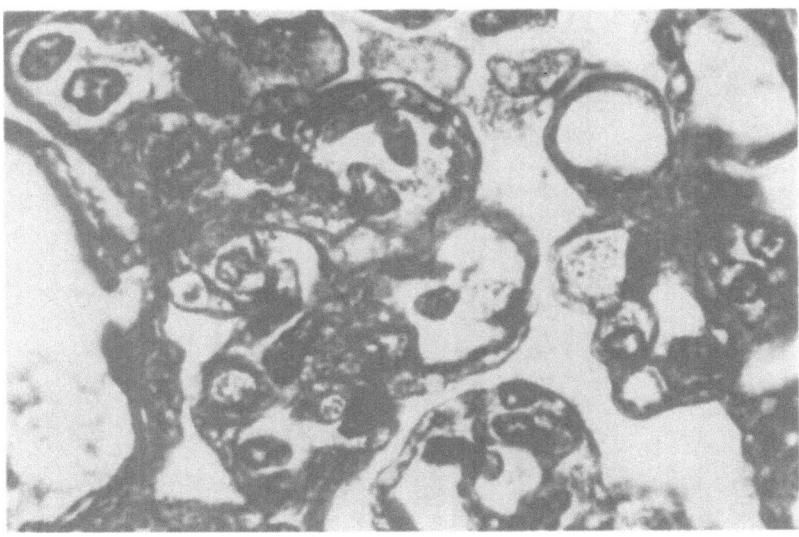

Figure 3. Membranoproliferative exudative GN: thickening of GBM with diffuse double-contours and areas of translucent material (Silver impregnation × 1000).

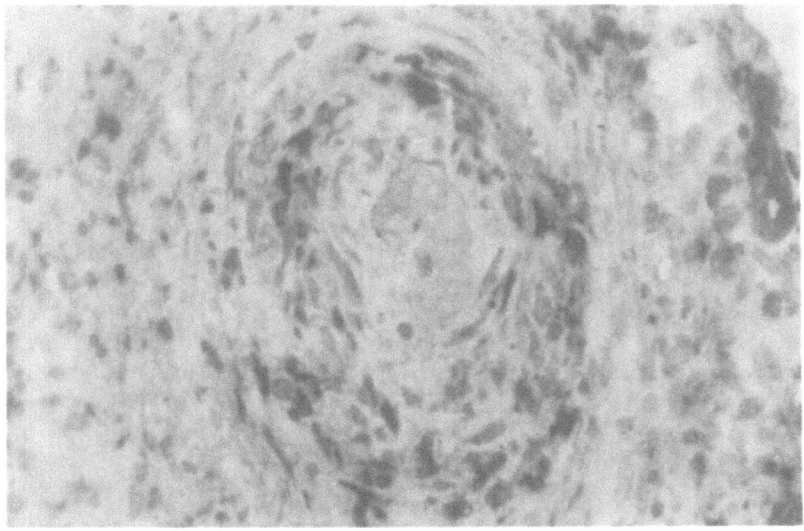

Figure 4. Severe perivascular monocyte infiltration in a case of EMC-GN (Non-specific esterase × 400).

vascular fibrosis and lympho-monocyte granulomatous-like reaction are more frequently seen in later stages [14].

Two other lesions, although not specific of EMC GN, are frequently present: interstitial infiltration of lympho-mononuclear cells and fibrosis of the medio-intima of medium-size arteries [2, 4].

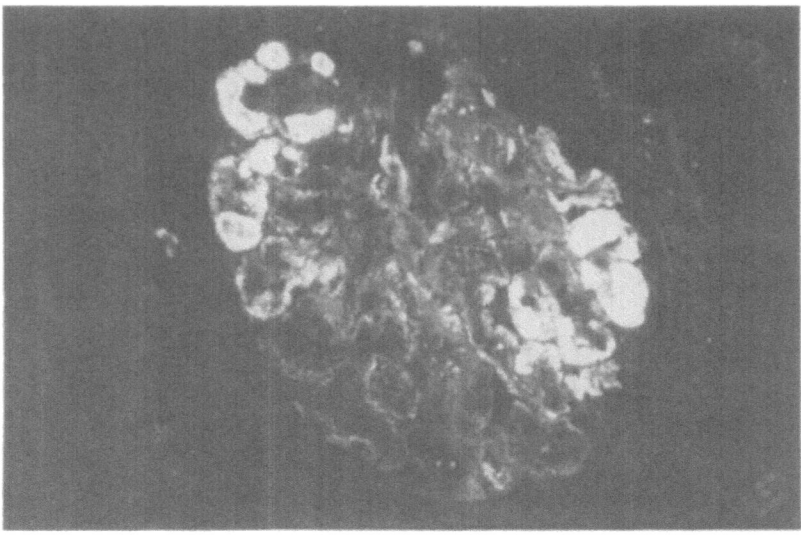

Figure 5. Membranoproliferative exudative GN with prevalent thrombi intense staining of intraluminal thrombi at immunofluorescence (Anti-IgM × 250).

Results

122 renal biopsies performed in 100 EMC patients during the years 1971-1984 have been reviewed. The above described main lesions were variably associated in the different patients, giving patterns which allowed further classification in 5 histological and immunohistological groups.

1. *Membranoproliferative exudative GN with prevalent thrombi* (18 pz.)

Characterized at light microscopy (LM) by marked intracapillary hypercellularity with massive infiltration of monocytes (50–60 monocytes per glomerulus were counted as an average), huge and diffuse endoluminal thrombi (always in more than 50% of glomeruli), diffuse double-contours and high prevalence of vasculitis (61% of cases). At IF intraluminal thrombi stained intensely for IgG and IgM; a faint segmental staining of peripheral loops was rarely found (Fig. 5).

2. *Membranoproliferative exudative GN without prevalent thrombi* (41 pz.)

Characterized at LM by intracapillary severe hypercellularity but with less important monocyte infiltration (about 30 monocytes per glomerulus as an average), and by widespread double-contours of peripheral capillary walls.

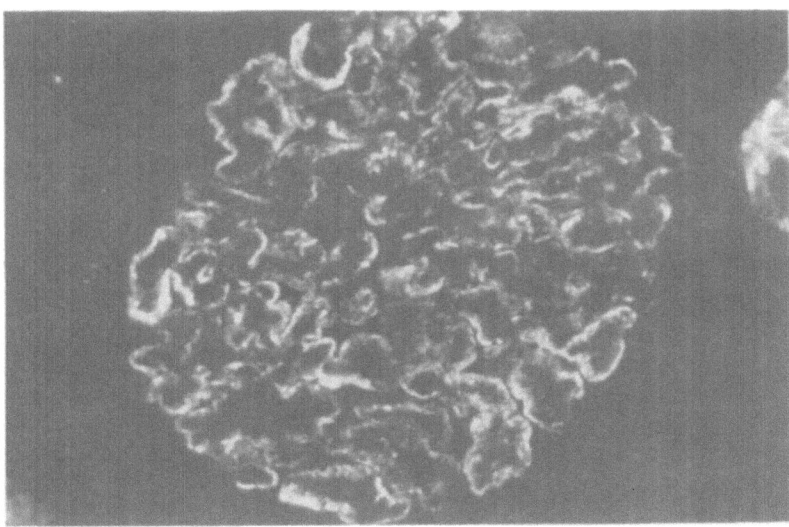

Figure 6. Membranoproliferative exudative GN without prevalent thrombi: diffuse staining of peripheral loops at immunofluorescence (Anti-IgG × 250).

In nearly half of these patients small endoluminal thrombi were also present (always in less than 30 % of glomeruli). Vasculitis was seen in 17 % of cases. IF pattern was characterized by intense diffuse subendothelial staining of peripheral loops and, when present, of thrombi with anti-IgG and anti-IgM sera (Fig. 6).

3. *Mild membranoproliferative exudative GN* (18 pz.)

This group showed less marked lesions than the previous ones: the histological pattern at LM was characterized by a segmental intracapillary hypercellularity with moderate monocyte infiltration (10 monocytes per glomerulus), segmental double contours, rare endoluminal thrombi in about one third of patients and vasculitis in 22 % of cases. IF showed faint segmental staining of some peripheral loops and of rare small intraluminal thrombi.

This group may represent a later stage of group 1 and group 2, with partial regression of histological lesions.

4. *Lobular membranoproliferative GN* (10 pz.)

At LM a typical pattern of lobular GN was present with prevalent mesangial cell proliferation, mesangial matrix expansion and areas of centrolobular sclerosis. Also in this group however, a few intracapillary monocytes were present (about 8 monocytes per glomerulus as an average), whereas in idiopathic lobular membranoproliferative GN we never found intracapillary monocytes [10].

Vasculitis was present in 30% of cases. At IF a diffuse staining of capillary walls was found, with the 'peripheral lobular' pattern typical of lobular GN.

5. *Minimal change GN or meseangial GN* (13 pz.)

At LM this heterogeneous group is characterized by minimal lesions or by segmental mesangial proliferation without monocyte infiltration and GBM alterations. IF was negative (1/3 of cases) or showed faint segmental parietal deposits of immunoglobulins. This group also could represent the final stages of groups 1 and 2.

As regards other histological features it seems interesting to point out that in all groups of EMC-GN we found a very low incidence of obsolescent glomeruli, of extracapillary proliferation (crescents, when present, were always segmental and never circumferential), and of marked interstitial or vascular fibrosis, suggesting a rather poorly aggressive appearance of this GN even in patients with a long history of renal disease (Table I).

As regards IF findings, in all histological groups the deposits were mainly stained by IgG, IgM and C3. Earlier complement components and fibrinogen were found in a lower percentage of cases [8]. No significant differences

Table I. Prevalence of less frequent histological lesions in different groups of EMC-GN

Group	Obsolescent glomeruli (mean %)	Crescentic glomeruli (mean %)	Marked interstitial fibrosis (mean % of PTS)	Marked vascular fibrosis (mean % of PTS)
MPET (18 pts)	4,6	2,8	11	5
MPE (41 pts)	4,7	1,3	7	7
MMPE (18 pts)	11,9	1,8	27	11
LMP (10 pts)	7,5	3	20	40
MC (13 pts)	5,5	0	0	0
Total (100 pts)	6,2	1,7	10	10

MPET : Membranoproliferative exudative GN with prevalent thrombi
MPE : Membranoproliferative exudative GN without prevalent thrombi
MMPE: Mild membranoproliferative exudative GN
LMP : Lobular membranoproliferative GN
MC : Minimal changes or mesangial GN

in the positivity for the various antisera was found in the 5 groups (Table II). IF staining with anti-HBsAg antisera has also been seen in the glomeruli of some patients, but we already demonstrated that this is a non-specific staining, due to some interference of the Rheumatoid factor IgM anti-IgG present in the kidney in EMC [17].

Twenty-two repeat biopsies were performed in 19 patients (Table III): monocyte infiltration, as well as the amount of intraluminal thrombi, was reduced or completely disappearaed in 5/5 patients with MPET, in 4/7 cases of MPE and in 1/4 cases of MMPE. On the other hand 3 patients showed an

Table II. Prevalence of if positivity for various antisera in different groups of EMC-GN (%)

Group	IgG	IgA	IgM	C_3	C_4	C_{1q}	F
MPET (15 pts)	80	53	100	80	20	40	46
MPE (36 pts)	83	44	94	86	17	33	30
MMPE (17 pts)	52	47	94	76	5	29	23
LMP (6 pts)	100	50	100	100	0	33	50
MC (10 pts)	60	40	80	70	0	30	0
Total (84 pts)	75	46	94	82	12	33	30

MPET : Membranoproliferative exudative GN with prevalent thrombi
MPE : Membranoproliferative exudative GN without prevalent thrombi
MMPE: Mild membranoproliferative exudative GN
LMP : Lobular membranoproliferative GN
MC   : Minimal changes or mesangial GN

Table III. Histological features in 22 serial biopsies in EMC-GN (re-biopsy or post-mortem examination).

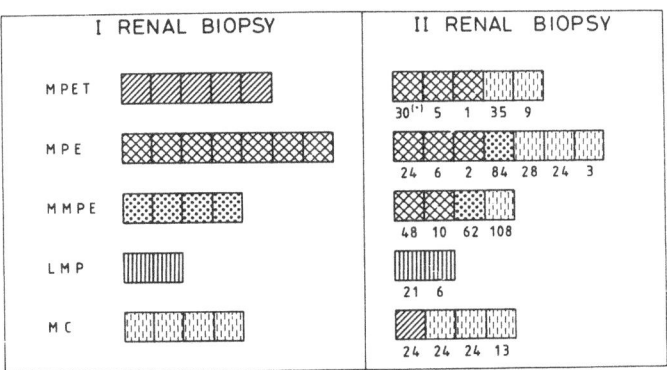

MPET	MEMBRANOPROLIFERATIVE EXUDATIVE GN WITH PREVALENT THROMBI
MPE	MEMBRANOPROLIFERATIVE EXUDATIVE GN WITHOUT PREVALENT THROMBI
MMPE	MILD MEMBRANOPROLIFERATIVE EXUDATIVE GN
LMP	LOBULAR MEMBRANOPROLIFERATIVE GN
MC	MINIMAL CHANGES OR MESANGIAL GN
(•)	INTERVAL BETWEEN BIOPSIES (IN MONTHS)

exacerbation of their nephropathy with more severe lesions. In both cases of LMP GN, the picture was unmodified at the second biopsy.

This data confirms other reports that histological lesions in EMC GN may change with time, either with partial or complete remission or with subsequent 'poussée' of acute exacerbations [1, 2, 14].

Conclusion

The most frequent histological pattern in EMC-GN is that of membrano-proliferative exudative GN characterized by: the deposition of cryoglobulins at the subendothelial level and/or in the capillary lumen (endoluminal thrombi) [1–4]. These two patterns of deposition seem to be mediated by two different pathogenetic mechanisms: A) *In vivo* acute endoluminal precipitation of cryoglobulins, as a consequence of their physico-chemical features. B) More chronic immunological deposition of cryoglobulins along the capillary walls, as a consequence of their immune-complex nature [1, 18].

A marked exudative component due to massive glomerular infiltration by monocytes is also highly characteristic, related to acute or chronic precipitation of cryoglobulins in the glomeruli [10–13]. Whatever the mechanism of recruitment, monocytes could play a role both in phagocytosing intraglomerular cryoglobulins and in inducing tissue damage through their phlogogenic properties [10, 19–23]. Partial or total reversibility of the above described lesions is frequent, with disappearance of monocyte infiltration and of GBM alterations: subsequent bouts of recurrences may also occur, probably associated with new intense deposition of cryoglobulins at the glomerular level [1, 2, 10, 14]. Glomerular obsolescence and interstitial fibrosis are usually mild even in patients with a long history of renal disease and progression to end-stage chronic Kidney lesions is quite infrequent [1, 2].

Acknowledgements

The Authors wish to thank mrs Stefania Nava for technical help and mrs Mascia Marchesini for typing the manuscript. Part of the work has been supported by Grant n° 84.01985.94 from Consiglio Nazionale delle Ricerche (Rome, Italy).

References

1. D'Amico G, Ferrario F, Colasanti G, Bucci A: Glomerulonephritis in essential mixed cryoglobulinemia. Proceedings of XXI EDTA-ERA. London: Pitman, pp 527–548.

201

2. Tarantino A, De Vecchi A, Montagnino G, Imbasciati E, Mihatasch MJ, Zollinger HU, Barbiano di belgioisoso G, Busnach G, Ponticelli : Renal disease in essential mixed cryoglobulinemia. Long-term follow-up of 44 patients. Quart J Med 197:1-30, 1981.
3. Zimmerman SW, Dreher WH, Burkholder PM, Goldfarb S, Weinstein AB: Nephropathy and mixed cryoglobulinemia: evidence for an immune complex pathogenesis. Nephron 16:103-115, 1976.
4. Cordonnier D, Vialtel P, Renversez JCh, Chenzis F, Favre M, Tournoun... A, Barioz C, Bayle F, Dechelette E, Denis MC, Couderc Pb: Lésions rénales chez 18 malades porteurs de cryoglobulines mixtes IgM-IgG de type II. Actualités Néphrologiques de l'Hôpital Necker. Paris: Flammarion, pp 219-241, 1982.
5. Feiner H, Gallo G: Ultrastructure in glomerulonephritis associated with cryoglobulinemia. Amer J Pathol 88:145-161, 1977.
6. Bartlow BG, Oyama JH, Ing TS, Miller AW, Economou SG, Rennie IDB, Lewis EJ: Glomerular ultrastructural abnormalities in a patient with mixed IgG-IgM essential cryoglobulinemic glomerulonephritis. Nephron 14:309-319, 1975.
7. D'Amico G, Ferrario F, Colasanti G, Bucci A, Bestetti Bosicio M: Glomerulonephritis in essential IgG-IgM mixed cryoglobulinemia. La Ricerca (Clin Lab) 10:59-65, 1980.
8. Barbiano di Belgioioso G, Tarantino A, Colasanti G, De Vecchi A, Bertoli S, Bartolomeo F, D'Amico G, Ponticelli C, Minetti L: Immunohistological patterns in mixed IgG-IgM essential cryoglobulinemia glomerulonephritis. In: Leaf, Giebisch, Bolis, Gorini: Renal pathophysiology. New York: Raven Press 245-252, 1980.
9. Maggiore Q, Bartolomea F, L'Abbate A, Misefari V, Martorano C, Caccamo A, Barbiano di Belgioioso G, Tarantino A, Colasanti G: Glomerular localization of circulating antiglobulin activity in essential mixed cryoglobulinemia with glomerulonephritis. Kidney Int 21:387-394, 1982.
10. Ferrario F, Castiglione A, Colasanti G, Barbiano di Belgioioso G, Bertoli S, D'Amico G: The detection of monocytes in human glomerulonephritis. Kidney Int 28:513-519, 1985.
11. Monga G, Mazzucco G, Barbiano di Belgioisoso G, Busnach G: The presence and possible role of moncyte infiltration in human chronic proliferative glomerulonephritides. Light microscopic, immunofluorescence and histochemical correlations. Amer J Pathol 94:271-284, 1979.
12. Monga G., Mazzucco G, Coppo R, Piccoli G, Coda R: Glomerular findings in mixed IgG-IgM cryoglobulinemia. Light electron microscopy, immunofluorescence and histochemical correlations. Virchows Arch B Cell Pathol 20:185-196, 1976.
13. Tarantino A, Ponticelli C: Kidney involvement in essential cryoglobulinemia. In: Bacon and Hadler: The kidney and rheumatic disease. London: Butterworth pp 128-149, 1982.
14. Morel-Maroger L, Méry JP: Renal lesions in mixed IgG-IgM essential cryoglobulinemia. Proceedings of 5th Int Congr Nephrol Basel: Karger, pp 173-178, 1972.
15. Verroust P., Méry JP, Morel-Maroger L, Clauvel JP, Richet G: Les lesions glomerulaires des gammopathies monoclonales et des cryoglobulinemies idiopathiques IgG-IgM. Actualités Néphrologiques de l'Hopital Necker. Paris: Flammarion, pp 167-202, 1971.
16. Gorevic PD, Kassab HJ, Levo Y, Kohn R, Meltzer M, Prose P, Franklin EC: Mixed cryoglobulinemia: clinical aspects and long term follow-up of 40 patients. Amer J Med 69:287-308, 1980.
17. Maggiore Q, Bartolomeo F, L'Abbate A, Misefari V: HBsAg glomerular deposits in glomerulonephritis: fact or artifact. Kidney Int 19:579-586, 1981.
18. Tarantino A, Montagnino G: The pathogenesis of essential cryoglobulinemia. In: Remuzzi and Bertani: Glomerular injury 300 years after Morgagni. Milano: Wichtig, pp 245-254, 1983.
19. Striker GE, Mannik M, Tung MY: Role of marrow-derived monocytes and mesangial cells in removal of immune complexes from renal glomeruli. J Exp Med 149:127-136, 1979.

20. Holdsworth SR, Neale TJ, Wilson CB: Abrogation of macrophage-dependent injury in experimental glomerulonephritis in the rabbit. Use of antimacrophage serum. J Clin Invest 68:686–698, 1981.
21. Unanue ER: Secretory function of mononuclear pagocytes. Amer J Pathol 83:396–415, 1976.
22. Nathan CF, Murray HW, Cohn ZA: The macropahage as an effector cell. N Engl J Med 303:622–626, 1980.
23. Dubois CH, Foidart JB, Hautier MB, Dechenne CA, Lemaire MJ, Mahieu PR: Proliferative glomerulonephritis in rats: evidence that mononuclear phagocytes infiltrating the glomeruli stimulate the proliferation of endothelial and mesangial cells. Eur J Clin Invest 11:91–104, 1981.

17. Clinical and histological correlations in essential mixed cryoglobulinemia (EMC) glomerulonephritis

GIOVANNI BARBIANO DI BELGIOJOSO,
ALBERTO MONTOLI, ANTONIO TARANTINO,
FRANCO FERRARIO, PATRICIA MALDIFASSI,
ANNA BALDASSARI and LUIGI MINETTI

In EMC the clinico-pathological correlations of renal disease, even in large series, have been poorly investigated [1]. An acutely presenting renal disease with severe proteinuria, hematuria and sudden rise of serum creatinine has been described associated with a histological pattern of diffuse proliferation and monocyte infiltration, massive deposition of intraluminal thrombi occluding capillary lumina. Patients with a chronic clinical syndrome showed a proliferation and a monocyte exudation of various degree with diffuse subendothelial deposits [2–5]. These patients had often a nephrotic syndrome (NS), but sometimes exhibited only proteinuria and microscopic hematuria. In these chronic cases a heavier proteinuria was found to be correlated with a more intense monocytes infiltration [6]. Also immunofluorescence patterns of intraluminal or parietal deposition was in relation with the kind of clinical presentation [7, 8].

In this paper we correalte the clinical syndromes with the histological patterns, examining also the influence of main morphological lesions on symptoms.

All patients were submitted to renal biopsy and 18 patients had a second or third biopsy. The criteria of diagnosis of EMC and other clinical parameters employed to select the patients have been reported elsewhere [4] and have been exactly the same for the three Nehrological Units where the study has been performed. The procedures for light and immunofluorescence examination of renal biopsy specimen have been described in detail in previous report [4].

The classification of histological pictures has been presented in this issue by dr. Ferrario and co-workers. As it was described, histological groups, according to their progressive severity were as follows: 1) Minimal changes (13 cases); 2) lobular membranoproliferative (MP) glomerulonephritis (GN) (10 cases); 3) mild MP exudative GN (18 cases); 4) MP exudative GN (41 cases); 5) MP exudative GN with prominent intraluminal thrombi (18 cases).

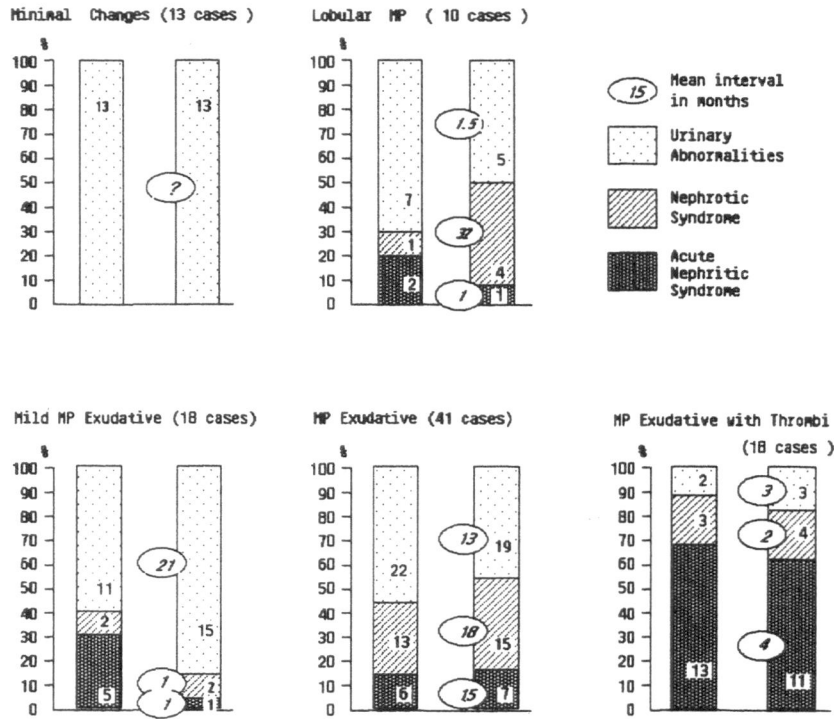

Figure 1. Incidence of clinical syndromes at onset of disease (left columns) and at time of biopsy (right columns) in single histological groups. Data are exposed as absolute numbers within columns and as percent (height of columns). The mean interval is indicated in the circle. For the group with minimal changes the interval was often difficult to assess and is indicated with a question mark.

Clinical syndromes at onset and at biopsy have been classified into the three main clinical syndromes, typical of glomerular diseases: urinary abnormalities (UA) (55 cases) for isolated proteinuria exceeding 0.2 g/24 hrs or proteinuria and microscopic hematuria; NS (19 cases at onset and 25 at biopsy) for proteinuria greater than 3 g/24 hrs, serum albumin concentration lower than 3 gr/dl and edema; acute nephritic syndrome (ANS) (26 cases at onset and 20 at biopsy) for severe proteinuria, hematuria usually macroscopic, hypertension and sudden rise in serum creatinine, sometimes complicated by an acute oliguric renal failure.

At time of observation, renal insufficiency, defined as plasma creatinine over 1.5 mg/dl, was present in 47 cases, hypertension in 84, hematuria in 89 patients.

The composition of cryoglobulins and other clinical parameters will be presented in a separate paper of this issue by dr. Tarantino and co-workers.

The clinical syndrome for each one of the five histological groups at time of onset and of observation is illustrated in Fig. 1. Data are exposed as number of cases and percent (height of columns), comparing onset and biopsy observation. The mean interval between the two times of observation for subgroups with the same clinical syndrome at biopsy is indicated within circles. For minimal changes all cases had only urinary abnormalities in both times; the interval, because of the often minimal urinary alterations, was difficult to assess for this group.

For lobular MP group, at biopsy we observed that cases were mainly divided between UA and NS. Some nephrotics, who have a longer mean interval from onset (32 months) had started with other syndromes, mostly proteinuria.

The three groups with exudative changes are shown in the lower part of the figure.

The mild MP showed a clear-cut prevalence of urinary abnormalities, with a longer mean interval between onset and biopsy. Nevertheless, some cases had started with ANS and shifted to proteinuria and hematuria later on.

Exudative MP have a prevalence of NS and UA, but ANS were also present (15% of cases). There is not a striking difference between onset and biopsy and the first two clinical syndromes show a much longer interval than the last one.

The exudative group with thrombi has a strong prevalence of acute forms, and a short mean interval for all subgroups. Only 3 out 18 cases had always a NS with a short interval. The 3 cases with UA at biopsy had an ANS 3 months before and two patients with proteinuria at onset developed ANS at biopsy, and this explains the mean longer interval (4 months).

The extension of systemic involvement was evaluated in patients with different glomerular lesions. The histological groups were compared for the presence of less or more than three symptoms. Considered symptoms were: purpura, arthralgias, weakness, weight loss, Raynaud's phenomenon, hepatomegaly, splenomegaly, abdominal pain and polyneuropathy.

We observed that the incidence of cases with more than three of the above mentioned symptoms increased with the severity of glomerular involvement: the groups with exudative lesions had values of 28%, 41% and 78% in mild MP, MP exudative and MP exudative with thrombi, respectively. The difference was significant ($p < 0,001$).

Plasma creatinine levels at time of biopsy showed mean higher values for lobular MP and diffuse exudative MP, while all cases of MP with thrombi were abnormal, with a very wide range. As a whole, in 54 out of 100 cases creatinine was above normal. Comparison between single groups was not significant, but if the evaluation was performed on the overall population through analysis of variance, a significant difference was found.

There was not a significantly different distribution of cryocrit among histological groups. The wide range of values can account for this lack of correlation, which was true also for clinical syndromes.

Serum complement levels showed the well known pattern of EMC-GN [9], with C4 very strongly depressed expecially in more severe cases (62/72 cases) and C3 frequently reduced (39/89). These variations were not significantly different in histological groups.

Taking into account the main histological lesions, independently from histological grouping, we looked for correlations between the presence of marked lesions (+ + or + + +) and the clinical syndromes. The distribution of cases is illustrated in Table I. The presence of monocytes was much more frequent in NS and ANS than in UA, and the difference was highly significant. The same was true for thrombi and vasculitis, even if this last parameter was less significant. Also double contours and interstitial infiltrates were significantly more frequent in the last two clinical syndromes than in the first one.

Some of the main histological lesions belonging to glomeruli, interstitium and vessels were studied in three groups of patients divided according to their creatinine levels, in order to evaluate the localization of histological damage in relation to decrease of renal function (Table II). Obsolescent glomeruli were more frequent in the second group, with moderate renal insufficiency, thrombi and vasculitis in the third one. The difference was highly significant. Interstitial infiltration was more frequent in the second group, fibrosis in the second and third group. The other vascular changes did not differ significantly.

Table I. Distribution of lesions in clinical syndromes.

	Mesangial proliferation ++/+++	Monocytes ++/+++	Double contours ++/+++	Subend. deposits ++/+++	Thrombi ++/+++	Interest. infiltr. ++/+++	Vasculitis present
Urinary abnormalities (54 cases)	25 (46%)	23 (43%)	26 (48%)	3 (5%)	4 (7%)	3 (6%)	10 (18%)
Nephrotic syndrome (26 cases)	20 (77%)	21 (81%)	20 (77%)	0 —	5 (19%)	8 (31%)	7 (27%)
Acute nephritic syndrome (20 cases)	10 (50%)	16 (80%)	16 (80%)	1 (5%)	13 (65%)	5 (30%)	10 (50%)
	n.s.	$p < 0.001$	$p < 0.01$	n.s.	$p < 0.001$	$p < 0.01$	$p < 0.01$

Table II. Correlation between renal function and some histolgical parameters (Biopsies and re-biopsies = 122 cases).

Plasma creatinine mg/dl ↓	Glomeruli		Intersitium		Vessels		Vasculitis
	Obsolescent >20%	Thrombi ++/+++	Infiltration ++/+++	Fibrosis ++/+++	Arteriolar hyalinosis ++/+++	Arterial fibrosis ++/+++	
I <1.4 (67 cases)	3 (4%)	5 (7.5%)	2 (3%)	4 (6%)	10 (15%)	7 (10%)	8 (12%)
II 1.5–3 (37 cases)	10 (27%)	10 (27%)	15 (40%)	8 (22%)	9 (24%)	7 (19%)	14 (38%)
III >3 (18 cases)	2 (11%)	10 (56%)	4 (22%)	4 (22%)	3 (16%)	2 (11%)	9 (50%)
Total cases (122 cases)	15 (12%)	25 (20%)	21 (17%)	16 (13%)	22 (18%)	16 (13%)	31 (25%)
	$p < 0.001$	$p < 0.0001$	$p < 0.0001$	$p < 0.005$	n.s.	n.s.	$p < 0.001$

Repeat biopsies performed in 18 pts, showed that at second biopsy clinical syndromes had improved in 5 pts (4 with ANS and one with NS at first biopsy).

Histological pattern was also improved (4 cases) or unchanged (1 case). 11 pts were unchanged in their clinical picture, while histology showed an improvement in 7 cases, a similar picture in 3 cases and a worsening in one. Most of the cases that improved histologically had UA at the first biopsy, those unchanged were UA or NS. Two patients worsened both in clinical syndrome and in histological pattern (they had UA at presentation). This correlation shows that one-half of the patients (9/18) had a parallel course for clinical and histological pattern. For the majority of the remainers, the histological pattern improved earlier than the clinical one.

From the examination of our results we can conclude with a few comments.

Clinicopathological correlations confirmed for each histological group a corresponding prevailing clinical syndrome. Besides minimal changes, which constantly showed UA, lobular MP can be considered as a chronic condition with either proteinuria or NS. This last one sometimes develops later during the course of the disease.

Mild MP exudative GN is characterized by a moderate proteinuria, quite often following an episode of ANS. Cases with a diffuse MP exudative GN have a quite heterogeneous clinical pictures, all three syndromes being represented.

The classification of some cases of ANS in this group (instead of the group with thrombi) could be explained by a removal of thrombi by the time biopsy was performed.

Cases belonging to MP exudative with prevalent intraluminal thrombi have mainly an ANS, even though some patients with NS were observed. Nevertheless, ANS and NS may present with overlapping features, when a sudden onset of heavy proteinuria without hematuria is accompanied by a moderate increase of creatinine.

Chronic versus acute onset of disease, examined together with histological and immunohistological picture, this last one characterized by strong and exclusive thrombi deposition of IgG and IgM, may represent different mechanisms of glomerular injury.

Severe episodes of ANS are often reversible, with disappearance of thrombi at repeat biopsies. For these cases a mechanism of less specific immunoglobulins trapping into capillary lumina, due to their physico-chemical properties rather than the classical mechanism of immune-complexes deposition is probably operating [2]. This is in agreement with the observation of faint C3 deposition within thrombi [7]. For chronic cases, with parietal deposition of immunoglobulins and C3, presumably, the immune-complexes mechanism plays an important role, causing proteinuria and NS.

The histological features suggestive of either one of the two mechanisms are not correlated with cryocrit values or with hypocomplementemia, even though C4 was more deeply depressed in cases with more severe glomerular involvement.

Monocytes, thrombi and vasculitis were more prominent and frequent in cases with ANS and severe function impairement. Nevertheless, these main lesions were reversible and histological regression, eventually obtained by therapy, was more rapid than the clinical improvement.

Monocytes infiltration, though representing a factor of tissue damaging and of acute impairement of renal function, is a mechanism of cryoglobulins removal from glomerular structures, due to monocytes phagocytosing properties; therefore it is not a long-distance bad prognostic factor. Episodes of acute renal failure make part of the natural history of the disease, without a relevant influence on the evolution towards chronic renal failure, which is not, fortunately, a frequent event in EMC.

Summary

One hundred cases of EMC with renal involvement were studied for clinico-pathological correlations. All were submitted to renal biopsy and 18 had a second or third biopsy. Histological diagnosis was minimal changes in 13 cases, lobular membranoproliferative (MP) GN in 10 cases, mild MP exudative GN in 18 cases, diffuse MP exudative in 41 cases and MP exudative with prominent intraluminal thrombi in 18 cases. Clinical syndrome at biopsy was urinary abnormalities (UA) in all cases of minimal changes, UA or nephrotic syndrome (NS) in lobular MP; UA was predominant in mild MP, UA, NS and acute nephritic syndrome (ANS) in MP exudative, ANS in MP exudative with thrombi. The extension of systemic involvement was more evident in cases with more severe glomerular involvement. Plasma creatinine, cryocrit level or complement profile were not significantly different in single histological groups. The main histological lesions that more clearly influenced the clinical syndrome were monocyte infiltration, thrombi and vasculitis. Repeat biopsies showed a good agreement between the histological and clinical variations. The histological regression often preceded the clinical improvement.

References

1. Gorevic PD, Kassab HJ, Levo Y, Kohn R, Meltzer M, Prose Ph and Franklin EC: Mixed cryoglobulinemia: clinical aspects and long-term follow-up of 40 patients. Am J Med 69: 287–308, 1980.

210

2. D'Amico G, Ferrario F, Colasanti G and Bucci A: Glomerulonephritis in essential mixed cryoglobulinemia. Proc EDTA-ERA 21:527–547, 1984.
3. Morel-Maroger L, Méry JP: Renal lesions in mixed IgG-IgM essential cryoglobulinemia. In: Villareal H. (Ed) Proc 5th Int Congr Nephrol. Vol I S Karger Basel pp 173–178, 1974.
4. Tarantino A, De Vecchi A, Montagnino G, Imbasciati E, Mihatsch HJ, Zollinger HU, Barbiano Di Belgioioso G, Busnach G and Ponticelli C: Renal disease in essential mixed cryoglobulinemia. Long Term follow-up in 44 patients. Quart J Med New Series 50:1–30, 1981.
5. Barbiano di Belgioioso G, Bertoli S, Tarantino A, Colasanti G, Bestetti-Bosisio M, Ferrario F, Montagnino G, Banfi G, Bucci A, Colussi G, Guerra L and Micoli G: Renal lesions in essential mixed IgG-IgM cryoglobulinemia. Study of 48 cases. Boll. Ist. Sieroter Milanese 60:316–327, 1981.
6. Ferrario F, Castiglione A, Colasanti G, Barbiano di Belgioioso G, Bertoli S and D'Amico G: The detection of monocytes in human glomerulonephritis. Kidney Int 28:513–519, 1985.
7. Barbiano di Belgioioso G, Tarantino A, Colasanti G, De Vecchi A, Bertoli S, Bartolomeo F, D'Amico G, Ponticelli C and Minetti L: Immunohistological patterns in mixed IgG-IgM essential cryoglobulinemia glomerulonephritis. In: Leaf A and Giebisch G. Renal Pathophysiology, Raven Press, New York pp 245–252, 1980.
8. Hill GS: Multiple myeloma, amyloidosis, Waldenström's macroglobulinemia, cryoglobulinemias, and benign monoclonal gammapathies. In: Heptinstall RH. Pathology of the Kidney. Third Edition. Little, Brown & Co. Boston, pp 993–1067, 1983.
9. Tarantino A, Anelli A, Costantino A, De Vecchi A, Monti G and Massaro L: Serum complement pattern in essential mixed cryoglobulinemia. Clin Exp Immunol 32:77–85, 1978.

18. Ultrastructural features in glomerulonephritis in essential mixed cryoglobulinemia

M.J. MIHATSCH and G. BANFI

Introduction

Renal disease in essential mixed IgG-IgM cryoglobulinemia (EMC, type II) as seen by lightmicroscopy and immunofluorescence is well described based on a large number of cases (see Ferrario F., this issue). A few reports, only, are dedicated to the electromicroscopic picture of glomerulonephritis in EMC [1-7, 11, 13]. EMC glomerulonephritis is characterized by three outstanding morphologic features:

1. Crystalloid structure of the glomerular protein deposits.
2. Hyaline thrombi.
3. Monocytes in large numbers.

These morphologic features are not met in all cases of EMC glomerulonephritis. The crystalloid structure of deposits is pathognomonic [6] whereas hyaline thrombi and monocytes can also be found in glomerulonephritis in SLE and in postinfectious endocapillary glomerulonephritis [13]. The present investigation focuses on the ultrastructural appearance of the three major morphologic characteristics in EMC glomerulonephritis.

Material and Methods

Twenty-five renal biopsies of patients with EMC were investigated by electron microscopy. The method of electron microscopic investigation is described elsewhere [13]. In most patients, serum cryoprecipitates were fixed in glutaraldehyd and investigated by electron microscopy. The clinical and light microscopic data of these patients are included in other contributions in this issue.

Results

A survey of a few systematically analyzed parameters in the 25 patients is presented in Table I. In all but one biopsy, membrano-proliferative glomerulonephritis at different stages of evolution is found: Mesangial proliferation, mesangial interposition and mesangial matrix increase are prominent in most cases. In one biopsy, minor glomerular abnormalities only are present.

Special attention will be paid to the morphologic features mentioned above and to related topics.

1. Crystalloid structure

The ultra-structure of the cryoglobulins in mixed IgG-IgM cryoglobulinemia type II is unique [6, 10]. It consists of cylinders which appear in cross sections as annular bodies. The crystalloid structure is usually found in hyaline thrombi but is also seen in osmiophilic deposits at different sites within the glomeruli as well as in the serum cryoprecipitates [1, 6] (Fig. 1).

Detailed ultrastructural studies of serum cryoprecipitates have shown that the cylinders are 100 or 1000 nm long and have a hollow axis. On cross-sections they appear as annular bodies, having a light center, a dense ring and a lighter peripheral protein coat. The external layer consists of five to eight round or ovoid condensations. The total diameter measures 62–63 nm [10]. This structure forms when a monoclonal IgM with anti-IgG activity is associated with a polyclonal IgG at an equal or slightly greater

Table I. Frequency and severity of different morphologic parameters.

	% of cases	Mean score
	++ − +++/ > +	
PMN	36/76	1,3
Monocytes	52/96	1,8
H. thrombi	40/72	1,4
Subepithelial deposits	8/44	0,5
Intramembranous deposits	8/28	0,4
Subendothelial deposits	68/96	2,1
Mesangial-BM deposits	16/64	0,8
Mesangial matrix deposits	0/ 8	0,1
Mesangial matrix	60/84	1,6
Mesangial proliferation	76/96	2,2
Mesangial interposition	71/96	2,1

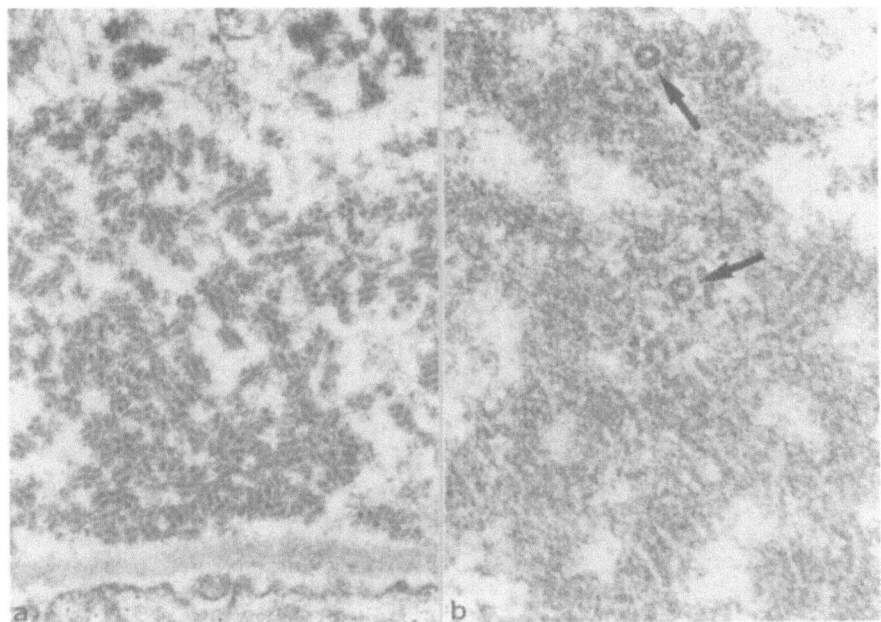

Figure 1. a) Ultrastructural appearance of crystalloid deposits in the glomerulus. BM-basement membrane. b) Ultrastructure of in vitro cryoprecipitate of IgG-IgM (tye II) cryoglobulins: Note cylinders of different length with hollow axis and in cross-section (Δ) annular bodies are present in the glomerulus and the cryoprecipitate without any difference. a: EM × 35'000 b: EM × 70'000.

ratio. Globular condensations with a diameter of 32 nm, which we have not identified in glomeruli, probably only consist of IgM [10].

The crystalloid structure found in mixed IgG-IgM cryoglobulinemia was never described to the best of our knowledge in cryoglobulinemia type I or type III. This enables the pathologist to make the diagnosis of mixed IgG-IgM cryoglobulinemia type II on the basis of the ultrastructural finding [6]. This fact is important for northern European countries and probably many other places in the world where mixed IgG-IgM cryoglobulinemia is rare whereas in countries with a high incidence of EMC the diagnosis is established by immunological methods before biopsy.

2. Hyaline thrombi

Hyaline thrombi by light microscopy represent either a) true hyaline thrombi i.e. extracellular protein deposits which obstruct glomerular loops or b) giant protein droplets (phagolysosomes) in monocytes (Figs. 2, 3) [6, 7, 11].

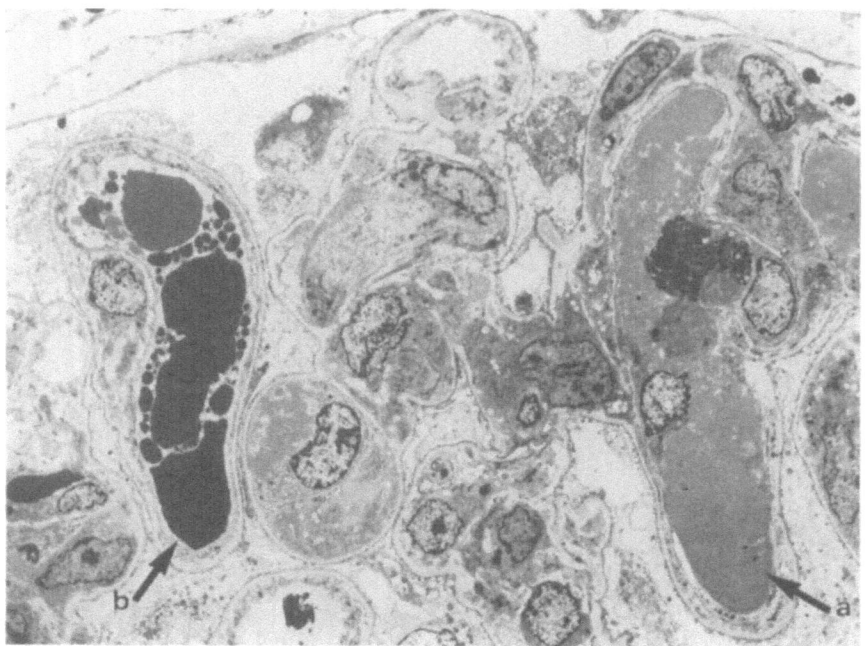

Figure 2. Glomerular segment with different types of hyaline thrombi: a) true hyaline trombus; b) protein droplets in monocytes. EM × 2100.

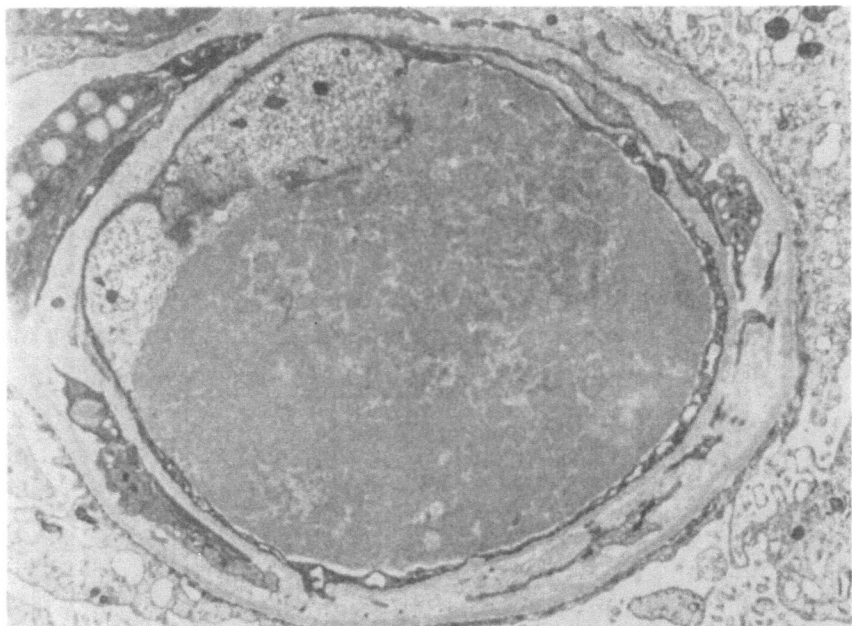

Figure 3. High magnification of a hyaline thrombus: the glomerular loop is completely occluded by a cryoglobulin thrombus. The endothelium is preserved. Note mesangial interposition and basement membrane doubling. EM × 7800.

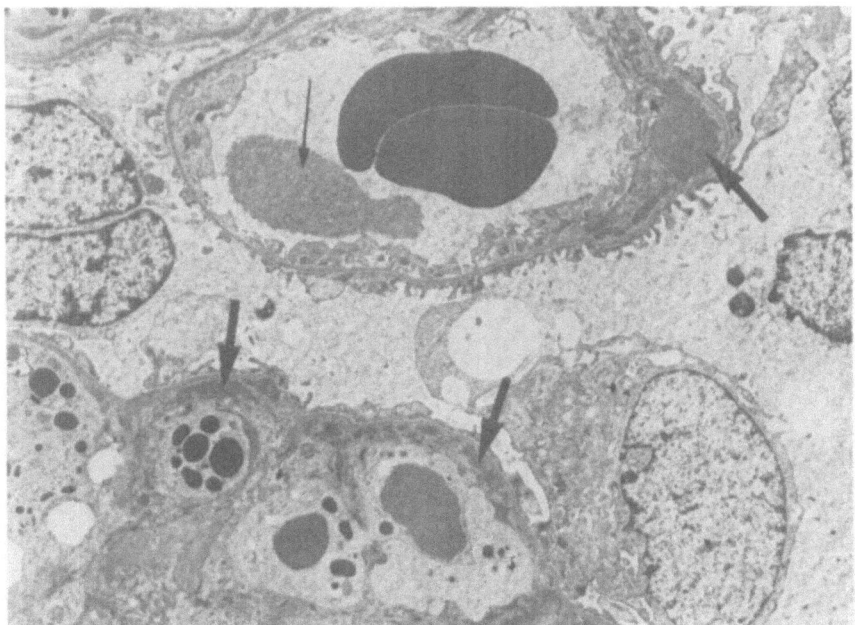

Figure 4. Two glomerular loops: one glomerular loop contains a so-called circulating deposit (△) besides numerous subendothelial and mesangial-basement membrane deposits (△), in the other loop, numerous monocytes (m) with protein droplets are seen, which are in immediate contact with the subendothelial deposits (△). EM × 5800.

Hyaline thrombi in the restricted sense are present in 72 % of the cases (Table I). The extent of hyaline thrombi is variable. In some cases they are very rare, in others abundant. In all cases, the hyaline thrombi show the characteristic crystalloid structure of the cryoglobulins. In some biopsies, only a few areas within the thrombi show this structure, whereas in others most of the thrombi are entirely made up of the crystalloid protein.

Side by side with hyaline thrombi or in adjacent glomeruli, plasma condensations (so-called 'circulating deposits') with typical crystalloid structure are found which are not obstructive (Fig. 4). The circulating deposits are also rarely found in postglomerular capillaries whereas hyaline thrombi are never seen in pre- or postglomerular capillaries in our cases [11].

Osmiophilic deposits must be distinguished from hyaline thrombi and circulating deposits. In mixed cryoglobulinemia, the deposits predominate in the subendothelial space. They may also be found in other locations e.g. subepithelial, mesangial space, etc., but mostly in small amounts (Table 1) (Fig. 4).

The crystalloid structure of deposits is best seen in subendothelial and subepithelial deposits, whereas mesangial deposits rarely exhibit the crystalloid structure. It may be speculated that the crystalloid structure is lost in the process of mesangial uptake.

216

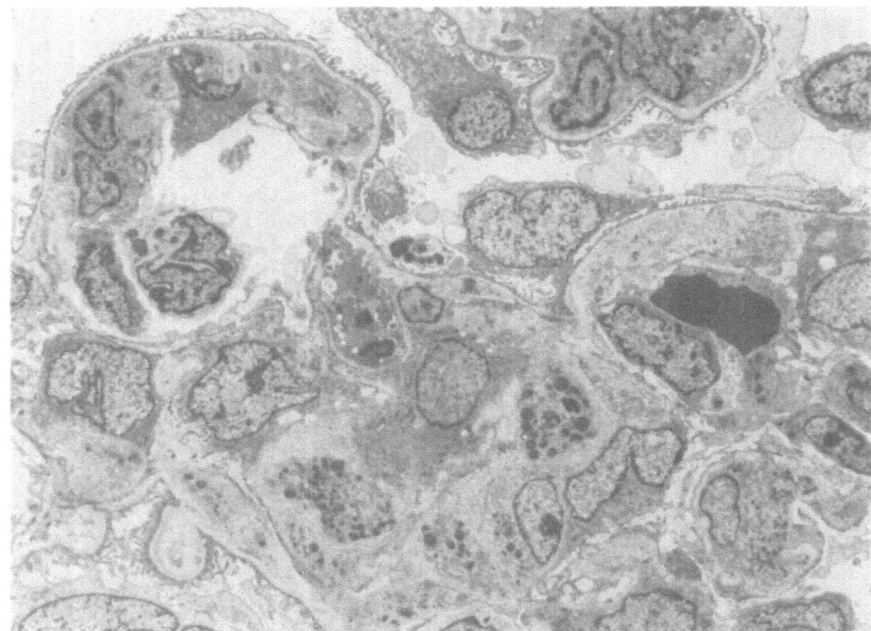

Figure 5. Glomerular segment with numerous monocytes and a polymorpho-nuclear leukocyte: Note monocytes covering the basement membrane which is denuded of the endothelium. EM × 3000.

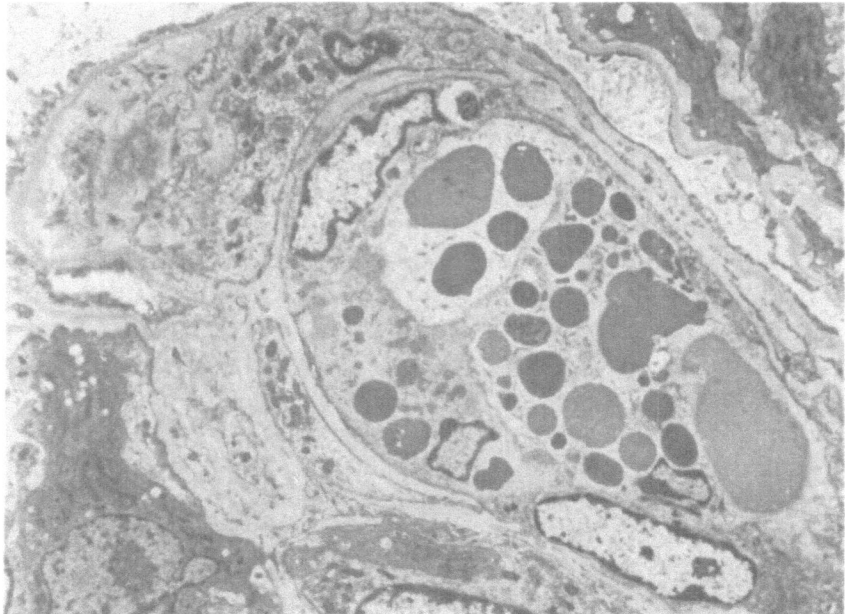

Figure 6. Glumerular loop with circumferential mesangial interposition and basement membrane reduplication: The residual loop lumen is filled with monocyte containing numerous protein droplets with different osmiophilia (phagolysosomes). EM × 6500.

Subendothelial deposits vary in their osmiophilia. In the more osmio-philic centre they show a distinct crystalloid structure which is lost in the more translucent periphery. These differences in osmiophilia may reflect deposit degradation.

3. Monocytes and polymorphonuclear leukocytes

Associated with hyaline thrombi and extensive subendothelial deposits, numerous monocytes and polymorphonuclear leukocytes (PMN) are found (Table I). The monocytes may occlude the glomerular loops or cover the inner aspect of basement membranes after endothelial destruction (Fig. 5). Both cell types are involved in the deposit degradation as suggested by the juxtaposition of these cells (Fig. 4) [6–8, 11]. A futher argument is the fact that the monocytes contain protein droplets of different osmiophilia (Fig. 6). Most of the intracellular protein droplets do not show a crystalloid struc-ture, indicating that the cryoglobulins loose their structure during phagocy-tosis.

Concluding remarks

Glomerulonephritis in EMC (type II) represents an excellent model for the study of the evolution of membrano-proliferative glomerulonephritis [6]. The recurrent character of the renal disease is often documented by the glomerular changes: Loops showing circumferential mesangial interposition, basement membrane reduplication with a hyaline thrombus in the residual capillary lumen indicating a recent recurrence of the disease (Fig. 3).

The crystalloid structure of deposits and the presence of phagocytes allows a detailed analysis of the function of the latters. For the monocytes, the phagocytic activity is clearly visible in form of the phagolysosomes con-taining cryoglobulines [6–8]. Immunelectronmicroscopic techniques as well as ultrastructural histochemical studies would allow, however, a better understanding of cryoglobulin-complex phagocytosis and degradation. Fur-thermore, studies are needed to explain the massive accumulation of mon-ocytes in cryoglobulinemic glomerulonephritis which is not seen in this extent in other forms of glomerulonephritis, indicating that other factors than complement derived chemotactic agents may also play a role [9].

The functional significance of the hyaline thrombi and the so-called cir-culating deposits is not clear [3–5]. It is doubtful if these thrombi occlud the glomerular loops in a way similar to fibrin thrombi or if they rather repre-sent sluggish flow of highly concentrated cryoglobulin-complexes containing plasma. It is assumed that these thrombi do not cause permanent loop

218

obstruction and are not an essential trigger for the development of glomerulonephritis [5]. The possibility that these thrombi occur during tissue processing due to cooling and fixation is not excluded. Experimental studies and intravital examinations should clarify the significance of these thrombi.

References

1. Cordonnier D, Martin H, Groslambert P, Micouin C, Chenais F and Stoebner P: Mixed IgG-IgM cryoglobulinemia with glomerulonephritis. Immunochemical, flurorescent and ultrastructural study of kidney and in vitro cryoprecipitate. American Journal of Medicine 59:867–872, 1975.
2. Cordonnier D, Vialtel P, Martin, H, Renversez JCh, Chenais F, Micouin C and Stoebner P: Cryoglobulines et glomerulonéphrites. Etude particulière des cryoglobulines mixte a composant monoclonal IgM. In: Actualités Néphrologiques de l'Hôpital Necker, Edited by J Hamburger, J Crosnier, JL Funck-Brentano, 349–385. Paris, Flammarion Medicine-Sciences 1977.
3. Farraggiana T, Parolini C, Previato G and Lupo A: Light and electron microscopic findings in five cases of cryoglobulinemic glomerulonephritis. Virchows Archiv A 384:29–44, 1979.
4. Feiner H and Gallo G: Ultrastructure in glomerulonephritis associated with cryoglubulinemia. American Journal of Pathology 88:145–155, 1977.
5. Feiner HD: Relationship of tissue deposits of cryoglobulin to clinical features of mixed cryoglobulinemia. Human Pathology 14:710–715, 1983.
6. Mihatsch MJ, Zollinger HU, Imbasciati E, Tarantino A, Banfi G and Amsler B: Glomerulonephritis bei essentieller IgG-IgM Kryoglobulinämie. Verh Dtsch Ges Path 62:352, 1978.
7. Monga G, Mazzucco G, Coopo R, Piccoli G and Coda R: Glomerular findings in mixed IgG-IgM cryoglobulinemia. Light, electron microscoic, immunofluorescence and histochemical correlations. Virchows Archiv B Cell Pathology 20:185–196, 1976.
8. Monga G, Mazzucco G, Barbiano di Belgiojoso G and Busnach G: The presence and possible role of monocyte infiltration in human chronic proliferative glomerulonephritis. American Journal of Pathology 94:271–284, 1979.
9. Rennke HG: Antibody induced glomerular injuty. Klin Wochenschr 63:862–867, 1985.
10. Stoebner P, Renversez JC, Groulade J, Vialtel P and Cordonnier D: Ultrastructural study of human IgG and IgG-IgM crystalcryoglobulins. Am J Clin Pathol 71:404–410, 1979.
11. Tarantino A, De Vecchi A, Montagnino G, Imbasciati E, Mihatsch MJ, Zollinger HU, Barbiano di Belgiojoso, G, Busnach G and Ponticelli C: Renal disease in essential mixed cryoglobulinaemia. Long-term follow-up of 44 patients. Quarterly Journal of Medicine 50:1–30, 1981.
12. Tubbs RR, Gephardt GN, Calabrese L, McMahon JT, Hall PM and Valenzuela R: Primary ultrastructural diagnosis of cryoglobulinemic glomerulonephritis. Arch Pathol Lab Med 105:474–477, 1981.
13. Zollinger HU and Mihatsch MJ: Renal Pathology in Biopsy, berlin, Heidelberg, New York, Springer-Verlag, pp 169-172, 1978.

19. Prognostic factors in essential mixed cryoglobulinemia nephropathy

TARANTINO A., MONTAGNINO G., BALDASSARI A.,
BARBIANO DI BELGIOJOSO G., COLASANTI G.,
MONTOLI A., BUCCI A. and PONTICELLI C.

Introduction

Kidney involvement in Essential Mixed Cryoglobulinemia (EMC) varies from 8 to 58% in the large series of patients [1–3] and is often regarded as an ominous prognostic sign [4].

We report here the outcome of 116 patients with EMC nephritis.

Patients and methods

The outcome of 116 patients followed by three Nephrology Units of Milan for 6 months to 18 years was analyzed.

Forty-five were males and 71 females. The mean age at the time of diagnosis of nephropathy was 52 ± 11 years. Cryoprecipitate typing was IgG alone in 4 patients, IgM alone in 1, polyclonal IgG and IgMk in 66n polyclonal IgG and IgM in 22, polyclonal IgG and IgMlambda in 3. In 17 patients light chains of both IgG and IgM were not characterized, while 3 had no cryoprecipitate typing. In most patients the disease was diagnosed at an age ranging from 58 to 64 years. The interval between the onset of disease and the appearance of renal involvement was less than 1 year in about 30% of patients and of 5–10 years in another 35% of patients.

An occasional faint positivity for antinuclear antibodies and anti-dsDNA antibodies was observed in 5 out of 60 and in 2 out of 34 patients respectively. Eighty-seven of 91 patients tested were HBsAg negative and 4 were HBsAg positive. An M-component was found at serum electroporesis in 14 out of 113 patients. In 19 patients a liver biopsy was performed: 9 had chronic persistent hepatitis (HBsAg positive in 1/9, HBsAg positive in 1/9), 3 chronic active hepatitis (HBsAg positive in 1/3), 5 liver cirrhosis (HBsAg negative in 5/5, HBsAg positive in 1/5). Two patients had no histological lesions and were not tested for Hepatitis B Antigen in their sera.

Six patients had a malignancy diagnosed either concomitantly or shortly before their admission to our Units. In a patient, a clinical and morphological diagnosis of discoid lupus was made on a skin biopsy 2 years before admission.

The overall incidence of extra-renal manifestations by recording their presence or absence through the whole course of the study period was: purpura 88%, hepatomegaly 88%, arthralgias 78%, weakness 67%, fever 56%, anemia 53%, splenomegaly 50%, Raynaud phenomenon 35%, peripheral or central nervous system involvement 31%, abdominal pain 27%, thrombocytopenia 26%, increase in liver enzymes 25%, weight loss 23%, pleurisy 23%. Thrombophlebitis, pericarditis, lung hemorrhage, lymphoadenopathy and Sicca Syndrome were rarely observed.

Statistical analysis was carried out with two tailed Student T test and correct chi-square test. Actuarial survival curves were calculated according to Peto & Pike method. Both patient and kidney survival curves were calculated: for the former, only patients' deaths were taken into account, while for the latter, both patients' deaths and kidney failures (defined by a plasma creatinine persistently higher than 3 mg/dl) were considered.

Results

The mean follow-up period was 119 ± 97 and 50 ± 47 months from the onset of the disease and from diagnosis respectively. During the follow-up twenty-seven patients died, 14 developed chronic renal failure (CRF), 6 of them required regular dialytic treatment (RDT). Three patients died while being in CRF and 2 on RDT owing to hyperkalimia and multiple myeloma respectively.

The survival curves from the onset of the disease and the time of diagnosis of the nephropathy are reported in Fig. 1.

For the first 5 years the two curves are identical, indicating that deaths only accounted for patients' loss. After this period, mortality still accounted for the majority of patient losses in spite of the fact that a certain number of patients is lost due to the appearance of CFR. At ten years from the onset of disease the probability of patient survival was 70%.

Thirty patients died, the major causes of death being cardiovascular disease, infections and liver failure (Table I).

We correlated the outcome of the disease with a number of clinical, laboratory and histological variables. No difference in sex and time interval between the onset of the disease and nephropathy was observed. We found a correlation between an unfavourable outcome and the presence of 4 or more extrarenal manifestations (Table II). Moreover, while patients with less than 4 signs had mostly purpura, fever arthralgias, weakness, hepatomegaly and

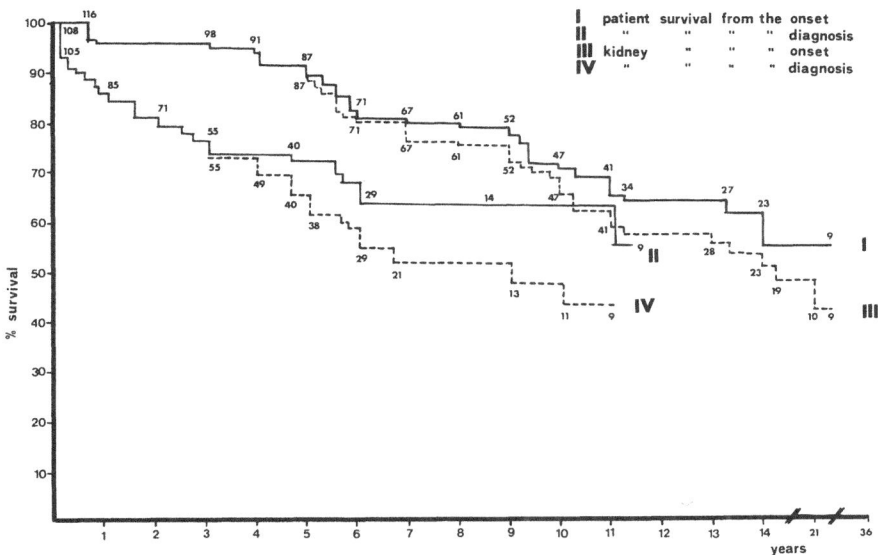

Figure 1. Actuarial patient and kidney survival curves.

Table I. Causes of death in 30 pts with EMC nephropathy.

A) Cardiovascular accidents	Cerebral haemorrhage	4
	Heart failure	3
	Intestinal infarction	2
	Myocardial infarction	2
	Pulmonary embolization	1
B) Infections	Sepsis	4
	Disseminated tubercolosis	1
	Listeria monocytogenes meningitis	1
	Pneumonia	1
	Peritonitis	1
C) Liver failure	HBsAg negative hepatitis	4
D) Neoplasia	Chronic lymphatic leukemia	1
	Non-hodgkin lymphoma	1
	Laryngeal cancer	1
E) Acute respiratory distress		1
F) Unknown		2

Interval between EMC onset and death 1–433 months (mean 170 ± 120).
Interval between renal disease diagnosis and death 1–120 months (mean 29 ± 34).

Table II. Correlation among clinical variables and patient and kidney survival (part 1).

Patients	Normal renal function	Death	CRF	P
A) Males	25	13	6	N.S.
B) Females	42	14	8	
Interval between the onset of the disaese and nephropathy				
A) 0–12 Months	16	10	4	
B) 13–60 Months	32	9	6	N.S.
C) 61 Months	19	8	4	
Extra-renal manifestations				
A) Less than 4 signs	54	14	10	
B) More than 4 signs	14	13	4	0.005
Hypertension				
A) Treatable hypertension	43	20	11	0.01
B) Refractory hypertension	13	6	3	0.02
C) Normotension	11	1	0	

Table III. Correlation among clinical variables and patient and kidney survival (part 2).

Patients	Normal renal function	Death	CRF	P
Presentingsyndrome				
Urinary abnormalities	45	11	6	
Nephrotic syndrome	13	7	3	0.02
Acute nephritic syndr.	10	9	5	0.02
Plasma creatinine levels				
Persistent stable				
Renal function	49	13	0	
Acute recurrent flare-ups	18	14	3	0.01
Progressive worsening	0	5	11	

Biochemical indices

Parameters	Serum concentration		P
	Surviving	Dead	
Cryocrit (%)	11.7 ± 11	22 ± 21	0.04
IgG (mg %)	1042 ± 536	660 ± 361	0.03
Pl. creat. (mg %)	1.63 ± 1.3	2.6 ± 2.0	0.003
Proteinuria (g/day)	1.75 ± 1.9	3.6 ± 3.8	0.003

splenomegaly, by contrast, the second group of patients showed polyneuropathy, abdominal coliky pain, pleurisy, thrombocytopenia, which could all be considered as indices of a more severe and/or generalized vasculitis. The presence of hypertension represented a bad prognostic sign. When comparing the presenting clinical signs of renal syndrome with patient outcome, we found that acute nephritic and nephrotic syndrome had the worst prognosis (Table III). However, taking into account patients who evolved into CFR and excluding deaths, no correlation was observed between the presenting syndrome and evolution towards CRF (data not shown). Moreover, patients with fluctuating plasma creatinine levels or acute exacerabations of renal disease had the worst prognosis.

Among the single biochemical parameters, such as cryocrit, Igs levels, rheumatoid factor activity, plasma creatinine values, degree of proteinuria and hematuria at the time of diagnosis, only cryocrit, plasma creatinine levels and proteinuria were positively correlated, while serum IgG levels were inversely correlated with death or CRF.

Finally, histological and immunohistological variables as well as the final picture of renal biopsy were compared with patient's prognosis. The extent and severity of interstitial fibrosis, tubular atrophy, IgM and IgA deposits had the major impact on the evolution of the disease, while severe exudative glomerulonephritis with and without intraluminal thrombi was predictive of the patient and kidney losses (Table IV).

Discussion

Some investigators have emphasized that the outcome of patients with EMC was influenced by some clinical parameters such as the appearance of

Table IV. Correlation among histological and immunohistological parameters and clinical outcome.

Histological pattern	Normal renal function	Death	CRF
A) Gnmp ex. thr.	9	5	4
B) Gnmp ex.	28	8	2
C) Mild gnmp ex.	9	5	4
D) Lobular gnmp.	5	5	0
E) Gn. prol. mes.	9	1	1

A	B	chi sq. = 3.45 p	0.05		A	C	chi sq. =	0 p = N.S.
A	D	chi sq. = 0.15 p = N.S.			A	E	chi sq. = 4.44 p = 0.025	
B	C	chi sq. = 2.09 p = N.S.			B	D	chi sq. = 1.11 p = N.S.	
B	E	chi sq. = 0.90 p = N.S.			C	D	chi sq. = 0.16 p = N.S.	
C	E	chi sq. = 4.44 p	0.02		D	E	chi sq. = 4.34 p	0.02

nephritis 'per se', cryoprecipitate composition and C3 serum levels. These assumptions were based on the observation that patients with EMC but without renal involvement had a mortality rate of 30%, while patients with renal disease presented a mortality rate of 70% [3]. Brouet et al. [5] showed that patients with Type II cryoglobulinemia had a course characterized by repeated exacerbations of their renal disease, while in patients with Type III cryoglobulinemia, a smouldering progression of kidney disease towards CRF was observed. In our series of 108 patients with EMC and nephritis, the survival rate was 70% at 10 years from the beginning of the disease. During the period of observation, 27 patients (25%) died. The reasons for this improved life expectancy were almost certainly multifactorial. Among them, we think that the selection criteria used to diagnose EMC and the early treatment of renal and extra-renal exacerbations [6] might have played a major role.

From this study, many clinical and morphological variables, assessed at the time of diagnosis, are implicated in predicting the final outcome of patients. Plasma creatine levels, cryoglobulin concentration, amount of urinary protein excretion, hypertension, immunoglobulin G levels are responsible for a bad prognosis. Moreover, the more severe the renal disease at diagnosis the worse the prognosis. This is also confirmed by morphological variables showing that patients with the most severe pattern of proliferative glomerulonephritis and intraluminal thrombi had the poorest prognosis. When comparing patients with more or less than 4 signs of extrarenal manifestations, we found that patients with more numerous systemic symptoms had the highest mortality rate. Moreover, in this group of patients, extrarenal symptoms were mainly represented by peripheral neuropathy, abdominal coliky pain, increase in liver enzymes and serositis. For this reason, we believe that, at least in these patients, widespread vasculitis might have a major impact on patients' prognosis.

Although only a minority of patients developed CRF (14/108; 13%), however it is possible that, due to the late appearance of CRF, a longer follow-up of our patients might eventually reveal a higher incidence of CRF.

Fourteen patients (13%) developed CRF and 6 of them required regular dialytic treatment. Interstingly enough, the presenting renal syndrome at diagnosis was not predictive of renal death.

In conclusion, our experience with EMC demonstrates that the appearance of renal disease is not necessarily correlated with a poor prognosis. Furtherly, two groups of patients can be identified: those having a restless course of their renal disease and a multisystemic involvement, and those having an apparently more benign course and fewer signs of systemic vasculitis. Whether these differences are correlated to the nature of the immunoglobulins involved in the cryoprecipitation phenomenon, to physicochemical characteristics or to other properties of cryoglobulins remains to be ascertained.

References

1. Bombardieri S, Paoletti P, Ferri C, Di Munno O, Fornai E, Giuntini C: Lung Involvement in Essential Mixed Cryoglobulinemia. Amer J Med 66:748–756, 1979.
2. Invernizzi F, Pioltelli P, Cattaneo R, Gavazzeni V, Borzini P, Monti G, Zanussi C: A Long-Term Follow-Up Study in Essential Cryoglobulinemia. Acta Haemet 61:93–99, 1979.
3. Pope RM, Fletcher MA, Mamby A, Shapiro CM: Essential Mixed Cryoglobulinemia Without Evidence for Hepatitis B Virus Infection. Ann Int Med 92:379–383, 1980.
4. Gorevic PD, Kassab HJ, Levo Y, Kohn R, Meltzer M, Prose P, Franklin EC: Mixed Cryoglobulinemia: Clinical Aspects and Long-Term Follow-Up of 40 Patients. Amer J Med 69:287–308, 1980.
5. Brouet JC, Clauvel JP, Danon F: Cryoglobulins: Clinicobiological Correlations. In: Cryoproteins (Colloque). Ed. Françoise Chenais. p 159–166, 1978.
6. De Vecchi A, Montagnino G, Pozzi C, Tarantino A, Locatelli F, Ponticelli C: Intravenous Methylprednisolone Pulse Therapy in Essential Mixed Cryglobulinemia Nephropathy. Clin Nephrol 19:221–227, 1983

Discussion Part V

WINEARLS (London): Dr. Ferrario, was there complement deposition in Kidney lesions? Was there any relationship with serum complement levels?

FERRARIO: Most of the biopsies showed IgG, IgM and C3 deposits in all histologic groups, while C4 and C1q deposits were present in a lower percentage. No relationship was present with the presence of hypocomplementemia.

NAISH: Dr. Ferrario, you showed that although there were a lower number of monocytes in the glomeruli of those patients who did not have intracapillary thrombi, there were still quite large numbers of monocytes there. Do you have any evidence for a difference in the function of those monocytes? Did you look at peripheral blood monocytes, or do you have any explanation for why there were monocytes there but no thrombi?

FERRARIO: I don't have a real explanation. I think that these cases could represent later stages of the disease. In fact some of these patients were biopsied later, during the phase of resolution of an acute nephritic syndrome.

CAMERON: This raises the questions of what the signal might be for the accumulation of monocytes. And also whether the monocytes were 'good', eating deposits or 'bad', causing damage.

FERRARIO: We studied about 500 idiopathic and systemic GN with the esterase method and found that the finding of a high number of monocytes (over 30 monocytes/glomerulus) was a marker of essential mixed cryoglobulinemia GN. Other GN show a less number of monocytes, even post-infectious or extracapillary GN. Since in idiopathic MPGN we never found monocytes, my opinion is that EMC-GN is not a 'true' mesangiocapillary glomerulonephritis: there are of course alterations of the capillary walls and diffuse double contours, but mesangial expansion is much less important than in idiopathic form. Monocyte infiltration seems to me an absolute marker of EMC-GN.

CAMERON: Using three monoclonal antibodies, including FMC 32, we found that the interposing cells in idiopathic mesangiocapillary GN are invariably monocytes and not mesangial cells.

SCHIFFERLI (Geneve): Dr. Ferrario, it is really striking that you found leukocytoclastic vasculitis in the skin and not in the kidney. This is difficult to understand if you consider a common pathogenesis. Could the monocytes reflect the chronicity of the lesion whereas skin lesions are fresh lesions? About the discrepancy between C3 deposits on one side and C4-C1q deposits on the other, I think that this is extremely interesting, because what is happening in the circulation has nothing or little to do with what is happening in immune deposits. Moreover, we have shown that skin deposits are capable of activating the alternative pathway of complement producing, probably, a strong inflammation by liberating the complement fragments which attract polymorphs' membrane cells.

CAMERON: This is interesting, but Dr. Ferrario and also Dr. Mihatsch confirmed that the vasculitic lesions within the kidney are very strongly infiltrated with monocytes, as you can see both by esterase and EM. And this occurs also in other forms of vasculitis such as in microscopic polyarteritis.

CORDONNIER: If I understand well, dr. Mihatsch you never found any structured deposits into the cytoplasm of monocytes?

MIHATSCH: I have the impression that in the moment of phagocytosis the deposits loose their typical structure. I have never seen in the kidney a phagocyted protein deposit in a monocyte with the typical structure as it is seen outside of the monocyte. So, I believe that during the process of lysosome digestion structure is lost.

GLASSOCK: My question concerns the mechanisms of the intracapillary precipitation in the kidney, since certainly it is occurring at something very close to body temperature. What is it about the glomeruli that makes them so vulnerable to the formation of these precipitates? Is it the fact that the protein concentration in the glomerular capillary is perhaps 20–30% higher than in peripheral capillary plasma? Does anyone wish to speculate about this mechanism?

FERRARIO: I think we face probably with two different pathogenetic mechanisms: the one which operates in the group of patients with prevalent thrombi and acute nephritic syndrome, with eventual disappearance of clinical and histological alterations and in which I think an acute precipitation occurs, possibly due to the physico-chemical properties of the cryoglobulins. The second involves the deposition of cryoglobulins along the capillary walls, as in lupus nephritis, possibly due to a more chronic immune complex deposition. But also in this type of deposition we have seen a disappearance of histological and IF lesions.

MIHATSCH: I think the problem of the hyalin thrombi is fairly difficult, because when you look at it by light microscopy there are many things looking like hyalin thrombi. You may have giant protein inclusions on monocytes, you may have true hyalin thrombi and you may have also giant deposits. True hyalin thrombi are those which occlude a glomerular loop but the endotelial cells are preserved. I could imagine that this is a transitory state, present just for only a very short time. This may be an explanation why these thrombi may vanish so quickly.

PETERS: This may be a heretical question to ask to the morphologists, but could they just tell me how they are confident that some of the material they see on electron microscopy isn't in fact some artefact caused by the fact that these samples are processed in a particular way?

MIHATSCH: We are looking always at artefacts and we tried to produce a constant artefact. We have always a shrinkage, for example.

PETERS: Shrinking is one thing, but the production of thrombus as a consequence of handling the specimen at room temperature is another.

D'AMICO: Can you explain to me why you should find at the same time also 100 monocytes?

MIHATSCH: In fact, when you find the thrombi, at the same time you find a large number of monocytes. The monocytes are present, there is no doubt about it, but in all these cases you will find also a large number of deposits.

TARANTINO: I think that cryoprecipitation is the first step in localization of cryoglobulins in the kidney. This may be due perhaps to filtration of the plasma through the glomerulus and may be dependent by some variations in pH and in the reactivity of IgM and IgG. Also I think that the charge of the two components of cryoprecipitate may be important for cryoprecipitation.

BARBIANO DI BELGIOIOSO: To answer Dr. Peters question I would comment that often we have to wait even seventy-two hours to obtain the precipitation of cryos in the serum: I think that 24 hours is a very little time to get precipitation as an artefact.

GIGLI: Dr. Mihatsch, you showed some very interesting ring structures in your electronmicroscopic findings. Did I understand you right that those are from cryoprecipitate and if they are not, what do you think they are?

MIHATSCH: They were the cross section of the cylinders.

D'AMICO: This is very similar to the picture that Dr. Abraham showed yesterday, but you didn't show any longitudinal section.

MIHATSCH: I think the cryoglobulins investigated by Dr. Abraham were different from the cryoglobulins we have investigated here.

D'AMICO: Dr. Mihatsch, you said that the same kind of precipitation of cryoglobulins may occur at intraluminal level and at subendothelial level. The two phenomena are strictly linked according to the scheme that you proposed. My impression is that the two phenomena can be separated. In the acute nephritic syndrome you find a large number of intraluminal thrombi and of monocytes, but at IF you don't find subendothelial parietal deposits. This is what we think could be a simple phenomenon of physicochemical abrupt precipitation in the lumen. In some other cases you find more subendothelial deposits, and less endoluminal precipitation (together with usually less acute clinical syndrome), and this seems a phenomenon more similar to what we find in immune-complex GN of systemic lupus. These two phenomena can be dissociated in some cases, at least according to the light microscopy and IF findings.

MIHATSCH: Since you have studied many more cases than I did, I must agree with you.

SCHIFFERLI (Geneve): I would like to come back to Dr. Glassock's question. One thing we have to realize is that the association and the precipitation of cryoglobulin is not the same phenomenon as the disassociation of it. I think that Dr. Abraham showed evidence that the build-up, for instance, of gels is probably not the same at all as the disruption of these gels. It must be much more difficult to disrupt than to build up and it is a general finding of everybody working with cryoglobulin that they do not disassociate always very quickly and efficiently; this is one of the problems in purifying them. Cryogels could form in the small capillaries of the skin and could be transported first to the kidney and then start to build up to larger aggregates. That is just one kind of explanation that I do not really believe in because there are now other cases described under the heading of immunotactoid glomerulopathy very recently by an American group: in this glomerulopathy you see the typical deposits of cryoglobulinemia without any circulating cryoglobulins. I was particularly interested in it because we saw such a patient and the pathologist came back to us and said 'just measure the cryoglobulinemia again'. We did it several times, but we never could find any. So I think that directly correlating the two, cryoglobulinemia and serum deposits, is perhaps wrong and there are specific phenomena occurring directly in the glomerulus without any evidence for cryoglobulins in the circulation.

SCHAINUK (Los Angeles): One of my questions is that these proteins seem to behave so much differently in the body than it does in a tissue and it may just be that cryoprecipitation in a tissue is just a means of identifying this protein which really acts by causing immunologic damage to the kidney.

The second thing that fascinates me is that the disease is so common in Italy: do we really not see this in other state or are you doing cryoglobulins test differently and we are missing it? Is there some genetic predisposition in more homogeneus population that you have here? Is there any other evidence of this genetic predisposition? In normal people here in Italy is there an abnormal percentage of serum cryoglobulins?

TARANTINO: I don't know why the EMC is so common in Italy. I think that a genetic factor may be important. There exists only a paper in literature which compares EMC and HLA antigen. But this work was done in Italy and I think that it doesn't explain why in another country EMC occurs with a so different frequence.

DAMMACCO: I just wanted to emphasize that maybe some kind of a genetic involvement may be indirectly suggested by the observations of some familial occurrences of cryoglobulins. I have described a family with four sisters, all affected by EMC. Furthermore I have another family situation in which the father and the daughter are affected by EMC.

D'AMICO: Maybe, to find if there is some genetic predisposition (we are doing some HLA studies, but they are not completed yet) we should ask our colleagues of dr Franklin group in New York, that saw so many American patients (dr Gigli can possibly answer) if many of them were of Italian origin.

DAMMACCO: I've been working in the Dr. Franklin's lab and I remember some of the family names of these patients and they were certainly not of Italian origin.

GIGLI: I agree. I think that the ethnic make up of New York City is very different and certainly our patients population was not primarily Italian. It was a very mixed population.

CORDONNIER: My question to the three pathologists is: what about interstitial tissue? As you know, there may be pleomórphic infiltrates, but we observed in three cases monomorphic infiltrates destroying the kidney and in one of such cases we were able to demonstrate that IgMk was predominantly localised on the surface of these B lymphocytes infiltrating the kidney. Have you seen any monomorphic infiltrate in your observations?

FERRARIO: No, we have not observed such infiltrates: preliminary data with monoclonal antibodies show the presence of OKT8 as well as OKM1 cells.

MIHATSCH: Most of the cases I have studied at EM had only very minor lymphocytic infiltrates and they were contributed usually by small, not activated lymphocytes, with a minority of monocytes.

CAMERON: We have done an extensive study of glomerular T cells in proliferative GN of other types (not of EMC), including idiopathic mesangiocapillary and, contrary to what has been reported from Australia, we found a very good correlation within the glomeruli with a number of T lymphocytes, particularly OKT8, and a number of monocytes.

GIGLI: This is exclusively a comment, but I would like to bring to your attention a new area that I think should be very relevant in nephrology, that is the function of complement receptors in the kidney. Only now they are investigated because of the availability of monoclonal antibodies, but I think that some of the questions that have been brought up of why the presence of one cell type versus another and what are they doing there, perhaps could be, in a speculative way, be answered by considering that there are complement receptors in the kidney which can bind complexes. Those complexes may be able to attack cells which can liberate factors responsible for attracting a given type of cells.

COLASANTI: In Dr. Peters' lab, some year ago, we studied 12 cases of EMC-GN for C3b receptors (not with monoclonal Ab) and we found a massive loss of receptors in those cases which presented also capillary walls lesions: there was a fairly good correlation between the lesions of the capillary walls and the loss of the receptors, but infiltration of monocytes was still present in those cases.

CAMERON: Some of you will remember the work of dr Kazatchkine, who described in Paris the fact that in lupus proliferative GN monocytic infiltration was particularly associated with the loss or down-regulation of the CR1 receptor. Of course, their patients had complement all over the place, so it was difficult to know what was going on. Very interestingly, a couple of years back we observed (and published) the same disappearance of of CR1 receptors associated with monocytic infiltration of the glomeruli in transplants, when there was no complement deposition visible. It may be that the presence of monocytes is associated with the loss of the CR1 receptor. It would be fascinating, when you get your monoclonal work going on your massive histology here, to look at the CR1 receptors in your patients and see if it correlates with the number of monocytes.

GIGLI: I also think they should look at the CR3 receptors.

CAMERON: Yes, if they can get an antibody.

GIGLI: They are available commercially.

MAGGIORE: Dr. Tarantino, I am wondering how much your large series is comparable to what reported by others as to cryoglobulin type and rheumatoid activity (I didn't catch how many of your patients had the rheumatoid activity in their cryoglobulins). Why did you include patients with cancer or lymphoma in EMC group? The second question is: how many and for how long patients received immunosuppressive treatment? I am asking this because with prolonged immunosuppressive therapy you could have shifted the renal death into a non-renal death. Do you think that the high incidence of infections, lymphoma and cancer could have been due to immunosuppressive therapy?

TARANTINO: Only one published series of patients (from New York) is really comparable to ours. The only difference being in the prognostic significance of GN and in the pathogenetic role of HBS Ag. All our patietns were treated with prednisone, many had repeated courses of immunosuppressive treatment, and others repeated courses of plasmapheresis also.

DAMMACCO: I think that the tumors which have been observed in some of these patients are possibly secondary to the immunosuppressive treatment also because of the type of the observed tumors (laringeal cancer, Waldenström's macroglobulinemia, Kaposi's sarcoma, lymphoma and multiple myeloma). These tumors are those more frequently found in immunosuppressed patients. It is well known that the prevalence of the tumors occurring in immunosuppressed patients is quite different from what we usually find in the normal population. This is exactly the experience which has been collected by the Israeli pannel in the U.S., from the Immunodeficiency Cancer Register or the Denver Transplantation and Tumor Register.

TARANTINO: I agree. In fact we described our two cases in detail just to underline the possibility that immunosuppressive therapy may play a role in the transformation of diseases in these patients.

CAMERON: It also does have some bearing on what is driving the proliferation of this particular clone of cells.

PONTICELLI: It is our impression that prolonged immunosuppressive therapy can have an important responsibility in predisposing to malignancy.

As we have no sufficient data to support the hypothesis that immunosuppression in these patients favourably influence the natural outcome of cryoglobulinemia, we are inclined at present to reserve therapy only for acute exacerbation.

D'AMICO: I think there is one aspect of our cohort of patients that should be stressed. In the series from USA patients with type II as well type III essential mixed cryoglobulinemia were described pointing out that some of them had renal disease. On the contrary, we have a cohort of patients that has been selected because of the existence of a renal damage. And it seems interesting enough to me that the great majority, I would say all the cases, that have been biopsied had a type II IgMk cryo, which means that probably the renal disease which we are describing today is not the nephropathy of EMC in general, but it is the glomerular disease which is produced by the precipitation of a monoclonal type II mixed cryoglobulinemia in the kidney.

TARANTINO: The only demonstration of K-chain on IgM is not sufficient to retain that IgM is monoclonal. Also in other diseases, like SLE or thiroiditis, oligoclonal antibodies were found: but when analyzed with isoelectrofocusing those antibodies have been demonstrated to be in fact polyclonal.

D'AMICO: I agree, but let's say that the patients we are speaking about are more similar to the 'old fashioned' type II cryo, 'less polyclonal' or oligoclonal, if you prefer, using the conventional method with which we classify a monoclonal component in cryo.

CAMERON: Could I ask Dr. Belgioioso about hypertension in these patients. I know we are almost totally ignorant of why any patient gets hypertension secondary to glomerular disease or to renal disease, in general. But this is a very striking incidence of hypertension in what is predominantly a rather old population. Have you any thoughts of what lesions, or what amongst the lesions, might be leading to this hypertension and why do you see such severe and important, and sometimes resistant, hypertension?

BARBIANO DI BELGIOIOSO: We have seen hypertension in 85% of our patients who presented also, very frequently, vascular lesions such as vasculitis, arterial hyalinosis and arterial fibrosis but given the so much elevated number of cases with hypertension, we did not find any correlation between vascular lesions and either the severity or the incidence of hypertension. The higher incidence of vascular lesions in this disease, in comparison with the primary GN, seems to me a quite interesting finding.

CAMERON: That would have to be very carefully age-controlled.

BARBIANO DI BELGIOIOSO: Yes, because the mean age was between fifty and sixty, and because in our experience, as in dr Gorevic one's, females were more frequently affected than males.

Part VI. Round table on different therapeutic regimens in the management of E.M.C. patients

20. Long term management of essential mixed cryoglobulinemia

DANIEL J. CORDONNIER, PAUL VIALTEL,
ELISABETH DECHELETTE, FRANÇOIS BAYLE,
JEAN-LOUIS ALIX, JEAN-PHILIPPE VUILLEZ,
FRANÇOIS KUENTZ and ELISABETH BORREL

Essential mixed cryoglobulinemia (EMC) is a rather rare clinical entity; the published series are short: for example Gorevic et al. have reported 40 cases of EMC registered over the period 1960–1078 in one institution [1], Tarantino et al. 44 cases registered in two institutions [2]; Invernizzi et al. 79 cases, of which 35 had been followed for 8 to 17 years [3]; D'Amico et al. 29 cases followed for 1 to 13 years [4].

The clinical presentation and course vary greatly from one patient to another. To make a prognosis is rather difficult since some patients may experience a dramatic and spontaneous resolution of the illness [5–7] whilst others a very severe outcome. Despite the fact that many investigations have been made into this fascinating disease, its physiopathology is still not completely understood and the treatment of acute manifestations still rather empirical. More importantly, the long term management has not formed the subject of specific papers.

Nevertheless, careful study of the literature, contacts with colleagues having experience of this problem and our personal knowledge has lead us to propose a medical approach to the treatment of chronic manifestations of EMC studying successively available methods and indications depending on different clinical presentations and developments. Our proposals will be illustrated by new or till now non published elements of observations made subsequent to our paper of 1982 [8]. An update of this study is given in Fig. 1.

Evaluating the type of the cryoglobulin and the evolution profile of the disease

Before proposing a plan of treatment it is essential for each patient to know when and how he contracted the illness, what were the symptoms presented initially and those which appeared subsequently and at what rate. The

238

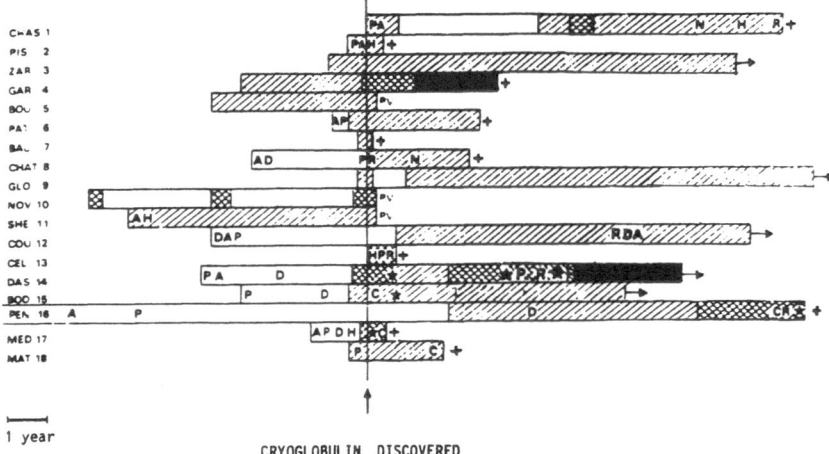

1 year

CRYOGLOBULIN DISCOVERED

Figure 1. Clinical course and evolution of nephropathy. *A,* arthralgia; *C,* cardiac trouble; *D,* Raynaud's syndrome; *H,* hepatic condition; *N,* péripheral neuropathy; *P,* purpura; *R,* respiratory failure; *PV,* patient lost for follow-up. *Asterisk,* series of six plasma exchanges; *plus,* decased; *arrow,* patient still followed up. Blank segments, period between the declaration of the first symptom and the discovery of the nephropathy; hatch marks, proteinuria and/or microscopic hematuria; crosshatch marks, nephrotic syndrome; solid segments, renal failure requiring hemodialysis. 18 patients up dated evolution profile [8].

search for infraclinical manifestations and those which are not clearly visible must be systematic. Raynaud's syndrome, peripheral neurologic involvement and arthralgias may be transient or slight enough to pass unnoticed by the patient. Purely biological hepatic or renal abnormalities should be looked for as a matter of course. One must also establish the long term persistance of the cryoglobulin and identify its type according to the classification of Brouet et al. [9]. Although no one to our knowledge, openly shares the view we have held since 1977 [10], we remain convinced that the prognosis of type III EMC is not the same as that for type II. The associated semeiology is slightly different. The occurence of glomerulonephritis is twice as frequent is sufferers of type II EMC as in those of the type III [10], and it is of the membrano proliferative type almost exclusively for carriers of type II EMC [8]. Such nephritis lead rarely to hemodialysis or to death per se [2] but they are linked with poorer prognosis [1]. Without significant prognosis value but of possible physiopathological interest is the fact that the ultrastructural appearances of the cryoprecipitates examined *in vitro* [12] and in tissues such as kidney, skin, liver or circulating cells [2, 4, 8, 11] are quite different of type II and type III EMC. In addition, the hepatic abnormalities are different in the two cases [13].

Guided by clinical studies and by the presence of a monoclonal component in cryoprecipitate, the physician must on several occasions during the development of the disease look for the cause of the EMC. Such a search might lead to replacement of the world 'secondary' and to an etiological treatment which may have for more chance of being effective. In this way one would carefully search for bacterial or parasitic infection especially in the case of type III EMC [14]; a benign or malignant dysglobulinemia, a Waldenström macroglobulinemia, and a lymphoma in the case of type II EMC.

The systematic search sometimes leads, even before clinical expression to the discovery of a radical transformation of the illness either into a hematopathy, which has been reported in at least 7 cases [2, 3, 9, 15, 16] or into systemic lupus erythematosus [17]. The distinction that we maintain exists between type II and III leads us to suggest that the IgM component of a EMC may be polyclonal and eventually becomes monoclonal some months or even years later, as is assumed to be the case in dysglobulinemias: one of our cases (CEL 13) is a clear demonstration in the respect: in a 56 year-old woman, a cryoglobulinemia IgM K-λ − IgG K-λ was linked to alcoholic cirrhosis of the liver and to a severe hypocomplementemic membrano-proliferative glomerulonephritis. The search for Hbs antigen was negative. The patient left the hospital refusing all treatment. Three months later an oedemato-ascitic decompensation lead to a second examination in the course of which cryoglobulinemia was detected this time of the type IgM K–IgG Kλ.

Together, such clinical and biological tests should be able to establish a development profile for each patient. We may compare two types of profile.

The first, benign, concerns patients for whom the cryoglobulinemia was detected by the appearance of one or several indicative symptoms of the illness; the latter may develop over many years, even decades with occasional arthralgias, purpuric blemishes or sicca syndrome; mild proteinuria or microscopic hematuria may also be present. During all this time and even during the symptomless periods each cryoprecipitate test is positive and the complement system remains activated; this profile accounts for 50–60% of cases [4].

The second, severe, development profile is observed in patients suffering from disturbing, painful, or debilitating symptoms occuring together or in successive outbursts: relapsing orthostatic, widespread, eventually necrotic purpura; severe Raynaud's syndrome, serious peripheral neuropathy [18] may be added to by renal dysfunction, threatening in its immediate (acute nephritic syndrome with severe hypertension) or subsequent functional prognosis (nephrotic syndrome with chronic renal failure) [1–10, 23]. There may be also a hepatic dysfunction (active chronic hepatitis) [1, 9, 13]. Finally certain manifestations may be very serious and may threaten life; angeitis [1–8], cardiopathy [19], pneumopathy [8, 9, 20].

An initiating factor must be searched for in every case. It will often be a case of infection, but occasionally may be the result of other factors such as pregnancy [21].

Various schematic development profiles have been summarised by other authors [1, 4, 7].

Currently available therapeutic methods

Minor remedies

These are usually spontaneously carried out by the patient. It may be useful to ask them for possible initiating factors in order to remedy the problem simply if possible. He or she realises that a particular act immediately precedes the onset of symptoms. Thus, patient COU 12 (Fig. 1) in our study suffers from acroparesthesias, acrocyanosis, a dry cough and dyspnea whenever she leaves the house in Winter or opens the freezer door. She has learned to keep herself covered up and to have her husband open the freezer. Another patient, BOD 15, noticed that drinking alcohol or coffee preceeded almost all outbursts of purpura and acroparesthesia and that abstaining from these drinks was beneficial.

Rest in bed is a easy way of improving certain situations in particular cutaneous disorders provoked by orthostatism.

Systematic search and eradication of sites of infection is a classical approach to the treatment of all auto-immune disorders and glomerulopathies. Even though we may not always be lucky enough to find and remove the cause of EMC we may all the same hope to reduce the risk of a deterioration of the situation.

Treatment of arterial hypertension. It does not differ notably from that for any glomerulopathy sufferer. However, it is interesting to note, as we did in 1979, that arterial hypertension may be suddenly or simply improved by plasma exchanges [22].

Corticosteroids may be administered according to two possible protocols.

1) Conventionally, the dosage varying between 0.5 and 2 mg/kg/day [1–5, 7, 15, 18], the treatment being either continuous or administered every other day.
2) Pulse therapy, in doses comparable to those used in the treatment of transplant rejection (5 to 15 mg/mg/kg/day) has been proposed for the cure

of bouts of nephropathy with certain success by De Vecchi et al. [23]. The mechanism of such a treatment remains unclair; nevertheless comparable results obtained in lupus do not appear to be attributable to a favourable effect on phagocytic function [24]. In addition, susceptibility to infection is greater in patients receiving this form of treatment.

Cytotoxics drugs. Their use is justified by the observation of antibody secreting clones in lymph nodes [15], the spleen [9, 15, 25] blood marrow [26] or kidney [8, 10]. Cyclophosphamide [27] azathioprine and chlorambucil are the drugs *most* frequently used. Far more rarely used are 6-mercaptopurine or melphalan [18]. The dose varies according to whether the product is used as the principal element of the treatment, or as a minor component intended to avoid rebound of antibodies after plasma exchange: in the latter case, cyclophosphamide for instance, is used at low doses: 0.5 mg/kg/day.

As well as the common side-effects of these products we should keep in mind the possibility of induced leukemia [27–29]. It is now certain, particularly when treating non-malignant illnesses that these treatments should be of as short a duration as possible, and, if practicable, discontinuous. The risk of leukemogenesis remains very low if patients are treated continuously for less than 6 months or with less than 1 gram of chlorambucil or 50 g of cyclophosphamide in total [30]. Finally we propose the use of chlorambucil at a daily dose of 0.25 mg/kg for one month and then for ten days over 4 to 6 months.

One is presently considering the use of strong doses of IV injected cyclosphosphamide for acute forms of lupus and related auto-immune disorders. The risk of pulmonary toxicity we feel is too high [31] to allow the use of this type of medicine in long term treatments of EMC at present. These precautions are all the more important when we consider that increasing number of cases reported in the literature concern patients of less than 40 years of age [1–4, 10, 23, 32].

Finally we should keep in mind the possibility of pseudoleukocytosis in EMC sufferers when leucocyte counts are made with certain electronic counters. This may occur at the time of diagnosis but also during development when such false information may hide leukopenia in a patient treated with immunosuppressive drugs [33]. Manual counts must be used in the monitoring of such therapies in EMC patients.

Antimalarials. They have anti-inflammatory and immunodepressive properties *in vitro* and *in vivo* which are now widely accepted and used. Their effect on leucocyte phagocytosis [34] should earn them an important place in the treatment of chronic forms of MEC, alone or added to non-steroïd anti-inflammatory drugs.

Plasma exchanges (PE) and related techniques (plasmapheresis, cryopheresis) proposed for the first time in the treatment of 2 cases of EMC by L'Abbate in 1977 [35], are now widely used for acute phases of the illness; they have also been proposed recently for the continuous treatment of certain forms of type II or III EMC whether it be with [8, 35, 36] or without [37–39] immunosuppressive drugs. One session usually leads to a very distinct reduction of the cryocrit which generally rises again over several days, even weeks. The use of a cytotoxic agent usually manages to delay this rise [40]. All authors agree that there is no correlation between the variations in the cryocrit and the different complement fractions in particular C_3 and C_4 which remain equal to their initial values.

The results vary considerably depending upon the indication for which they were stipulated (neuropathy, nephritis) and for the same type of symptoms from one case to another, certain patients being completely unaffected, others even showing a deterioration. The latter may, moreover, be due to the sudden precipitation of the cryoglobulin in the glomerular loops, probably a result of the cold plasma infusion. This complication should be anticipated and the plasma warmed before perfusion [41]. On the whole, however, the authors recognise the frequency with which the general condition of the patient improves and the minor symptoms (purpura, arthralgias) disappear. The return to normality of blood pressure, even the lasting accessibility to the treatment of hypertension, discussed earlier, is a positive factor in favour of this type of treatment. When the disease recurs, some have observed no perceptible effectiveness of a second series of exchanges. On the contrary, for others, results for a second series of exchanges are just as positive as those for the first [40].

In the absence of published controlled trials, it is only possible to give empirical advice on the type of membrane or replacement solute to be used, or the required frequency of sessions. For example we have recently proposed a randomised protocol for acute phases and the following months, the aim of which being to compare pulse steroïd therapy to P.E., both in association with intermittent chlorambucil therapy [42].

Besides the first clinical results, an important argument in favour of the use of P.E. rests on the observation that the half-life of a heat-or anti-D antibody-fragilised red blood cell was considerably shortened. This should be interpreted as a function of improvement of the reticulo-endothelial system [8, 22, 43].

Both morphologic (presence of cryoprecipitate in circulating phagocytic cells or Kupfer cells [8–13] and functional arguments (alteration of the expression of Fc receptors at the surface of phagocytic cells) [43–45] theoretically plays in favour of this interpretation. In fact there are few results which confirme this improvement.

P.E. do not cause a modification of the complement system, even when used in a prolonged manner [2, 37].

Antiplatelet agents have been proposed by Ponticelli following the observation of an acquired immune storage in EMC [4]. Indeed Cortellaro et al. had previously suggested that platelets might be able to phagocyte immune material in EMC, which would be followed by a release of vaso-actives amines and then platelet aggregation [46].

Conversely, Weinberger et al. failed to find any abnormalities in the platelet ultra-structure in four patient with EMC. They observed a thrombopathy with abnormal platelet aggregation and no tendancy towards thrombosis [32]. Thus, further studies are required in order to understand the hemostasis and coagulation abnormalities of these patients at different stages of the disease before any definite therapeutic proposals may be made.

Splenectomy was proposed in the 1970's and was successfully used in some cases as a complementary treatment after the failure of cytotoxics and corticoïds in patients with splenomegaly or pancytopenia [25].

Indications of the various therapeutic methods

The physician has two main objectives: to be effective and alter the course of the illness in the right direction, and to avoid iatrogenic complications; the two being compatible but requiring great caution, keeping always in mind the possibility of a spontaneous remission of some severe clinical disorders including renal failure [5–7].

In benign forms, the abstainment from therapy is the rule, only the 'minor remedies' described earlier may be applied. Plenty of rest in bed in particular should be prescribed in cases of outbreak of orthostatic purpura. Antimalarials, whether or not they are associated with acethylsalicylic acid or with non-steroidal anti-inflammatory drugs, may be prescribed in order to reduce the severity and distance between arthralgias. We would also have used these drugs in cases of Sjögren's syndrome.
If necessary, a conventional treatment of hypertension should be prescribed.

We followed the progress of such patients over many years, subjecting them to yearly clinical and biological surveillance examinations, whether or not they had a glomerular nephropathy (for example our patients ZAR 13, GLO 9, BOD 15).

In severely evolving forms, numerous therapeutic schemes have been proposed based on a still incomplete physiopathological understanding. To our knowledge none have been verified by controlled trials.

During acute outbreaks, we would use high doses of corticoïds, P.E. and immuno-depressors, according to methods discussed elsewhere in this book. When these outbreaks subside, what should we do? We know that this kind of treatment is able to improve either temporarily or lastingly the clinical symptoms, and to reduce the amount of circulating cryoglobulins, but do not alter the complement activation or the structure of the monoclonal IgM [Obs. CHAS 1 or MAT in 8, 18].

In cases of failure, even partial, replacing one of these methods for another has been proposed. It is true that a failure observed with one does not necessarily imply failure of all the others [18]. We feel however, having no experience of P.E. of very long duration, that cytotoxic and cortisone treatments should only be administered for short periods of time and within limits that avoid iatrogenic complications. Until we are in a position to establish randomised protocols whereby the way is clearer, we feel that we cannot do otherwise.

Individual cases

In certain patients, a symptom of a group of symptoms may be for the most part clinical, in others, the preoccupying problem may be biological, such cases must be discussed individually.

Disabling purpura

Certain cases of highly extended purpura are resistant to a period of rest and recur as soon as the patient resumes active life. Certain cases become more complicated, taking on a blistery or ulcerous and necrotic appearance. In such instances, we should resort to major therapeutic methods in particular P.E. For Invernizzi et al., the only clinical manifestations which could be closely connected to cryocrit were ulcers of the legs [3]. In a Grenoble patient however P.E. had no effect whatsoever and it was chlorambucil administered once a month from January to July 1980 which proved effective. Subsequently, 3 autumnal relapses were again treated successfully with 3 or 4 courses of chlorambucil. The last goes back to 1983 and there has been no relapse since.

Digestive necroses indicated by hemorrhages or an intestinal occlusion may be considered as mucous equivalents of cutaneous symptoms and in the least severe forms should be treated medically before resorting to surgical intervention [48].

Hepatopathies are not usually clinically manifest when this is the case, therapeutic attempts are made taking into account the results of the hepatic biopsy. If one has been able to detect by electron microscopy the cryoprecipitate in the Kupfer cells, and a periportal infiltrate, there may be a case for the use of P.E. in order to modify the macrophagic system [8].

Refractory arterial hypertension justifies all methods currently at our disposal in this area. In the most resistent cases may be a useful recourse since such hypertensions quite often accompany a nephropathy.

The long-term treatment of these *complex nephrotpathies* has already been the subject of numerous articles. We must considere separately acute (proliferative glomerulonephritis) or moderate (minor lesions) glomerular attacks, practically isolated (GLO 9 or COU 12), which do not noticeably modify development of the illness and those which are severe (membrano-proliferative GN) and associated with important vascular and interstitial lesions. In the first case, unless a nephrotic syndrome sets in no treatment should be attempted. On the contrary in the second, especially in cases of nephrotic syndrome and/or development towards renal insufficiency, one is tempted to use major therapeutic methods. Some report complete and long-lasting success after using corticoids and immunosuppressors [21] others insist upon the importance of P.E.

According to the results obtained with two patients put onto a program of peritoneal or hemodialysis, it seems that systemic manifestations disappear, but that biological symptoms are not altered, even after 2 years of hemodialysis (hypocomplementemia, cryoglobulinemia).

A very unusual problem was posed by the discovery of lymphomatous granulomas in the kidneys which occured in three cases (Obs. I_1 CRE. [10]) (Obs. II_2 PIS. and MAT. 18). The only therapy would suggest was the administration of immunosuppressors, without success.

Cardiopathies constitute a rare but serious problem. It is clear that patients suffering from EMC may also suffer from myocardial infarction or from rhumatismal cardiopathy.

We would like to draw attention to complex myocardiopathies whose origin is still not clear and which may be directly or indirectly associated with EMC [19]. One of our patients (MED. 17) died of this type of cardiopathy despite the use of P.E. and cyclophosphamide. The autopsy revealed numerous lymphocyte infiltrates of the myocardium but immunofluorescence did not reveal immune deposits.

Pneumopathies are not just iatrogenic and infectious complications of the treatments carried out. It has been shown in a case of alveolo-capillary block syndrome, an intravascular accumulation of the cryoprecipitate [20]. Such cases should also be improved by P.E.

Neuropathies affect 7 to 15% of patients suffering from EMC. They are rarely acute affecting one nerve only. They are most often subacute, motor-sensory and quite diffuse involving three different mechanisms which theoretically justify P.E. [38]. In the first case, a demyelinisation is observed with a perivascular mononuclear infiltrate. Antimyelin antibodies might be removed by P.E. which appear to be effective.
The second mechanism might involve obstruction of the vasa nervorum by the cryoprecipitate and the third a perivascularitis of the same vasa nervorum [1]. The number of published cases is still low. Our personal and as yet unpublished opinion is that P.E. which are very effective as a first treatment, see their effects diminish and finally disappear with subsequent returns of the pathological process.

Pregnancy may reveal EMC. In the only published case to date [21] the patient had a history suggesting cryoglobulinemia going back 7 years. A hematuria was noted at 32 weeks of pregnancy and a proteinuria at 39 weeks. The child was of normal weight and was born at the expected time. An attack of acute renal insufficiency with nephrotic syndrome occured in the mother four weeks latter. The clinical symptoms and histological indications were distinctly affected by the use of P.E., cortisone and cyclophosphamide.

Hematological modifications

A leucocytosis should firstly be verified by a cell count by hand to eliminate the possibility of a pseudoleucocytosis (cf. supra). It may be the manifestation of a leukemic which may have been proceeded over many years by manifestations of a EMC [16].
A leucopenia which would be related to immunosuppressive treatment or infection may suggest a lupus since this illness may occur ten years after the development of EMC [17].
Further-more, isolated or forming part of a pancytopenia, it may be the result of a precursor cell suppressive activity by the cryoglobulin. The depletion of the cryoglobulin by P.E. may result in an improvement of the blood count [47].

Conclusions

It is no possible to mention all the incidents which may occur in the course of the long-term follow-up of EMC and to detail what exactly should be their management.

Because of the relative rarity of EMC and in spite of the diversity of clinical and evolutive profiles, it is essential to accept randomised therapeutic protocols. Otherwise we shall remain for some time to come in empiricism and subjective evaluation, which, in 1985, are still the only means of interpreting the effects of our therapeutic methods, expensive as they are.

References

1. Gorevic PD, Kassab HJ and Levo Y: Mixed cryoglobulinemia: Clinical aspects and long term follow up of 40 patients. Am J Med 69:287–308, 1980.
2. Tarantino A, De Vecchi A, Montagnino G, Imbasciati E, Mihatsch MJ, Zollinger HU, Barbiano Di Belgiojoso, Busnach G and Ponticelli C: Renal disease in essential mixed cryoglobulinemia. Long term follow up of 44 patients. Quart J Med NSL 197:1–30, 1981.
3. Invernizzi F, Galli M, Serino G, Monti G, Meroni PL, Granatieri C and Zanussi C: Secondary and essential cryoglobulinemias. Frequency nosological classification and long-term follow up: Acta Haematol (Basel) 70:73–82, 1983.
4. D'Amico G, Ferrario F, Colasanti G and Bucci A: Glomerulonephritis in essential mixed cryoglobulinemia Proc Eur Dial Transplant Assoc Eur Ren Assoc 21:527–548, 1985.
5. Verroust P, Mery JPh, Morel-Maroger L, Clauvel JP and Richet G: Les lésions glomérulaires des gammapathies monoclonales et des cryoglobulinémies idiopathiques IgG-IgM: Act Nephrol Hôpital Necker (Flammarion Ed):167–202, 1971.
6. Marmy A, Beaufils M, Chevet D, Mignon F, Sraer JD and Richet G: Insuffisance renale aiguë des cryoglobulinémies. Etude de 13 cas: Submitted for publication, 1985.
7. Fontana A, Doll B and Joller H: IgG-IgM cryoglobulinemia with a purpura-arthralgia-arthralgia-nephritis syndrome: Schweiz Med Wochenschr 112:7-13, 1982.
8. Cordonnier D, Vialtel P., Renversez JC, Chenais F, Favre M, Tournoud A, Barioz C, Bayle F, Dechelette E, Denis MC, and Coudere P: Renal diseases in 18 patients with mixed type II IgM-IgG cryoglobulinemia: monoclonal lymphoid infiltration (2 cases) and membranoproliferative glomerulonephritis (14 cases): Adv Nephrol 12:177–204, 1983.
9. Brouet JC, Clauvel JP, Danon F, Klein M and Seligman M: Biologic and clinical significance of cryoglobulins: a report of 86 cases Am J Med 57:775–788, 1974.
10. Cordonnier D, Vialtel P, Martin H, Renversez JC, Chenais F, Micouin C and Stoebner P: Actualités nephrologiques de l'Hôpital Necker. Flammarion Med Sc Paris:349–385, 1977.
11. Cordonnier D, Martin H, Groslambert P, Micouin C, Chenais F and Stoebner P: Mixed IgG-IgM cryoglobulinemia with glomerulonephritis. Immuno-chemical fluorecent and ultrastructural study of kidney and in vitro cryoprecipitate. Am J Med 59:867–871, 1975.
12. Stoebner P, Renversez JC, Groulade J, Vialtel P and Cordonnier D: Ultrastructural study of human IgG and IgG-IgM crystalcryoglobulins. Am J Clin Pathol 71:404–410, 1979.
13. Zarski JP, Rougier D, Aubert H, Renversez JC, Cordonnier D, Stoebner P and Rachail M: Association of cryoglobulins and hepatic disease: incidence nature and immuno-chemical characteristics of cryoglobulinemia: Gastroenterol. Clin Biol 8:845–850, 1984.

248

14. Galli M, Monti G, Cereda UG, Del Giudice G, Fiorenza AM and Invernizzi F: Transient symptomatic cryoglobulinemia in gram- negative bacteria infections. Boll Ist Sieroter Milan 63:57–60, 1984.
15. Meltzer M and Franklin RC: Cryoglobulinemia: a study of 29 patients. Am J Med 40:828–836, 1966.
16. Raju SF, Chapman SW, Dreiling B and Tavassoli M: Hairy-cell leukemia with the appareance of mixed cryoglobulinemia and vasculitis: Arch Intern Med 144:1300–1302, 1984.
17. Perek J, Mittelman M, Eisbruch A and Djaldetti M: Systemic lupus erythematosus preceded by long-term cryoglobulinemia Ann Rheum Dis 43:339–340, 1984.
18. Ristow SC, Griner PF, Abraham GN, Shoulson I: Reversal of systemic manifestation of cryoglobulinemia. Arch Int Med 136:467–470, 1976.
19. Ouchi E, Suzaki T, Nunokawa T, Sato I, Sawai T: An autopsy case of mixed monoclonal cryoglobulinemia accompanied by hypertrophic cardiomyopathy. Rinsho Ketsueki 24:1723–1727, 1983.
20. Chejfec G, Lichtenberg, Letratanakul Y, Lange C, Baerwaldt M, Gould VE: Respiratory insufficiency in a patient with mixed cryoglobulinemia: Ultrastruct Pathol 2:295–302, 1981.
21. Goodman GJ, Ryan PF and Sinclair RA: Post partum nephrotic syndrome in mixed essential cryoglobulinemia Aust NZ J Med 13:633–635, 1983.
22. Cordonnier D, Godin M, Vialtel P, Rougier D, Arvieux J, Chenais F and Alibeu C: Effets de plasmaphéréses massives sur l'évolution d'une glomérulonéphrite chronique membrano-proliférative hypocomplémentaire associée à une cryoglobulinémie IgMK-IgGKλ (poster no 51): La riunione congiunte delle sociedad Española de Nefrologia, Société Française de Néphrologie, Societa Italiana di Nefrologia. Torino 26–27, 1979.
23. De Vecchi A, Montagnino G, Pozzi C, Tarantino A, Locatelli F and Ponticelli C: Intra-venous methylprednisolone pulse therapy in essential mixed cryoglobulinemia nephropathy. Clin Nephrol 19:221–227, 1983.
24. Boghossian SH, Isenberg DA, Wright G, Snaith ML and Segal AW: Effect of high dose methylprednisolone therapy on phagocyte function in SLE. Ann Rheum Dis 43:541–550, 1984.
25. Mathison DA, Condemi JJ, Leddy JP, Callerame MC, Panner BJ and Vaughan JH: Purpura arthralgia and IgM-IgG cryoglobulinemia with rhumatoid factor activity, response to cyclo-phosphamide and splenectomy. Ann Intern Med 74:383, 1971.
26. Gharavi AE, Campion G and Hughes GR: Use of anti-idiotypic antibodies to demonstrate rheumatoid factor producing bone marrow cells in essential mixed cryoglobulinemia: Ann Rheum Dis 43:651–652, 1984.
27. Germain MJ, Anderson RW and Keane WF: Renal disease in cryoglobulinemia type II: response to therapy. A case report and review of the literature: Am J Nephrol 2:221–226, 1982.
28. Horsman DE, Card RT and Skinnider LF: Waldenström macroglobulinemia terminating in acute leukemia: a report of three cases. Am J Hematol 15:484–488, 1983.
29. Pedersen-Bjergaard J, Ersbøll J, Migind-SØrensen H, Kieding Holesen S, Philip P, Salling-Larsen M, Shultz H and Nissen NI: Risk of acute nonlymphocytic leukemia and preleu-kemia in patients treated with cyclophosphamide for non-hodgkin's lymphomas. Ann Intern Med 103:195–200, 1985.
30. Kahn MF, Arlet J, Bloch-Michel H, Caroit M, Chaouat Y and Reiner JC: Le risque de leucose aiguë après traitement des rhumatismes inflammatoires chroniques et des connesc-tivites par les cytotoxiques à visée immuno-suppresive. Rev Rhum 46:163–167, 1979.
31. Weiss RB and Muggia FM: Cytotoxic drug induced pulmonary: up date 1980. Am J Med 68:259–266, 1980.
32. Weinberger A, Berliner S, Djaldetti M, Neri A, Creter D and Pinkhas J: Ultrastructural and functional studies of platelets from patients with essential mixed cryoglobulinemia: Isr J Med Sci 20:1087–1089, 1984.

33. Luzar MJ, Camisa C and Neff JC: Essential mixed cryoglobulinemia (Type II) with pseudoleukocytosis. Arthritis Rheum 27:353–355, 1984.
34. Jones CJP and Jayson MIV: Chloroquine: its effects on leucocyte auto and heterophagocytosis. Ann Rheum Dis 43:205–212, 1984.
35. L'Abbate A, Paciuci A, Bartolomeo F, Misefari V, Nobile F, Cerrai T and Maggiore Q: Selective removal of plasma cryoglobulins in cryoglobulinemia. Proc Eur Dial Transplant Assoc 14:486–487, 1977.
36. Schena FP, Manno C, Dimonte D, Carabellese S, Cazzato L, Paglionico N and Russo R: Plasma-exchange in the treatment of cryoglobulinemia. Ric Clin Lab 13:133–140, 1983.
37. Bombardieri S, Ferri C, Paleologo G, Bibolotti E, Camici M, Fosella PV, Pasero G and Moriconi L: Prolonged plasma exchange in the treatment of renal involvement in essential mixed cryoglobulinémia. Int J Artif Organs 6:47–50, 1983.
38. Chad D: The pathogenesis of cryoglobulinemic neuropathy. Neurology 1982 32:725–729, 1982.
39. Delaney VB, Fraley DS, Segal DP and Bruns FJ: Plasmapheresis as sole therapy in a patient with essential mixed cryoglobulinemia. Am J Kidney Dis 4:75–77, 1984.
40. L'Abbate A, Caccamo A, Misefari V, Bartolomeo F, Delfino D and Maggiore Q: Long term effect of cryoapheresis and cytostatic treatment in essential mixed cryoglobulinemia. Proc IXth Int Cong Nephrol Los-Angeles Astract:103a, 1984.
41. Evans TW, Nicholls AJ, Shortland JR, Ward AM and Brown CB: Acute renal failure in essential mixed cryoglobulinemia: precipitation and reversal by plasma exchange. Clin Nephrol 21:287–293, 1984.
42. Cordonnier D, Dechelette E, Lambert P, Alix JL and Bayle F: Proposition for multicentric randomized trial for severe mixed essential cryoglobulinemias (abstract). Ann Intern Med 135:26, 1984.
43. Lockwood CM: Cryoglobulinemia and renal disease. Kidney, Int 16:522, 1979.
44. Hamburger MI, Gorevic PD, Lawley JJ, Franklin EC and Franck MM: Mixed cryoglobulinemia: association with defective reticuloendathelial system Fc receptor function. Trans Amer Assoc Phys Cns 92:104, 1979.
45. Rocateflo D, Coppo R, Martina G, Malavasi F, Basolo B, Rollino C, Amore A and Piccoli G: Defective function with normal expressions of cell-surface Fc receptors in mixed cryoglobulinemia. Proc XXIInd Congress of Eur Dial Trans Assoc Eur. Ren Assoc Brussels Abstract:54, 1985.
46. Cortellaro M, Lambertenghi-Deliliers G, Cofranscesco E, Pogliani E, Pozzoli E, Imbasciati E and Praga C: Human platelet aggregation by mixed cryoglobulins. Acta Haematol 54:36–45, 1975.
47. Ginder PA, Midendorf DF and Abdou NI: Pancytopenia with mixed cryoglobulinemia. Evidence for anti-percursor cell activity of cryoglobulin-effects of plasmapheresis. J Clin Immunol 2:55–58, 1982.
48. Reyes CV and Chejfel G: Gangrene of colon associated with essential mixed cryoglobulinemia: case report. Mil Med 14:151–153, 1984.
49. Boschetti C, Cortellaro M, Invernizzi F, Massoro P, Rigolone A and Polli E: Treatment with sulfinpyrazone of essential mixed cryoglobulinemia. Boll Ist Sieroter Milan 64:55–58, 1985.

21. Effects of cryoapheresis on plasma cryoglobulins and renal function in patients with EMC glomerulonephritis

Q. MAGGIORE, A. L'ABBATE, F. BARTOLOMEO,
C. MARTORANO and S. CUTRUPI

Treatment of essential mixed cryoglobulinemia (EMC) remains a controversial issue. This is not surprising because EMC is a rare condition running a chronic course characterized by exacerbations and spontaneous remissions, and by a multisystemic involvement widely varying in type and severity from patient to patient and even, within the same patient, from time to time. Under such circumstances it appears exceedingly difficult to organize properly controlled clinical trials so as to objectively assess the value of the various forms of therapy that have been proposed so far. As expedient to overcome these difficulties we will rely on the evidence which, we believe, confers some biological plausibility to cryoapheresis – the therapeutic proposal this presentation will deal with. Cryoapheresis consists in the iterative removal of cryoglobulin from the blood [1]. Lacking controlled trials, a treatment aimed at removal of the circulating cryoglobulins would appear biologically plausible on the ground that cryoglobulins play a pathogenic role in the genesis of tissue damage. The evidence supporting the pathogenic role of cryoglobulins is largely circumstantial and has been reviewed in the previous sessions of this meeting. We thought that further information on this topic could be gained by seeking ex iuvantibus evidence on the role of these putative immunopathogens. For this purpose we tried to evaluate the effect of cryoglobulin removal on the clinical manifestations of EMC. In this presentation we will summarize the results of our studies dealing with the effect of cryoglobulin removal on cryoglobulin plasma levels, the efficacy of immunosuppressive drugs in restraining the post-apheretic cryoglobulin rebound [2], the relationship between cryoglobulin depletion and change in renal involvement [3]; finally, we will discuss the mechanisms underlying the possible therapeutic value of manouvres effecting cryoglobulin depletion.

Either the short term and long term studies were carried out on 11 patients with EMC. Main clinical and laboratory findings in patients when first seen in our Unit are shown in Tables I and II. Technics employed for determinations of serological variables have been published elsewere [2].

Effect of cryoapheresis on cryoglobulin plasma levels

One can easily accomplish the selective removal of cryoglobulins from blood taking advantage from their cold sensitivity. The technic has been published elsewere [1]. Cooling of 5–6 liters of plasma brings about a decrease in cryoglobulin levels ranging from 50 to 60% of the pretreatment values. Fig. 1 shows the average changes in cryocrit, cryo IgM and cryo RF after a single cryoapheretic session. Changes in the level of other plasma proteins, such as non cryo IgM, albumin, IgA, C3, are much smaller. Thus this procedure allows the nearly selective removal of cryoglobulins from blood. As shown in Fig. 2 the higher the concentration of cryoglobulin the larger the amount that can be removed with each cryoapheretic treatment. After each treatment, however, cryoglobulin plasma concentrations return to pretreatment values within about one week with a steeper rise in the 4 days immediately following the apheretic treatment (Fig. 1). To get a quantitative index of cryoglobulin rebound, we estimated the refilling rate of cryoglobulins in the intravascular space from the concentration increment observed during the 4 days following the cryoapheretic treatment. For

Table I. Presenting clinical and laboratory findings in 11 patients with EMC glomerulonephritis.

Clinical data	No.	Laboratory data	Mean	Range
Age mean (range)	52 (43–69)	Cryoglobulins (mg/ml)	5.9	3–11
Sex M/F	6/5	Cryocrit (%)	11.3	5–20
Purpura	11	RF titer (rec. $\times 10^3$)	2.0	0.4–6
Arthralgia	11	C3 (mg/dl)	48	25–70
Hepatomegaly	10	C4 (mg/dl)	9	2–22
Splenomegaly	7	C1q (% of normal values)	48	30–72
Hypertension	5	Proteinuria (g/24 h)	3	0.5–10
Nephrotic syndrome	4	Creatinine Cl. (ml/min)	45	10–120

Table II. Pathological features.

Data	No.
Renal biopsy	10
Membrano-proliferative GN	9
Mesangio-proliferative GN	1
Liver biopsy	6
Normal	1
Chronic hepatitis	3
Cirrhosis	2

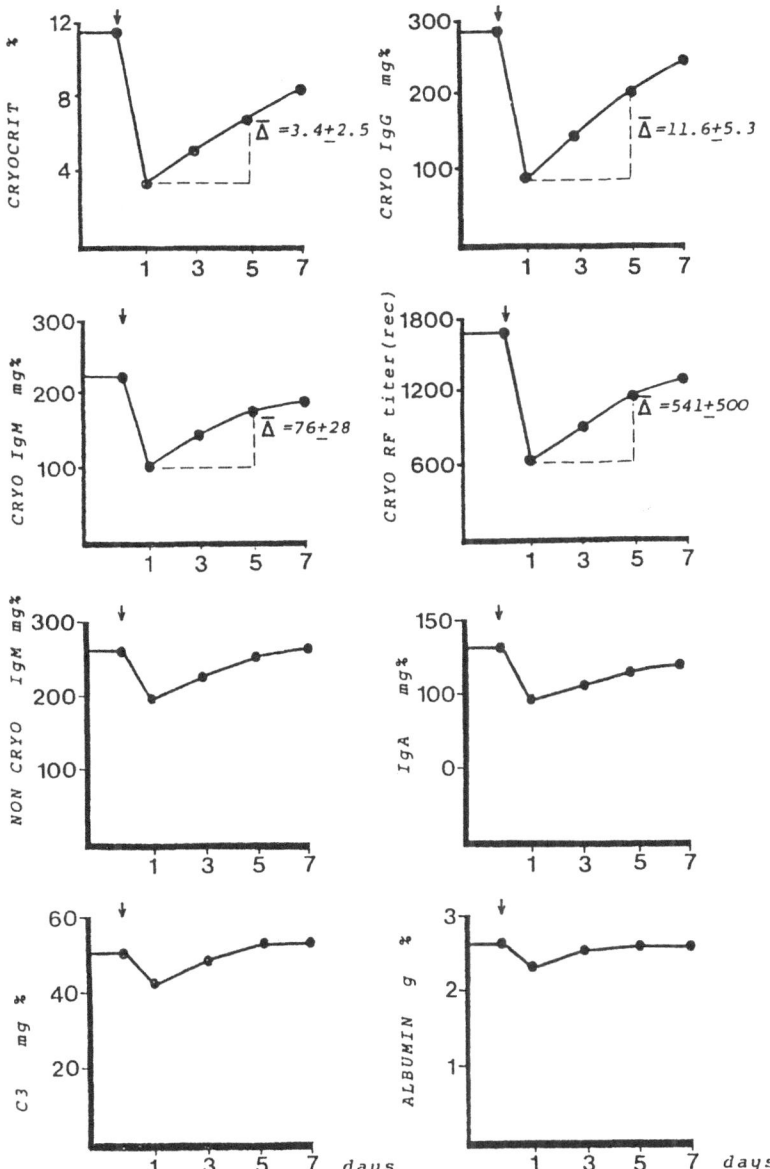

Figure 1. Effects of cryoapheresis on plasma levels of cryoglobulins and some other non-cryo proteins. Each point represents the average of 25 cryoapheresis carried out in 8 patients. Δ represents the average +SD change during 4 days.

example, the increment in cryo IgM plasma concentration averaged $76 \pm SD$ 28 mg % in 4 days or $19 \pm SD$ 10 mg % per 24 hrs. As implied by the wide standard deviations of these averages, post-apheretic plasma increment in

254

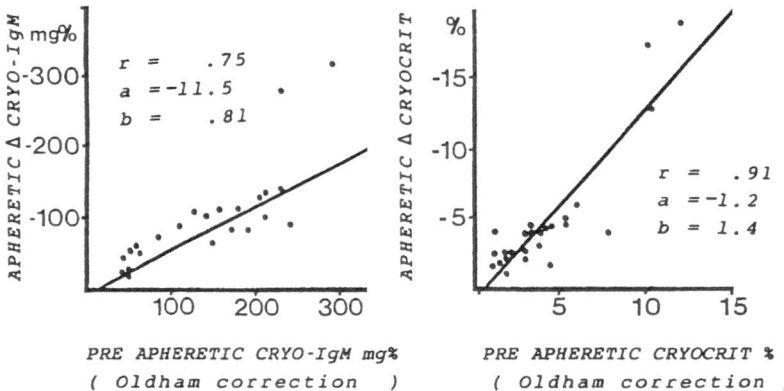

PRE APHERETIC CRYO-IgM mg%
(Oldham correction)

PRE APHERETIC CRYOCRIT %
(Oldham correction)

Figure 2. Relationship between pretreatment cryoglobulin plasma levels and decrease in cryo-globulinemia brought about by cryoapheresis.

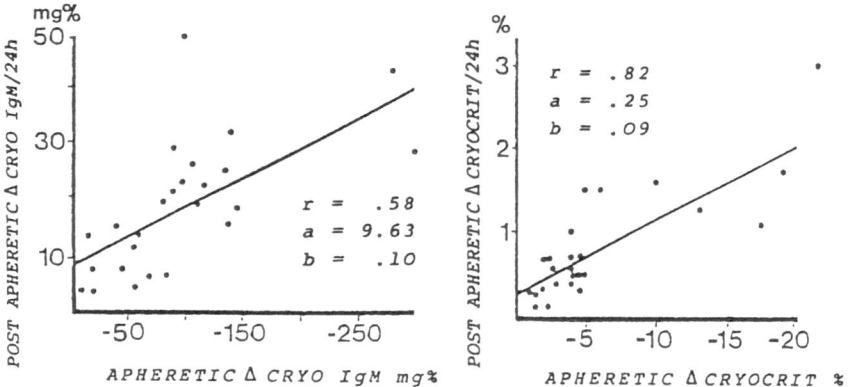

APHERETIC Δ CRYO IgM mg%

APHERETIC Δ CRYOCRIT %

Figure 3. Relationship between cryoglobulin decrease caused by cryoapheresis and post-apher-etic cryoglobulin rebound.

cryoglobulin varied widely from patient to patient. This variability is largely accounted for by the amount of cryoglobulin removed with each cryoapher-esis. As shown by the significant linear relationship illustrated in Fig. 3, the larger the removal of cryoglobulins effected by each cryoapheresis, the faster the plasma refilling rate of these abnormal proteins.

Likewise, the higher the pretreatment cryo IgM plasma levels the faster the cryoglobulin rebound (Fig. 4). In other words, the more efficient is the cryoapheretic procedure, the more rapid the plasma refilling with these abnormal proteins will be. As a corollary of these observations, repetition of cryoapheretic treatment did not appreciably affect the plasma refilling rate of cryoglobulins (Fig. 5). Thus the response to apheretic treatment in EMC is unlike that described in some patients suffering from vasculitis, SLE, or

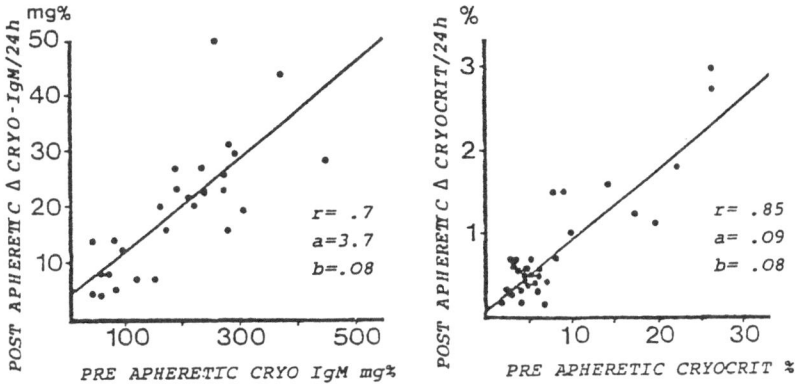

Figure 4. Relationship between pretreatment cryoglobulin plasma level and post-apheretic cryo-globulin rebound.

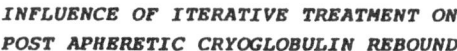

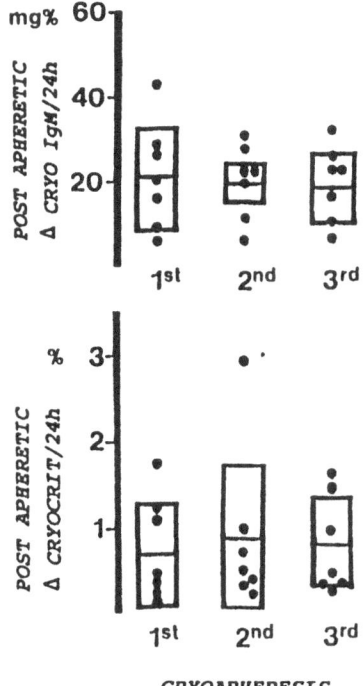

Figure 5. Post-apheretic cryoglobulin rebound after each of three cryoapheresis carried out at weekly intervals in 7 patients. Rectangles represent average + SD.

256

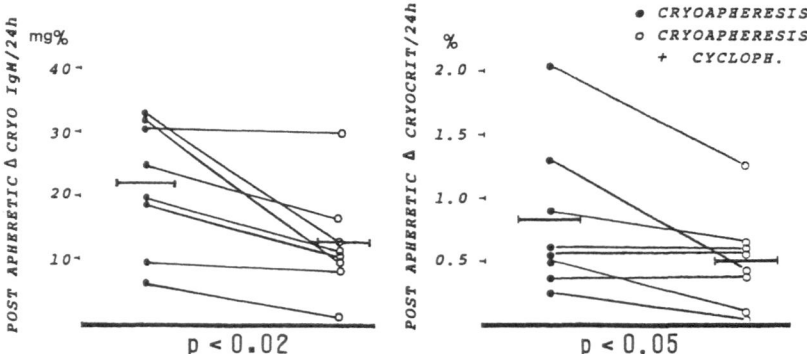

Figure 6. Effect of immunosuppressive treatment on post-apheretic cryoglobulin rebound. Each point denotes the average of all cryoapheresis received by each patient either before (●) and during (○) the immunosuppressive treatment.

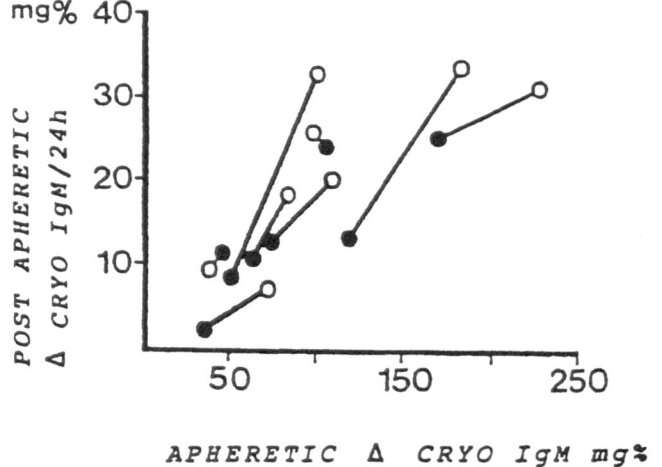

APHERETIC Δ CRYO IgM mg%

Figure 7. Effect of immunosuppressive treatment on the relationship between apheretic cryo-IgM decrease in plasma levels and its post-apheretic rebound. Each point denotes the average of Cryoaphereses received by each patient either before (○) and during (●) the immunosuppressive treatment.

rapidly progressive GN [4, 5]. In these patients apheretic treatments were followed by the progressive decrease in the level of circulating IC, due to improvement of their endogenous clearance. In EMC patients the rebound phenomenon quickly offsets the effect of apheretic treatment on cryoglobulin levels, probably because the abnormal synthesis is much more important in sustaining the high cryoglobulin levels than saturation of clearance process. Under these circumstances, it is hardly to be expected that iterative treatment will lead to a sustained reduction in plasma cryoglobulin levels,

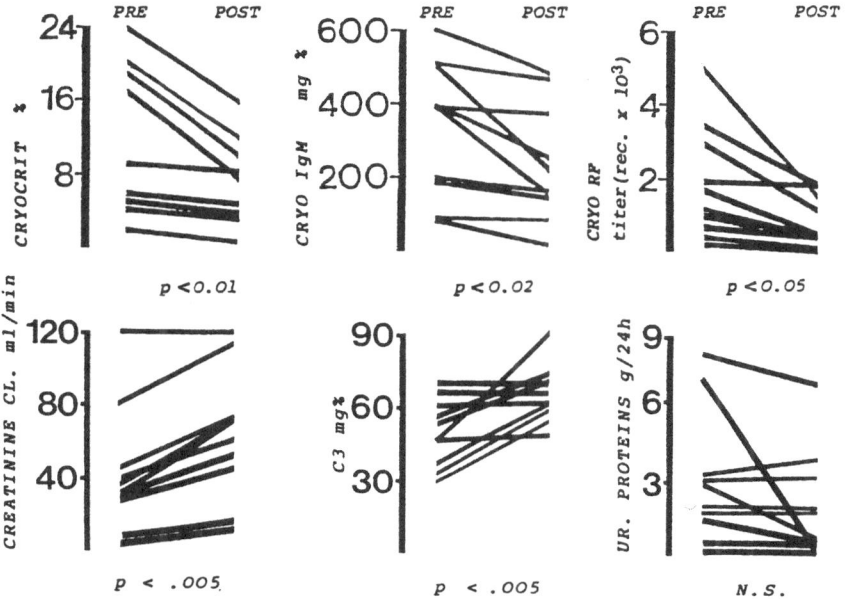

Figure 8. Changes in relevant serological variables and creatinine clearance after combined treatment.

unless carried out on a long term basis and at short intervals [6]. From this consideration it follows that we should complement the apheretic procedures with treatments capable of blunting the synthesis of the abnormal proteins.

Effect of immunosuppressive treatment on cryoglobulin rebound

To restrain the rebound phenomenon and in this way slow the frequency of cryoapheretic treatment we administered cytostatic drugs, adopting various regimens as indicated in Table III. Combined treatment was given to 10 patients for periods ranging from 2 to 4 months. One further patient died

Table III. Immunosuppressive treatments associated with cryoapheresis.

	No. of patients
— Cyclophosphamide (2 mg/kg/day) and Prednisolone (20 mg/day) for 2–4 months	8
— Arabinoside-C (200 mg/day for a weeak) and Cyclophosphamide (350 mg at the 3rd and 4th day)	4
— Methylprednisolone pulses (3 i.v. doses of 1 g)	2

258

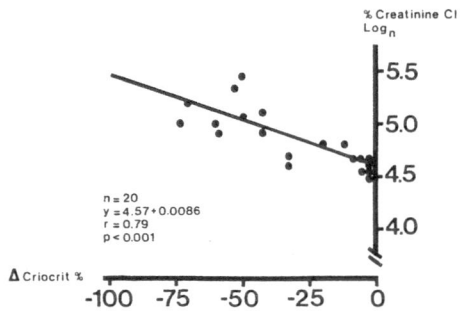

Figure 9. Relationship between % cryocrit changes and $\log_n$ % creatinine changes observed after one or more courses of combined treatment. Data obtained after the repetitive treatment have been included in the analysis as independent values.

for acute liver failure 15 days after the start of the treatment cycle and has not been included in the analysis.

With cytostatic treatment the post-apheretic increase of cryoglobulin was reduced by an average of 59%, though with wide variation from patient to patient (Fig. 6). This effect was evident even when the rebound was evaluated in relationship with the depletion effected with each cryoapheresis (Fig. 7). Thus for each degree of apheretic cryoglobulin depletion, plasma refilling rate of cryoglobulin was slower during the combined treatment than during the off drug period. As a result of this effect, iterative cryoapheresis at weekly intervals plus cytostatic drugs led to a sustained decrease in cryoglobulin levels after 2-4 months in 6 of 10 patients so treated (Fig. 8). Although this study is open to criticism due to its unbalanced cross-over design, we believe nonetheless, it provides very suggestive evidence that reduction in cryoglobulin level resulted mainly from the immunosuppressive treatment. Our studies leave unanswered the question, however, whether or not similar results could be attained without the apheretic treatment. Clearly, this question can be convincingly answered only by controlled trials comparing the combined treatment with immunosuppressive treatment alone.

Effects of combined treatments on renal involvement

At the end of one treatment cycle, lasting 2-4 months, creatinine clearance increased from an average pretreatment value of 45 ± 33 to 62 ± 36 ml/min. The low C4 levels did not change significantly, while C3 levels increased from 52 ± 12 to 65 ± 11 mg%. Proteinuria decreased in only 2 of the 5 patients who had protein excretion exceeding 2 g/24 hrs (Fig. 8). In general whenever cryocrit decreased by more than 25%, creatinine clearance im-

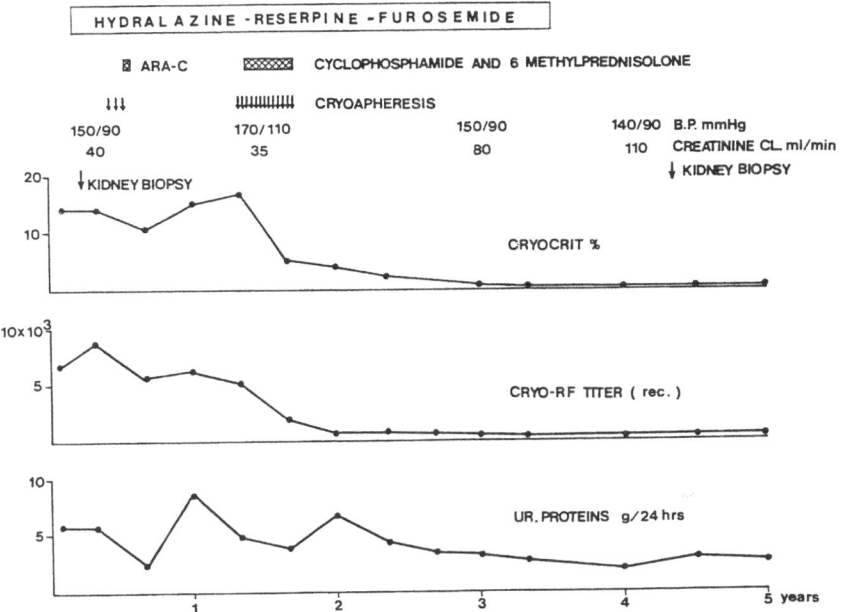

Figure 10. Long term changes in relevant variables in patient CC who received two courses of combined treatment.

proved with a significant relationship between the cryocrit decrease and creatinine clearance increase (Fig. 9). On one patient cryoglobulin levels decreased by 80% after 4 months of combined treatment and were no longer detectable after 1 year. Concurrently, creatinine clearance increased from 40 to 110 ml/min and arterial hypertension reverted to normotension without hypotensive drugs (Fig. 10). Repeat renal biopsy at this stage showed improvement of histological renal damage from membranoproliferative with hialine thrombi (Fig. 11) to mild mesangioproliferative lesions (Fig. 12a). Even more striking was the disappearance of the glomerular immunodeposits after treatment (Fig. 12b). Fig. 13 shows the changes in renal function in each of the 10 patients followed up over periods of time ranging from 2 to 9 years. It appears that the deranged renal function, when present, had a slowly progressive course over the years. Following each treatment cycle, indicated by the arrows, renal function improved in 7 over 10 patients with increase in creatinine clearance ranging from 20 to 135%. In two patients the improvement in creatinine clearance recurred when the treatment cycle was reiterated. Thus in this limited series of patients a wide spectrum of responses was observed ranging from none to complete remission, the improvement in renal function being always associated with a substantial decrease in cryoglobulins levels.

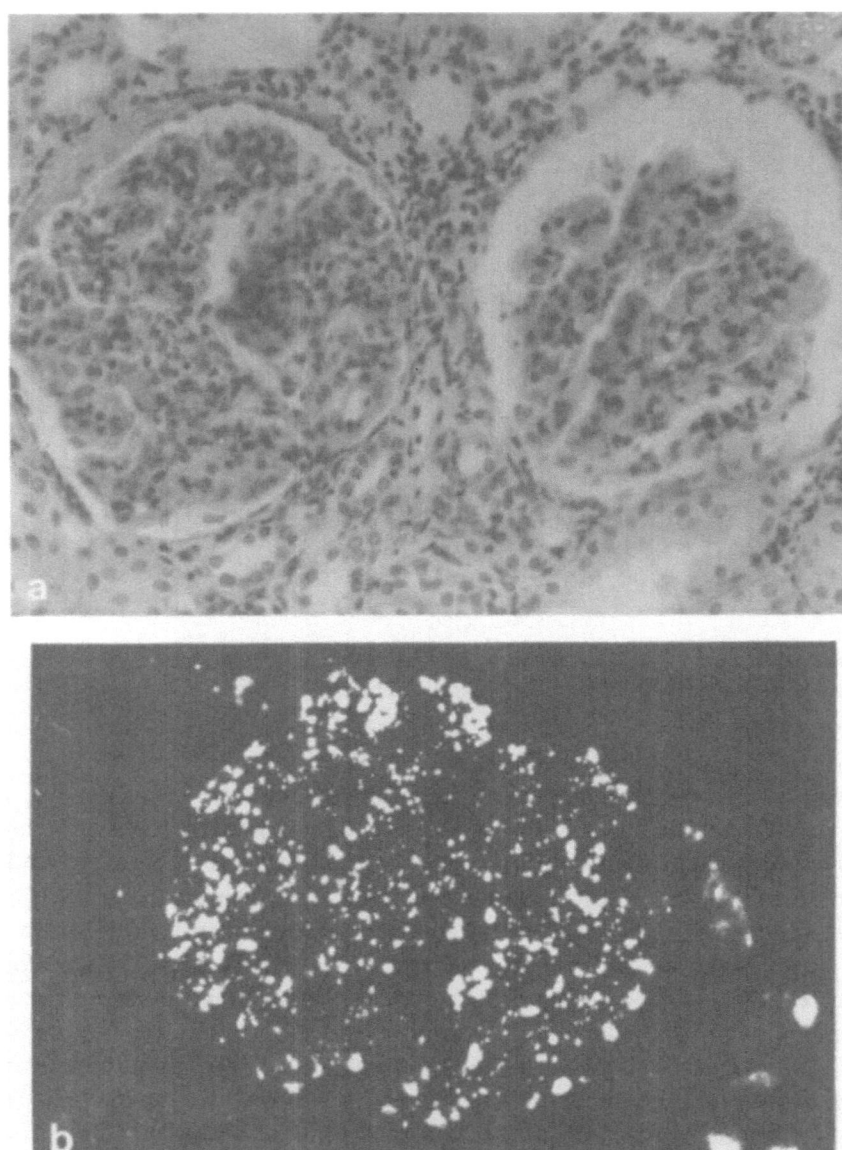

Figure 11. Pre-treatment kidney biopsy of patient C.C. showing (a) conspicuous hypercellularity, hyalin thrombi and subendotelial deposits, (b) glomerular deposits of RF activity demonstrated by means of a fluoresceinated preparation of aggregated IgG.

Mechanism of therapeutic effect of cryoglobulin depletion

The close temporal relationship between decrease in cryoglobulin level and increase in creatinine clearance together with the statically significant corre-

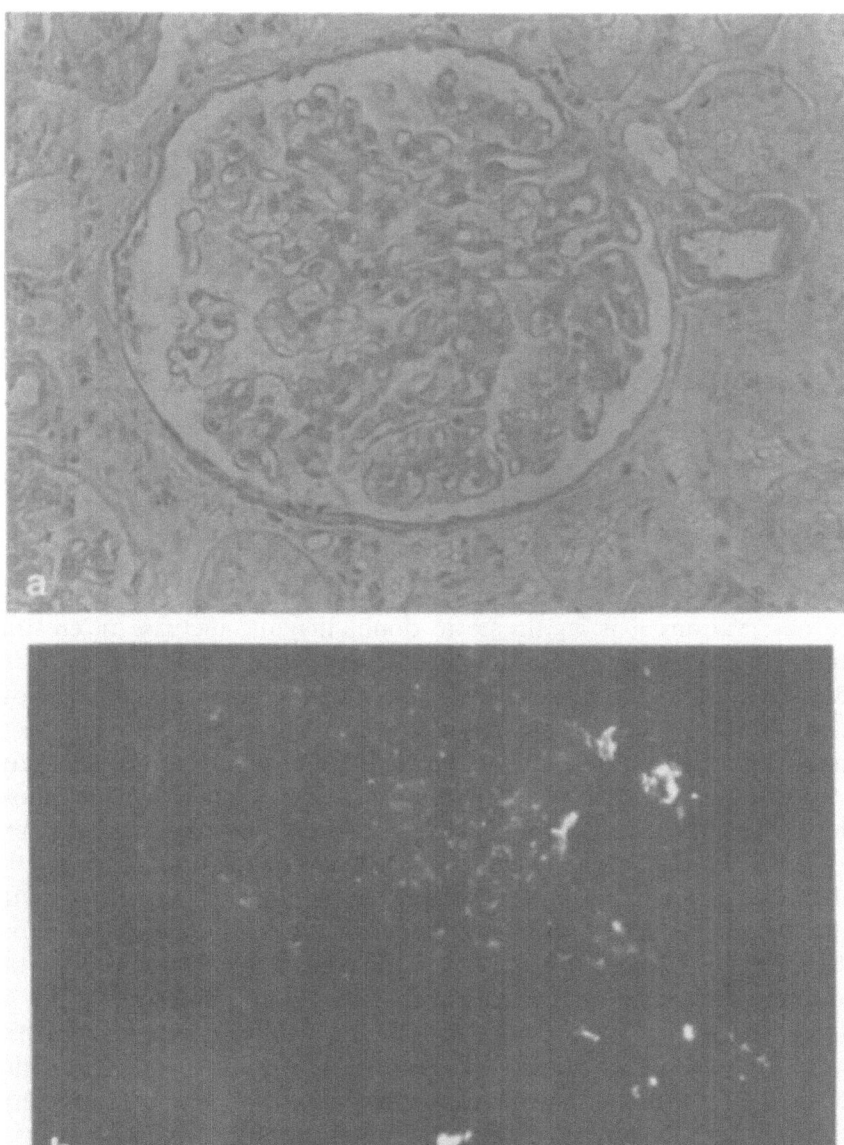

Figure 12. Post-treatment kidney biopsy of patient C.C. showing (a) mild proliferation of mesangial cells, (b) disappearance of glomerular deposits of RF activity. Deposits of IgG, IgA, IgM, C1q, C3 found in the pretreatment biopsy, were no longer detected in this biopsy.

lation between their quantitative changes suggest that the improvement in renal function resulted from cryoglobulin depletion brought about by the combined treatment. This conclusion, however, is at variance with previous observations stressing the lack of correlation between cryoglobulin levels

262

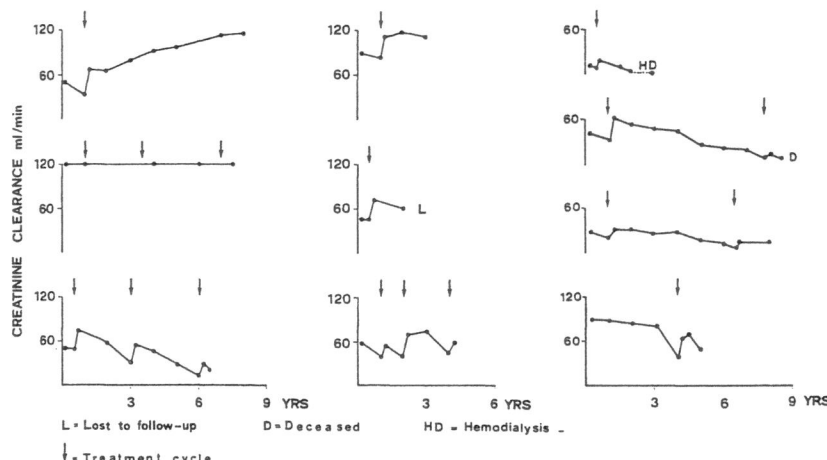

Figure 13. Long term changes in creatinine clearance in patients receiving one or more courses of combined treatment. Each arrow indicates one treatment cycle.

and the presence and severity of renal involvement [7]. On the basis of these observations it is legitimate to doubt that the increase in creatinine clearance was causally related to the decrease in cryoglobulin levels. Our studies do not allow to dispel this doubt. When viewed at the light of other circumstantial evidence, however, a causal relationship between the two phenomenon appears plausible. Cryoglobulins probably comprise a family of structurally and functionally different proteins, some of which endowed with nephropathogenic potential. Among these the best known is the monoclonal RF. Ford et al. have demonstrated that circulating RF can bind to IC deposited in glomeruli, there acting as an immunosorbent to entrap further circulating IC [8]. In a study published a few years ago we showed that IgM endowed with RF activity participate in the formation of glomerular immunodeposits in patients with EMC glomerulonephritis [9]. The ability of RF to act as an amplifier of IC deposition can be demonstrated also *in vitro*, on human kidney specimens. Fig. 14a shows binding of fluoresceinated RF to glomerular immunodeposits in a patient with a membranous GN; Fig. 14b shows the tissue specimen from the same patient treated with unfluoresceinated RF and then with a fluoresceinated aggregated IgG. The bright fluorescence indicates that the aggregated IgG are bound by RF that had reacted with glomerular immunodeposits. Control sections not treated with RF fail to bind the aggregated IgG. This IF pattern reaction can be easily demonstrated in tissue specimens obtained from patients with membranous GN and LE nephritis having IgG glomerular deposits but not in those obtained from patients suffering from non immunological renal disease. Overall these observations suggest that RF might act at least as a secondary pathogenic factor by its linking to IgG complexes already depo-

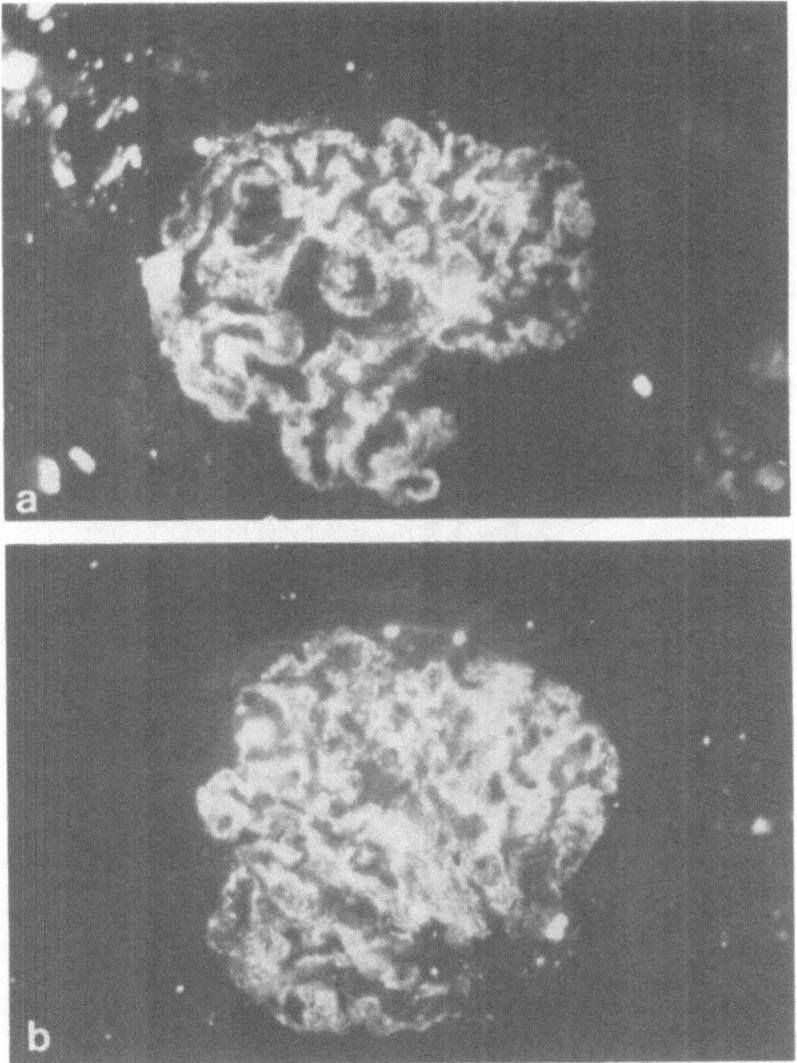

Figure 14. Glomerular staining with fluoresceinated RF (a) and with fluaresceinated aggregated IgG after pretreatment with unfluoresceinated RF (b) in kidney tissue sections of a patients with MGN having glomerular IgG deposits.

sited in glomeruli and promoting further deposition of circulating IC. We can assume, although the evidence is far from being compelling, that the greater the amount of IC deposited in tissue, the more severe the tissue damage will be. Conversely, depletion of circulating RF such as that effected by cryoapheresis should bring about a decrease in the amounts of RF and IC deposited in glomeruli, thereby attenuating the degree of renal damage. Even though the assemblage of all these pieces of circumstantial evidence may appear suggestive, overall it is still too evanescent to allow elusion of controlled clinical trials aimed at assessing the therapeutic value of cryoapheresis.

Acknowledgement

Partially supported by C.N.R. specialized subproject on 'Plasma Treatment'.

References

1. L'Abbate A, Paciucci A, Bartolomeo F, Misefari V, Nobile F, Cerrai T and Maggiore Q: Selective removal of plasma Cryoglobulins in cryoglobulonemia. Proc Eur Dial Transpl Assoc 14:486, 1977.
2. L'Abbate A, Maggiore Q, Caccamo A, Bartolomeo F and Misefari V: Suppression of postapheresis autoantibody rebound in cryoglobulinemia and cold agglutinin hemolytic anemia. J Intern Art Organs 6:5-1, 51, 1983.
3. L'Abbate A, Maggiore Q, Caccamo A, Misefari V, Bartolomeo F, Delfino D, Cutrupi S and Pagnotta G: Long term effects of cryoapheresis and cytostatic treatment in essential mixed cryoglobulonemia. J Intern Art Organs 8:5-2, 19, 1984.
4. Lockwood CM, Worlledge S, Nicholas A, Cotton C and Peters DK: Reversal of impaired splenic function in patients with nephritis or vasculitis (or Both) by plasma exchange. New Engl J Med 300:524, 1979.
5. Wei N, Klippel JH, Huston DP, Hall RP, Lawley TJ, Balow JE, Steinberg AD and Decker JL: Randomised trial of plasma exchange in mild systemic lupus erythematosus. Lancet i:17, 1983.
6. Bombardier S, Maggiore Q, L'Abbate A, Bartolomeo F and Ferri C: Plasma exchange in essential mixed cryoglobulinemia. Plasma Therapy 2:101, 1981.
7. Gorevic PD, Kassab HJ, Levo Y, Kohn R, Meltzer M, Prose P and Franklin EC: Mixed cryoglobulinemia: clinical aspects and long-term follow-up of 40patients. Am J Med 69:287, 1980.
8. Ford PM and Kosatka I: The effect of human IgM rheumatoid factor on renal glomerular immune complex deposition in passive serum sickness in the mouse.. Immunol 46:761, 1983.
9. Maggiore Q, Bartolomeo F, L'Abbate A, Misefari V, Martorano C, Caccamo A, Barbiano G, Tarantino A and Colasanti G: Glomerular localization of circulating antiglobulin activity in essential mixed cryoglobulinemia with glomerulonephritis. Kidney Int 21:387, 1982.

22. Treatment of renal disease in essential mixed cryoglobulinemia

C. PONTICELLI, G. MONTAGNINO, R. CAMPISE,
A. BALDASSARI and A. TARANTINO

The onset of renal disease generally worsens the prognosis of essential mixed cryoglobulinemia (EMC), particularly in patients who present an acute nephritic syndrome and in those with heavy proteinuria [1, 2]. Corticotherapy, immunosuppression, anticoagulation and plasmapheresis have been used with conflicting results in patients with EMC glomerulonephritis, so that at present there is no agreement about the optimal therapeutic approach and some investigators even prefer not to treat this condition [1].

In this paper we report our experience with intravenous high-dose methylprednisolone (MP) pulse therapy for the management of acute nephritic episodes with renal dysfunction and we present a pilot study on the effects of captopril on proteinuria in patients with EMC glomerulonephritis.

MP pulse therapy in EMC nephritic syndrome

By reviewing the literature [3–24], we have found that of 11 patients, with nephritic syndrome and renal function impairment, who received supportive treatment alone, 4 (36%) died or showed progressive renal failure, in 2 (18%) renal insufficiency remained stable, while spontaneous improvement occurred in the other 5 (45%) patients. This outcome was very similar to that reported in 27 patients with EMC and acute renal disease who were treated with oral corticosteroids either given alone or in combination with cytotoxic agents. In fact, 10 (37%) of them died or had progressive impairment of renal function, in 4 (15%) renal failure persisted unchanged and an improvement of renal function occurred in the other 13 (48%) patients. Therefore the efficacy of corticotherapy and immunosuppression in influencing the natural outcome of acute nephritic episodes in EMC is still unconvincing. Some reports, however, pointed out that a combination of corticosteroids and cytotoxic agents can offer some advantages over the use of these agents given alone [24].

266

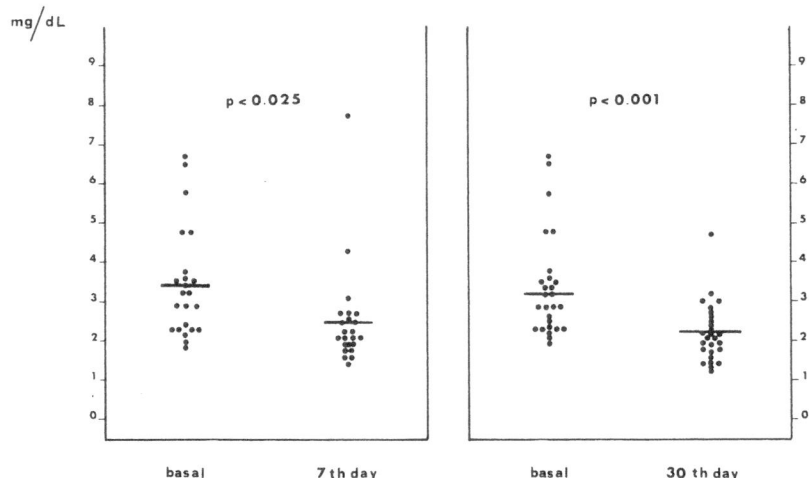

Figure 1. Effect of MP therapy on plasma creatinine.

Since 1977, we administer i.v. high-dose MP pulse therapy in most cases of renal and/or extra-renal exacerbations of EMC [20, 25].

Up to now, we have treated with MP megadoses 27 episodes of acute renal function deterioration which occurred in 16 EMC patients. Nine patients were women and 7 men, their age ranging between 31 and 68 years (mean 50.0 ± 8.5), at the time of their first episode of nephritic syndrome. Cryoprecipitable immunoglobulins were IgG-IgMk in 15 patients and monoclonal IgGk in one. Renal function deterioration was defined as an increase of at least 30% over the basal values of plasma creatinine leading to levels of 2 mg/dl or more. In all the episodes except 3 a proteinuria greater than 1 g per day was present. All the patients had arterial hypertension. Many patients also complained of extra-renal symptoms of different severity at the moment of nephritic syndrome (arthyalgias 10 cases, purpura 9, weakness 6, fever 5, abdominal colic 2). Treatment consisted of 3 consecutive pulses of i.v. MP, 1 g each, given every 24 hours. Subsequently, 0.4 mg/kg/day oral MP was given and gradually decreased to 0.1-0.2 mg/kg/day within 3–6 months. In several cases oral steroid was associated with a cytotoxic agent (azathiprine 1-2 mg/kg/day, cyclophosphamide 1-2 mg/kg/day or chlorambucil 0.1 mg/kg/day).

MP pulse therapy had a dramatic effect on extra-renal symptoms. Fever disappeared within a few hours, arthralgias, abdominal pain and leg ulcers promptly improved while weakness and purpura reversed more slowly. Plasma creatinine decreased within 7 days in 23 of 27 episodes, the cumulative mean levels reducing from 3.3 ± 1.3 to 2.5 ± 1.2 mg/dl ($p < 0.02$). One month after MP pulse therapy, plasma creatinine levels were lower than the basal values in all the cases except 3 in which renal function maintained almost unchanged. The cumulative mean plasma creatinine levels decreased from 3.3 ± 1.3 to 2.2 ± 0.7 mg/dl ($p < 0.001$) (Fig. 1). Proteinuria reduced from the basal values of 4.0 ± 2.8 g/day to 3.5 ± 2.4 after one week and to 3.2 ± 2.2 g/day after one month, but these differences were not significant. The basal cryocrit level was 29.1 ± 30.0 percent before MP pulse therapy, it was 25.3 ± 30.4 after one week and decreased to 18.4 ± 25.9 after one month. Again these differences were not significant.

Although this study was non controlled and although it is well known that some cases of acute renal failure in EMC patients can spontaneously heal, nevertheless the fact that in most cases of nephritic episodes renal function improved within a week from MP pulse therapy seems to us a good proof that this form of treatment is actually of benefit in cases of acute deterioration of renal function.

From a theoretical piont of view, high-dose MP therapy influence the outcome of EMC flare-ups and in particular the evolution of acute nephritic episodes by one or more of the following mechanisms: reduced immune complex formation [26], decrease of vasoactive inflammatory products [27], modification of glomerular plasma flow rate [28], vasodilatation [29], monocytopenia and reduced macrophage accumulation in the glomeruli [30], inhibition of the amplification pathway of complement [31], antioxidation being MP a powerful free radical scavenger [32].

MP pulse therapy can be made even in outpatients, is economic and almost free from side effects. We feel that whenever an acute nephritic episode occurs in a patient with EMC, MP pulse therapy should be given, as early as possible, as the first treatment reserving plasmapheresis to the few non responder patients.

Effects of captopril on proteinuria

There is no convincing evidence that the currently available therapy can interfere with proteinuria in patients with EMC nephritis. Some sporadic decreases of urine protein excretion during corticotherapy or immunosuppression seem more related to spontaneous fluctuations than to an actual therapeutic effect. For this reason we do not treat EMC patients with isolated proteinuria by corticosteroid or cytotoxic agents. On the other hand, we stress the importance of treating arterial hypertension, one of the most common symptoms of EMC which can predispose to cardiovascular disease. After the inhibitor of converting enzyme, captopril, has been made available in Italy, we used this agent in some patients with EMC and arterial hypertension. We were surprised to note that proteinuria decreased or even disappeared after the introduction of captopril. Therefore we decided to analyze the behaviour of proteinuria, plasma creatinine and cryocrit in

PROTEINURIA

g /24 hrs

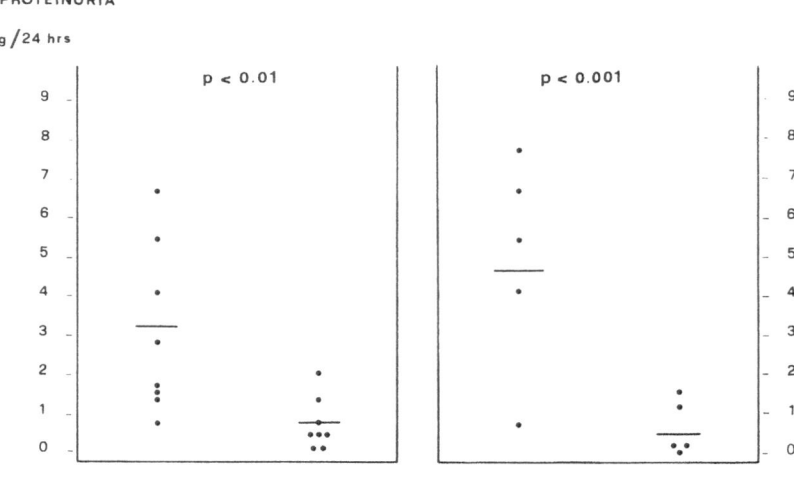

Figure 2. Effect of Captopril therapy on proteinuria.

those patients with EMC nephritis to whom captopril had been prescribed for managing arterial hypertension.

Twelve patients (9 women and 3 men, aged 45–71 mean 57.5 ± 9.6 years) were given captopril, at doses of 75–150 mg daily, generally in combination with other antihypertensive agents. Seven patients were followed for at least 3 months and 5 for at least 12 months after the introduction of captopril. Ten patients obtained a good control of hypertension, while two patients remained severily hypertensive. Plasma creatinine levels remained almost unchanged in most patients, but in one case plasma creatinine raised from 2.6 to 4.1 mg/dl after 12 months. Mean cryocrit levels did not modify during captopril administration.

Proteinuria decreased from 3.0 ± 1.9 g/day to 0.7 ± 0.7 g/day after 3 months ($p < 0.01$), but one patient who was free from proteinuria developed a relapse of proteinuria (6 g daily) 7 months after starting captopril. In the 5 patients followed for 12 months mean proteinuria levels fell from 4.8 ± 2.6 to 0.6 ± 0.7 g/day ($p < 0.01$) (Fig. 2).

The behaviour of proteinuria in these patients was considerably different than that observed in 15 other EMC hypertensive patients with a basal proteinuria greater than 1 g/day who did not receive captopril. In these latter patients the mean values of proteinuria (basal levels 2.5 ± 1.2 g/day) did not reduce either after 3 months (3.5 ± 1.9) or after 12 months (2.4 ± 1.9). The outcome of proteinuria was similar in the 8 patients who showed a hypertension resistant to the therapy and in the 7 patients who achieved a good control of hypertension during the follow-up (Fig. 3).

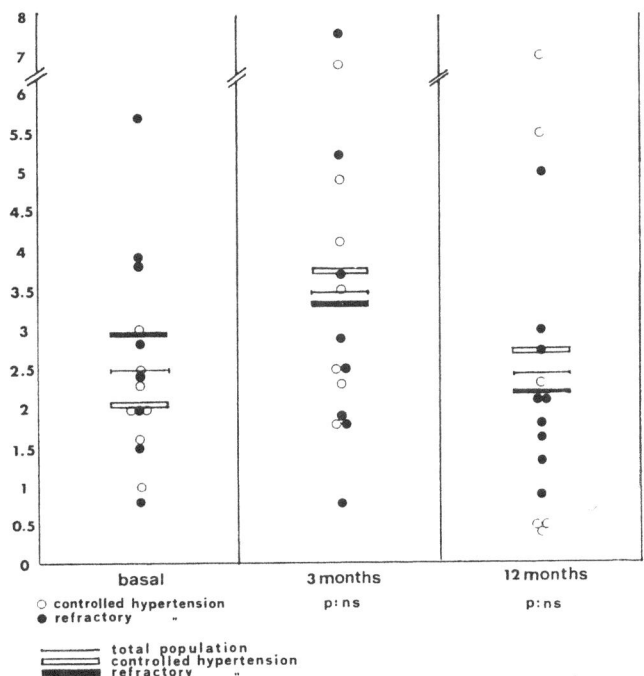

Figure 3. Outcome of proteinuria in EMC hypertensive pts. not given Captopril.

Since 9 of 12 captopril-treated patients did not receive corticotherapy or immunosuppression during the follow-up and since the other 3 patients did not change their previous therapy, it would seem that captopril actually produced an antiproteinuric effect. This effect is unlikely to be related to the control of arterial hypertension. In fact the two patients with bad control of hypertension showed a great decrease of proteinuria after captopril. Moreover, the outcome of proteinuria in hypertensive EMC patients who were treated with other antihypertensive drugs was similar either in the group in which a good control of hypertension was obtained or in the group of patients with resistant hypertension. One might rather speculate that captopril may operate as an immunoregulator or an antiinflammatory agent. As the drug can stimulate T suppressor lymphocytes [33] it could interfere with the production of autoanti-idiotypic antibodies [34] which are probably important for the pathogenesis of EMC. On the other hand, captopril may exert an antiinflammatory effect either by removing hydroxyl radicals or by blocking the kinins, which allows increased production of prostaglandins [35].

We are fully aware that these results are preliminary, uncontrolled and that the observation concerns a small group of patients followed for a short period. Further studies are therefore required and we are starting now with a controlled prospective study in order to verify the possible role of captopril as antiproteinuric agent in EMC.

References

1. Gorevic PD, Kassab HJ, Levo Y, Kohn R, Meltzer M, Prose P and Franklin EC: Mixed cryoglobulinemia. Clinical aspects and long-term follow-up of 40 patients. Am J Med 69:287–308, 1980.
2. Tarantino A and Ponticelli C: Kidney involvement in essential cryoglobulinemia. In: The Kidney and rheumatic disease. Bacon PA and Hadler NM, (Eds), Butterworth Scientific, London pp 128–149, 1982.
3. Meltzer M and Franklin EC: Cryoglobulinemia. A study of twentynine patients. Am J Med 40:828–856, 1966.
4. Golde D and Epstein W: Mixed cryoglobulins and glomerulonephritis. Ann Intern Med 69:1221–1227, 1968.
5. Feizi T and Gitlin N: Immune complex disease of the kidney associated with chronic hepatitis and cryoglobulinemia. Lancet ii:873–878, 1969.
6. Goldberg LS and Barnett EV: Essential cryoglobulinemia. Arch Intern Med 25:145–150, 1970.
7. Kaplan NG and Kaplan KC: Monoclonal gammopathy, glomerulonephritis and the nephrotic syndrome. Arch Intern Med 125:696–699, 1970.
8. Lapes MJ and Davis JS: Arthralgia-purpura-weakness cryoglobulinemia. Arch Intern Med 126:287–289, 1970.
9. Franklin EC: Cryoglobulinemia. Am J Med Sci 262:50–57, 1971.
10. Mathison DA, Condemi JJ, Leddy JP, Callerame ML, Panner BJ and Vaughan JH: Purpura, arthralgia and IgM-IgG cryoglobulinemia with rheumatoid factor activity. Ann Intern Med 74:383–390, 1971.
11. Martinez JS and Kohler PF: Variant 'Goodpasture's syndrome'? The need for immunologic criteria in rapidly progressive glomerulonephritis and hemorrhagic pneumonitis. Ann Intern Med 75:67–76, 1971.
12. Verroust P, Méry JP, Morel-Maroger L, Clauvel JP and Richet G: Les lésions glomérulaires des gammopathies monoclonales et des crioglobulinémies idiopathiques IgG-IgM. In: Actualités Néphrologiques de l'Hôpital Necker. Ed. Hamburger J, Crosnier J, Funck-Brentano JL, Flammarion, Paris pp 167–202, 1971.
13. Skrifvars B, Tallqvist G and Tornroth T: Renal involvement in essential cryoglobulinemia. Acta Med Scand 194:229–234, 1973.
14. Bartlow BG, Oyama JH, Ing TS, Millwer AW, Economou SG, Rennie IDB and Lewis EJ: Glomerular ultrastructural abnormalities in a patient with mixed IgG-IgM essential cryoglobulinemic glomerulonephritis. Nephron 14:309–319, 1975.
15. BengtssonU, Larsson O, Lindstedt G and Svalander C: Monoclonal IgG cryoglobulinaemia with secondary development of glomerulonephritis and nephrotic syndrome. Q J Med 175:491–503, 1975.
16. Scully RE and McNeely BU: Case records of the Massachusets General Hospital. N Engl J Med 292:1285–1290, 1975.
17. Zimmerman SW, Dreher WH, Burkholder PM, Goldfarb S and Weinstein A: Nephropathy and mixed cryoglobulinemia: evidence for an immune complex pathogenesis. Nephron 16:103–115, 1976.

18. Cordonnier D, Vialtel P, Martin H, Renversez JCh, Chenais F, Micouin C and Stoebner P: Cryoglobulines et glomérulonéphrites. Etude particulière des cryoglobulines mixtes à composant monoclonal IgM. In: Actualités Néphrologiques de l'Hôpital Necker. Hamburher J, Crosnier J, Funck-Brentano JL (Eds), Flammarion, Paris, pp 349–385, 1977.

19. Nightingale SD: Familial cryoglobulinemia. J Hopkins Med J 140:267–270, 1977.

20. Ponticelli C, Imbasciati E, Tarantino A and Pietrogrande M: Acute anuric glomerulonephritis in monoclonal cryoglobulinaemia. Brit Med J 1:948–949, 1977.

21. Lockwood CM: Lymphoma, cryoglobulinemia and renal disease. Kidney Int 16:522–530, 1979.

22. Ogihara T, Saruta T, Saito I, Abe S, Ozawa Y, Kato E and Sakaguchi H: Finger print deposits of the kidney in pure monoclonal IgG kappa cryoglobulinaemia. Clin Nephrol 12:186–190, 1979.

23. Tarantino A, De Vecchi A, Montagnino G, Imbasciati E, Mihatsch MJ, Zollinger HU, Barbiano di Belgioioso G, Busnach G and Ponticelli C: Renal disease in essential mixed cryoglobulinaemia. Q J Med 197:1–30, 1981.

24. Germain MJ, Anderson RW and Keane WF: Renal disease in cryoglobulinemia type II: response to therapy. Am J Nephrol 2:221–226, 1982.

25. De Vecchi A, Montagnino G, Pozzi C, Tarantino A, Locatelli F and Ponticelli C: Intravenous methylprednisolone pulse therapy in essential mixed cryoglobulinemia nephropathy. Clin Nephrol 5:221–227, 1983.

26. Ooi YM, Ooi BS and Vallota EH: Circulating immunecomplexes after renal transplantation. Correlation of increased ^{125}I-C1q binding activity with acute rejection characterized by fibrin deposition in the kidney. J Clin Invest 60:611–619, 1977.

27. Fauci AS, Dale DC and Balow JE: Corticosteroid therapy: mechanism of action and clinical consideration. Ann Intern Med 84:304–309, 1976.

28. Bayliss C and Brenner BM: Mechanism of the glucocorticoid induced increase in glomerular filtration rate. Am J Physiol 234:166–170, 1978.

29. Najslett A, McGiff JC and Colina-Chourio J: Interrelations of the renin-kallikrein-kinin system and renal prostaglandins in the conscious rat. Circulation Res 43:799–807, 1978.

30. Holdsworth SR and Bellomo R: Differential effects of steroids on leukocyte-mediated glomerulonephritis in rabbit. Kidney Int 26:162–169, 1984.

31. Weiler JM and Packard BD: Methylprednisolone inhibits the alternative and amplification pathways of complement. Infect Immunol 38:122–126, 1982.

32. Anderson DK and Means ED: Iron-Induced lipid peroxidation in spinal cord: protection with mannitol and methylprednisolone. J Free Rad Biol Med 1:59–64, 1985.

33. Delfraissy JF, Galanaud P, Balavoine JF, Wallon C and Dormont J: Captopril and immune regulation Kidney Int 25:925–929, 1984.

34. Gundgrandsson T, Hansson L, Herlitz H, Lindholm L and Nilsson LA: Immunological changes in patients with precious malignant essential hypertension Lancet i:406–407, 1981.

35. Martin MFR, Surrall KE, McKenna F, Dixon JS, Bird HA and Wright V: Captopril: a new treatment for rheumatoid arthritis? Lancet i: 1325–1327, 1984

23. Long term treatment of mixed cryoglobulinemia (MCG)

DAVID GELTNER

Until recently, MCG patients suffering from severe complications were treated with cytotoxic agents and steroids. With the introduction of plasmapheresis (PP) new hope has been offered to patients with autoimmune diseases in general and MCG patients in particular.

Plasmapheresis is a relatively new technique introduced into medicine in the last few decades in order to eliminate from the blood one or more factors causing severe disease. The subject was reviewed and indications summarized by Shumak and Rock recently [1], (Tables I, II). These data demonstrate the widespread use of that technique in medicine today.

Table I. Disorders in which the efficacy of therapeutic plasma exchange can be monitored by measurement of a pathogenic substance in plasma.

Disorder	Pathogenic substance
Hyperviscosity syndrome	Monoclonal immunoglobulin
Cryoglobulinemia	Cryoglobulin
Cold antibody-type autoimmune hemolytic anemia	Red-cell autoantibody
Factor VIII deficiency unresponsive to factor VIII	Antibody to factor VIII
Post-transfusion purpura	Platelet antibody (anti-Pl^{Al})
Preparation for ABO-incompatible marrow transplantation	Antibody to A or B antigen
Maternal alloimmunization to Rh(D) antibody	Antibody to Rh(D) antigen
Familial hypercholesterolemia	Low-density lipoproteins and cholesterol
Poisoning	Drug
Myasthenia gravis	Autoantibody to acetylcholine receptor
Fabry's disease	Ceramide tribexoside
Refsum's disease	Phytanic acid
Goodpasture's syndrome	Antibody to basement membrane
Pemphigus	Autoantibody to epidermal cell-membrane glycoproteins

Table II. Established indications for therapeutic plasma exchange.

Disorder	Clinical indications
Hyperviscosity syndrome	Relief of acute syndrome
Cold antibody-type autoimmune hemolytic anemia	Life-threatening hemolysis unresponsive to other management
Goodpasture's syndrome	At diagnosis in conjunction with immunosuppression

PP is a modern version of blood-letting used in patients' treatment during many centuries. It was used early in this century by Fleig [2] and Abel [3], and later in 1955 by Waldenstrom and Willert [4] for the treatment of hyperviscosity syndrome in a patient with macroglobulinemia.

Fahey and his group reported a successful treatment of the same disease in 1960 and 1963 [5, 6].

The next step in the waning interest in PP was the introducing of cell separators which enabled performance of the procedure in an elegant and efficient way. In 1973 Grey and Kohler reported a patient [7] with cryoglobulins causing severe neuropathy and urticaria, treated successfully by PP, but found later to suffer from multiple myeloma (MM). In 1979 two different groups, working separately, contributed to our understanding the mechanism of action of PP in immune complex disease [8, 9]. Delayed clearance of IgG-coated red blood cells has been found in patients with SLE, probably because of a defect in the splenic Fc receptor. The receptor was 'blocked' by immune complexes without a possibility to clear them and then deal with the newly-formed immune complexes. This defect was found to be specific for immune complexes and not for albumin. The authors therefore believed that the rationale for use of PP in patients with IC diseases was to enhance the clearance of immune complexes by the spleen, i.e. 'unblocking' the ailing Fc receptor. It was also noticed that relatively small amounts of PP were needed in order to 'unblock' the Fc receptor and that its effect lasted much longer after PP was stopped.

This defect in Fc receptor was also found in MCG patients with nephritis only [10]. So far few studies have been published about the use of PP in patients having all types of cryoglobulins. In 1974 Brouet et al. [11] published a review about 86 patients with cryoglobulinemia of which eight were treated with PP. None of them had MCG. Betourne et al. [12] described two patients: one had MCG and the other MM. They both showed a spectacular improvement after PP. McLeod et al. [13] described three patients of whom only one was suffering from MCG (the other two – MM, and Waldenstrom macroglobulinemia) treated with PP with good results. Bombardieri et al. [14] reported of 3 patients suffering from renal failure due to MCG who were treated with PP and improved (two had PP alone). Berkman and Orlin [15] reported 5 patients suffering from symptomatic cryoglobulinemia. Two had MCG. PP improved their clinical condition, and in one PP was discontinued without return of symptoms. As could be seen in Table III, so far only 7 case reports of MCG patients treated with PP have been published.

We decided to study patients with MCG only, because we believed that the nature of cryoglobulins in that disease is different from type I or III immunoglobulins, since MCG patients' cryoglobulins are being composed purely from immune complexes and thus behave differently than cryoglobulins in MM or Waldenstrom's macroglobulins.

Our results were summarized in part elsewhere [16] and included 5 patients, all suffering from MCG. Later we studied another 3 patients. The first five patients were studied in New York University Medical Center and the work was carried out under the supervision of E.C. Franklin.

Patients

Five patients (3 women, 2 men) ranging in age from 48 to 68 were chosen for treatment. Four had progressive renal disease with azotemia, 2 were hypertensive, 2 had severe and 2 mild neurologic complications, and 3 had severe vasculitic ulcers. All had a long history of clinical symptoms and 3 had prior therapy with prednisone alone (Table III).

Protocol and methods

Three patients received prednisone 1 mg/kg, chlorambucil at a dose necessary to maintain a white blood cell (WBC) count of 3,000–4,000/mm^3, and plasmapheresis 1 to 2 liters twice a week except for patient CL who was treated only once a week. One patient was started on intravenous cyclophos-

Table III. Summary of MCG patients treated with PF.

Author	No. of patients
Berkman et al.	2 (Ref. 15)
McLeod et al.	1 (Ref. 13)
Betourne et al.	1 (Ref. 12)
Bombardieri et al.	3 (Ref. 14)
Present study	8 (Part in ref. 16)

phamide (1,000 mg) every 3 weeks instead of chlorambucil and was then switched to cyclophosphamide (150 mg) by mouth and later to chlorambucil. One patient received only prednisone and plasmapheresis because of pancytopenia due to chronic liver disease. Treatment was continued until significant improvement occurred or the onset of complications necessitated cessation of treatment. Plasmapheresis was done on a Haemonetics Model 30, and blood lines were kept at room temperature. Replacement solutions consisted of 5 % albumin or normal saline.

Cryocrit

Cryocrit was carried out on serum clotted at 37 °C and kept in graduated 10-ml centrifuge tubes stored at 4 °C for 72 hours. After centrifugation for 10 minutes at 3,000 rpm, the results were expressed as the percentage of the volume occupied by the precipitate.

Clinical scoring

Clinical scoring ranged from + 3 (severe systemic manifestations) to 0 (no symptoms).

Case reports

Effects of treatment

NE, a 58-year-old white woman with a 7-year history of purpura, ulcerations and paresthesias of the lower extremities, had MCG IgM (κ), IgG in August 1978. HBsAg and HBsAb were negative; rheumatoid factor was positive, C3, 91 mg/dl and C4, 9 mg/dl (normal is 80–120 and 15–45 respectively). Blood pressure was 110/70 mm Hg, and splenomegaly and stasis changes up to 6 cm below the knees were noted. Foot drop was greater on the right than on the left side and sensation was decreased distally from the midcalf. Pertinent laboratory findings at the onset and throughout the course of the disease are shown in Table I and Fig. 1.

She was started on prednisone 60 mg/day without marked improvement. When she developed multiple ulcerations above both ankles and worsening proteinuria (3.0 gm/24 hours) (start of Fig. 1), she was started on plasmapheresis, 1–2 liters twice a week and prednisone 50 mg/day. Six weeks later chlorambucil was added. Within 3 months the ulcerations were healing and the edema above the ankles had resolved. Paresthesias significantly im-

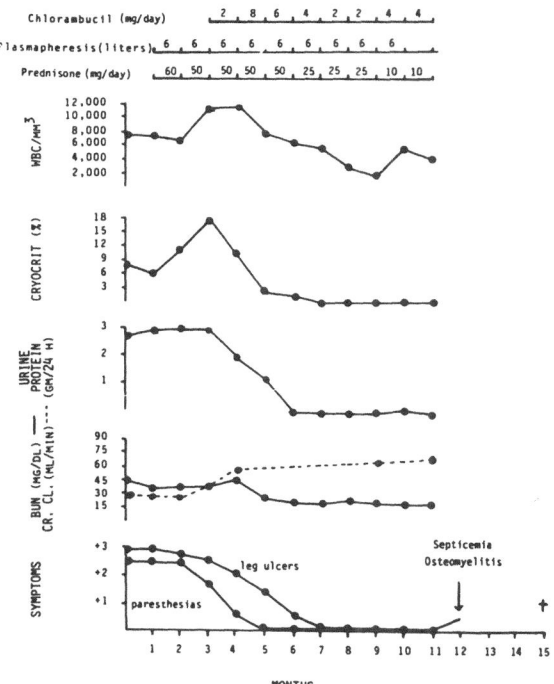

Figure 1. Effect of treatment on patient NE.

proved; C3 was 90 mg/dl and C4, 9 mg/dl. Roentgenograms of the feet revealed osteoporosis but no osteomyelitis. Plasmapheresis was discontinued after 10 months. The patient had decided to discontinue chlorambucil and prednisone. A month later she developed Salmonella septicemia and osteomyelitis of the left lateral malleolus due to reulceration; an above-the-knee amputation was ultimately necessary. Several months later the septicemia reappeared and she died. No autopsy was performed. Salmonella was again grown from the wound.

GA, 50-year-old white women with a 4-year history of paresthesias, purpura, and myalgias of the lower extremities had been treated with multiple anti-inflammatory agents (prednisone 20 mg/day and cyclophosphamide) without relief. When seen at New York University Medical Center, she had MCG IgM (κ), IgG. HBsAg was negative and rheumatoid factor was positive. In June 1978, blood pressure was 100/600 mm Hg. She had palpable purpura to the midthigh bilaterally, chronic stasis changes, multiple ulcerations above both malleoli, a left foot drop, peripheral sensory neuropathy (left > right), and splenomegaly. The cryocrit was between 18 and 20%. She was started on prednisone 50 mg and intravenous cyclophosphamide 1,000 mg every 3 weeks. After 3 months without improvement, she was

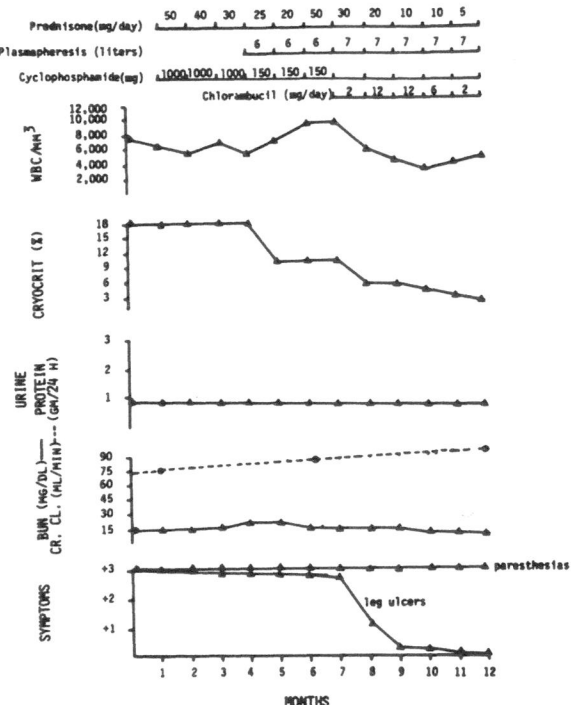

Figure 2. Effect of treatment on patient GA.

switched to oral cyclophosphamide (150 mg/day), and plasmapheresis (about 1–2 liters twice a week) was started. Three months after the introduction of cyclophosphamide, no improvement was noted and chlorambucil was introduced instead of cyclophosphamide. C3 was 70 mg/dl and C4, 5 mg/dl. Pertinent laboratory values throughout the course of treatment are shown in Fig. 2 and Table I.

Three months after initiation of plasmapheresis, cryocrit had fallen to 9%; C3 was 85 mg/dl; C4, 9 mg/dl. Paresthesias persisted without much improvement, but there was progressive healing of vasculitic ulcers. All medications were stopped after 12 months of treatment. Followup showed a recurrence of her ulcerations and worsening paresthesias after she stopped all treatment for 2½ months. Healing of the ulcers was again achieved by another course of therapy (not shown in Fig. 2).

SA, a 68-year-old Mediterranean-born man with a 10-year history of asymptomatic purpura, was found to be anemic in September 1976. One month later he had hematuria, pedal edema, and markedly abnormal renal function. Renal biopsy revealed diffuse proliferative glomerulonephritis. A MCG IgM(κ), IgG was found. HBsAg was negative; HBsAg and rheumatoid factor were positive; C3 was 110 mg/dl; C4, 10 mg/dl. He was started on

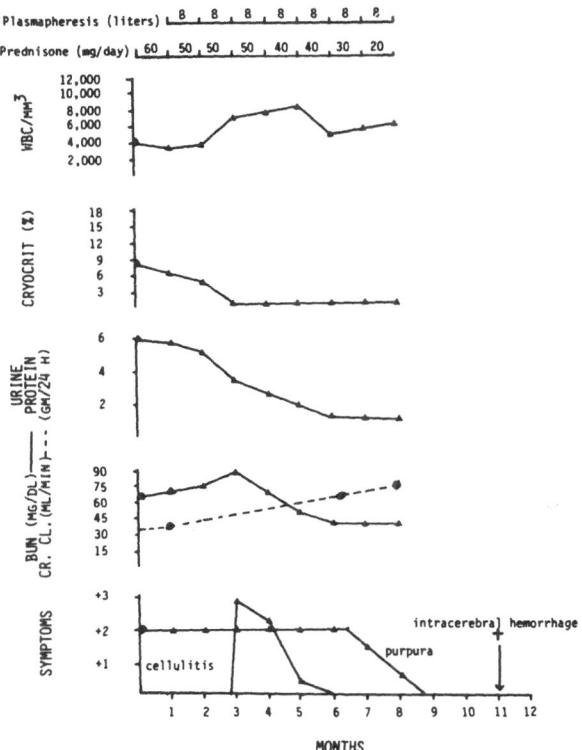

Figure 3. Effect of treatment on patient SA.

prednisone 60 mg/day and plasmapheresis (1,000 ml twice a week); the patient improved and was sent home on the same treatment with gradual reduction of prednisone (Fig. 3). This was accompanied by a fall in cryocrit, improvement in renal function and disappearance of purpura (Fig. 3). After 7 months of therapy, plasmapheresis was discontinued but prednisone was maintained at 20 mg/day. He was lost to followup for 2 months and then was admitted to a local hospital for an intracranial hemorrhage which resulted in death 2 days later.

FO, a 48-year-old black man with a history of alcoholism and intravenous drug abuse has been on methadone for the past 8 years. After 12 years of recurrent purpura starting in 1966, MCG was discovered IgM (κ), IgG, HBsAg was negative, but HBsAg was positive. Rheumatoid factor was positive. Skin biopsy revealed leukocytoclastic angiitis. Liver biopsy showed lymphocytic and plasma cellular infiltrates. A renal biopsy revealed subacute diffuse membranoproliferative glomerulonephritis (Table I). In July 1978 he was started on prednisone 60 mg/day because of decreasing renal functiond. Prednisone was tapered and discontinued by October 1978 as he

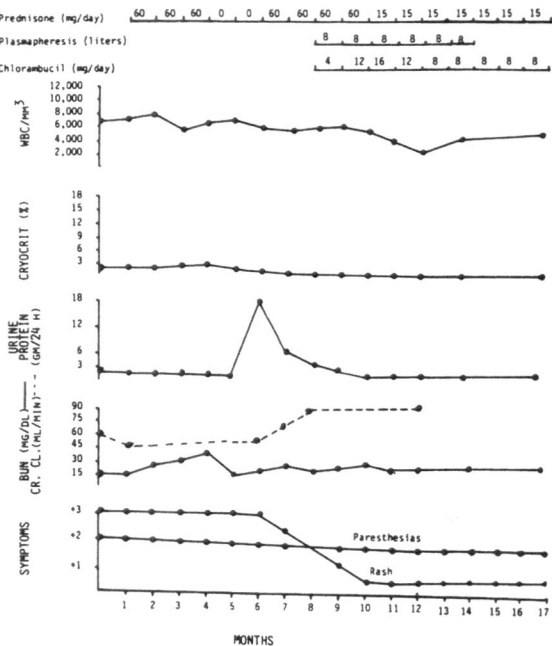

Figure 4. Effect of treatment on patient FO.

showed marked improvement. Three months later nephrotic syndrome developed and the skin showed multiple palpable purpuric lesions and areas of hyperpigmentation. Blood pressure was 170/120 mm Hg and there were signs of congestive heart failure and cardiomegaly. Liver and spleen were palpable. C3 was 90 mg/dl; C4, 9 mg/dl; electrocardiography showed normal sinus rhythm with non-specific T-wave changes. Chest roentgenograms showed cardiomegaly and congestive heart failure. Due to his deteriorating renal function, he was started on diuretics, digitalis, antihypertensive medication, and prednisone (60 mg/day). Two months later, because of lack of response, chlorambucil (4 mg) and plasmapheresis (1 liter twice a week) were started. Over the next 2 months, chlorambucil was raised to 16 mg/day and prednisone tapered to 15 mg/day. There was no evidence of congestive heart failure or nephrotic syndrome, but chronic signs of purpura persisted. Four months after initiation of chlorambucil and plasmapheresis, C3 was 121 mg/dl; C4, 32 mg/dl and renal function had improved (Fig. 4). Chlorambucil was lowered to 12 and then 8 mg/day, as the WBC count fell to 3,000 to 4,000/mm^3. Three months later he had no fever, ulcerations, adenopathy or infections; C3 was 130 mg/dl; C4, 44 mg/dl. Plasmapheresis was stopped after 6 months and prednisone and chlorambucil were stopped after an additional 3 months. The patient is still free of symptoms 6 months later and has had no complications. A summary is shown in Fig. 4.

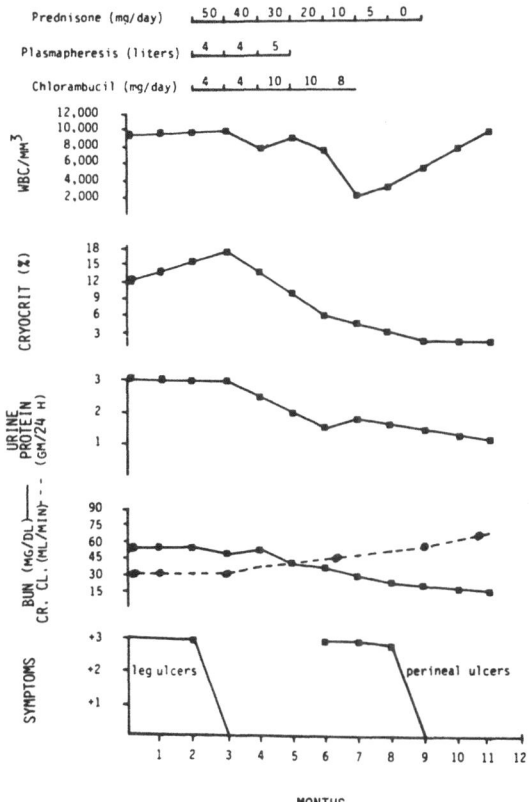

Figure 5. Effect of treatment on patient CL.

CL, a 52-year-old Hispanic woman with a 3½ year history of cutaneous ulcerations developed purpura and proteinuria in 1978 and was found to have MCG IgM (κ), IgG, HBsAg and HBsAg were positive. Rheumatoid factor was positive. A renal biopsy revealed membranoproliferative glomerulonephritis (Table I) and there was laboratory evidence of renal dysfunction (Fig. 5). Three months later physical examination revealed hypertension (150/100 mm Hg), hepatomegaly, chronic stasis changes, and two vasculitic ulcers. Two months later prednisone 50 mg/day was started; plasmapheresis 2 liters/week and chlorambucil 4 mg/day. Foot ulcers and renal function improved rapidly and the patient did well until 4 months later when she developed mouth and perineal ulcers. Because the WBC count was 1,800 per mm³, chlorambucil was discontinued. Within 6 weeks the white blood cell count rose to 5,000 per mm³ and the ulcers healed. Blood pressure was within normal limits. Prednisone was stopped 2 months later when renal function showed marked improvement. No futher vasculitic ulcers

Table IV. Summary data of live patients with MCG.

Patient (sex)	Age	Duration of MCG (years)	Organ involvement	Kidney biopsy	Prior treatment	Duration of treatment (mths)	Followup period* (months)	Reason for discontinuation of treatment	Complications
NE (F)	58	7	Kidney, skin, nerves, blood vessels	Subacute proliferative glomerulo-nephritis	Prednisone	10	14	Plasma-pheresis, improvement; others, patient decision	Osteomyelitis, septicemia; death
GA (F)	50	4	Nerves, skin, blood vessels	–	Prednisone	11 Plasmapheresis, 8	24	Improve-ment	Leukopenia
SA (M)†	68	10	Liver, kidney	Diffuse proli-ferative glo-merulonephritis	–	7	11	Plasma-pheresis, improvement	–
FO (M)†	48	13	Kidney, skin	Diffuse mem-branoproli-ferative glo-merulonephritis	Prednisone	Plasmapheresis, 6 Prednisone, 11 Chlorambucil, 9	20	Improvement	–
CL (F)†	52	3.5	Kidney, skin	Membrano-prolif-erative glomeru-lonephritis	–	Prednisone, 6 Plasmapheresis, 3 Chlorambucil, 5	15	Improvement	Leukopenia

* Includes treatment time   † HBsAb positive

occurred and the patient remains asymptomatic with only minimal protein-uria.

All patients showed remarkable clinical and laboratory improvement. Cryocrits decreased from a mean of 12% to 2%. As can be seen in Table IV, the renal disease improved in all 4 patients with a fall in BUN from 42 mg/dl to 24 mg/dl and 24-hour urine protein from 6 gm to 1 gm. Creatinine clearance rose from mean of 43 ml/min to 67 ml/min. The deep vasculitic ulcers on the lower extremities of 2 patients healed completely. No new purpuric lesions were seen and in most the old ones faded. On the other hand the complement levels showed no significant change (except in patient NE) and no improvement was seen in the motor defect consequent to the neuropathy.

The mean period of treatment until improvement was 3 months and the mean followup was 16.6 months. Patients FO and CL are essentially symptom-free. Two patients died; SA died 2 months after discontinuation of plasmapheresis and no information is available on his other medications. The other patient (NE) stopped medication on her own. A few weeks later osteomyelitis of the left ankle developed and an above-the-knee amputation was necessary. Death was due to a cerebrovascular hemorrhage. Since the osteomyelitis developed under a healing vasculitic ulcer, it is not clear whether it was a complication of the treatment or whether the discontinuation of all medications stopped the healing process and caused the ulcer to spread to the bone. Patient GA continues to require analgesic therapy for severe pain in the lower extremities. Osteomyelitis developed under a cutaneous ulcer 6 months after cessation of treatment which improved under antibiotic treatment. Recently triple therapy was resumed because of worsening of the ulcers and again resulted in healing of the ulcers. In addition to these 2 patients with osteomyelitis, patient CL developed significant leukopenia ($1800/mm^3$) and at the same time a perineal ulcer which healed after cessation of chlorambucil therapy. The other 3 patients were studied in Kaplan Hospital, Rehovot, Israel. They suffered from severe dermal vasculitis or mild nephritis. We strictly kept 2 months of prior treatment with no

Table V. Mean values of laboratory data in 5 patients before and after combined treatment.

Test	Mean value	
	Before treatment	After treatment
Cryocrit (%)	12	2
24-hour urine protein (gm)	6	1
BUN (mg/dl)	42	24
Creatinine clearance (ml/min)	43	67

Table VI. Six months follow-up of 3 MCG patients treated with plasmapheresis protocol*.

Patient and sex	Age	Disease duration	Organ involvement	Cryocrit (%)			Bun (mg %)			Urine protein (gr/24 h)			Leg ulcers			Prednisone		Chlorambucil	
				0	2M	6M	0	2M	6M	0	2M	6M	0	2M	6M	2M	6M	2M	6M
KF (F)	56	15	Skin Kidney	15	3	4	35	25	30	3	1	2	+4	+3	+1	40	20	4	3
ZL (F)	50	12	Skin	20	2	5	40	25	30	1	0.5	1	+4	+3	0	35	20	4	2
HB (F)	60	8	Kidney	12	2	5	60	20	25	3	1	1	+4	+3	0	35	15	4	2

* For protocol details see text
M – Months

more than 40 mg of prednisone and 4 mg of chlorambucil. No more than 1.5 liters of PP was done weekly for 6 weeks and patients were followed up for 6 months and received replacement therapy by normal saline.

As shown in Table VI all patients demonstrated marked improvement in all parameters summarized. There was no deterioration in their clinical situation at the end of 6 months period, in spite of the discontinuation of PP after 6 weeks. In contrast, prednisone and chlorambucil were tapered gradually. The fluids we used for replacement were normal saline and no complications occurred. The results of our limited study support the evidence published before, that the main role PP plays in IC disease is 'unblocking' the macrophages Fc receptor and thus enables to change small volumes for limited periods of time.

It is of importance to emphasize that PP is not an unharmful procedure. Many complications were described and summarized [17]. Among them 23 deaths out of 10,000 procedures performed annually, signs of citrate toxicity such as nausea, vomiting, chills, syncope and various cardiac arrhythmias. More serious complications as pulmonary emboly, epilepsy, metabolic alkalosis, cerebral spasm, hypertensive crisis and disseminated intravascular coagulations have also been described. Not all of the side-effects are well explained but there was a direct correlation between the occurrence of side-effects, the volume of plasmapheresis and the replacement fluid. That subject was reviewed very thoroughly by V. Jones et al. [18]. The fluids generally used for replacement are normal saline, 5% albumin, plasma and fresh frozen plasma (FFP). Most complications are related to the latter two for obvious reasons. The indications for plasma use are only when large volumes of PP are being performed but it could be avoided in most patients. The only indication for FFP is thrombotic thrombocytopenic purpura. In view of these data we think that the protocol suggested by us for the long-term treatment of MCG patients with PP is almost hazardless because of the small volume exchanged and low frequency of performance.

We therefore conclude our two steps study:

1. MCG patients not responding to moderate doses of prednisone and chlorambucil should undergo plasmapheresis treatment.
2. A six-weekly course of 1.5 liters of exchange per week is suggested.
3. Good clinical and laboratory results are expected during 6 months.
4. PP enables us to reduce hazardous treatment such as prednisone and cytostatic treatment.
5. Further evaluation including more patients and control group is indicated.

References

1. Shumak KH and Rock GA: Therapeutic plasma exchange. N Engl J Med 310:762–771, 1984.
2. Fleig C: Autotransfusion of washed corpuscles as a blood washing procedure in toxemia: Hetero-transfusion of washed corpuscles in anemia. Bull Mens Acad Sci Let Montpellier 1:4–9, 1909.
3. Abel JJ, Rowntree LG and Turner BB: Plasma removal with return of corpuscles (plasmapheresis). J Pharmacol Exp Ther 5:625–641, 1914.
4. Waldenstrom JG: Plasmapheresis — blood letting revived and refined. Acta Med Scand 208:1–4, 1980.
5. Schwab PJ and Fahey JL: Treatment of Waldenstrom macroglobulinemia by plasmapheresis. N Engl J Med 263:574–579, 1960.
6. Solomon A and Fahey JL: Plasmapheresis therapy in macroglobulinemia. Ann Int Med 58:789–800, 1963.
7. Grey HM and Kohler PF: Cryoimmunoglobulins. Sem Hematol 10:87–112, 1973.
8. Lockwood CM, Worlledge S, Nicholas A, Cotton C, Peters DK: Reversal of impaired splenic function in patients with nephritis or vasculitis (or both) by plasma exchange. N Engl J Med 300:524–530, 1979.
9. Frank MM, Hamburger MI, Lawley TJ, Kimberly RP and Plots PH: Defective reticuloendothelial system Fc receptor function in systemic lupus erythematosus. N Engl J Med 300:518–523, 1979.
10. Hamburger MI, Gorevic PD, Lawly TJ, Franklin EC and Frank MM: Mixed cryoglobulinemia: Association of glomerulonephritis for defective reticuloendothelial Fc receptor function. Trans Assoc Am Physicians 93:104–112, 1979.
11. Brouet JC, Clauvel JP, Danon F, Klein M and Seligman M: Biological and clinical significance of cryoglobulins. A report of 86 patients. Am J Med 57:775–788, 1974.
12. Betourne CL, Buge A, Decky H, Doria M, Dournon E and Rancurel G: The treatment of peripheral neuropathies in case of IgA myeloma and one of mixed cryoglobulinemia. Nouv Presse Med 9:1369–1371, 1980.
13. McLeod BC and Sassetti RJ: Plasmapheresis with return of cryoglobulin depleted autologous plasma (cryoglobulinpheresis) in cryoglobulinemia. Blood 55:866–870, 1980.
14. Bombardieri S, Maggiore Q, L'Abbate A, Bartolomeo F and Ferri C: Plasma exchange in essential mixed cryoglobulinemia. Plas Ther Transfus Technol 2:101–109, 1981.
15. Berkman EM and Orlin JB: Use of plasmapheresis and partial plasma exchange in the management of patients with cryoglobulinemia. Transfusion 20:171–178, 1980.
16. Geltner D, Kohn RW, Gorevic P and Franklin EC: The effect of combination therapy (steroids, immunosuppressives and plasmapheresis) on 5 mixed cryoglobulinemia patients with renal, neurologic and vascular involvement. Arth Rheum 24:1121–1127, 1981.
17. Editorial: Hazards of apheresis. Lancet II:1025–1026, 1982.
18. Jones JV, Cumming RH, Bacon PA, Evers J, Fraser ID, Bothamley J, Tribe CR, Davis P and Hughes GRV: Evidence for a therapeutic effect of plasmapheresis in patients with SLE. Quat J Med 192:555–576, 1979.

Discussion Part VI

PETERS: From the presentations the impression emerge that there are treatments effective in the control of the acute phases of this disease, when there is an acute precipitation of cryoglobulins in the kidneys, in the skin, and maybe in the nerves as well. But it is much more difficult to evaluate what patients should be treated in the long term. I would like to hear dr Glassock's comment whether Captopril has some specific effect on efferent arteriole constriction in these patients which may alter the hemodynamics of the glomerulus as it is known to occur, for example, in some patients with malignant hypertension and heavy proteinuria. That finding struck me as being particularly interesting and very challenging.

GLASSOCK: If the hypertension is renin-dependent and if angiotensin II is affecting the efferent arteriole, captopril therapy would be expected to increase glomerular plasma flow which would then have an effect on proteinuria by diminishing the diffusive forces for transglomerular passage of proteins. I doubt that this would result in the complete disappearance of proteinuria. Therefore, if you had a number of cases in which the proteinuria disappeared, it is probably due to mechanisms other than just a hemodynamic effect.

PETERS: One could envisage that those hemodynamic effects could influence the processes of glomerular cryoprecipitation or whatever it is that is going on there.

GLASSOCK: Yes, if glomerular plasma flow increased one would anticipate that post-glomerular plasma protein concentration would fall and therefore cryoglobulin concentration would fall. If such concentration is a factor in glomerular precipitation. I would agree with your statement.

PONTICELLI: I think that to clarify this point a controlled trial should be made comparing Captopril, and other converting-enzyme inhibitors, in order to evaluate whether the antiproteinuric effect is related to the hemodynamic effect or to a possible interference of Captopril with the immune system. First of all i'd like to confirm on a large series that Captopril is really antiproteinuric in cryoglobulinemic patients and then we can design another trial.

CORDONNIER: To dr. Ponticelli two questions: did you attempt to compare captopril with enalapril, since sulfidril group may have some effect? and second, what did it happen when you stopped captopril? Did the proteinuria recur?

PONTICELLI: As far as the first question is concerned: no, we didn't yet. We are planning to do it in the future. We stopped Captopril in one patient who had an increase of proteinuria. Another patient, who withdrew by his own the drug, showed an increase of proteinuria up to 6 gr/day.

MAGGIORE: If the antiproteinuric effect of captopril lies in its action on arterioles I would expect a decrease of GFR, as it happens in patients with renal artery stenosis. Was this change in fact associated with decreasing in creatinine clearance?

PONTICELLI: No we didn't observe changes in creatinine clearance in our patients, with the exception of one patient who already had renal failure.

COLASANTI (Milan): Dr. Ponticelli, what about the use of captopril in other proteinuric situations?

PONTICELLI: Generally, we are careful in using captopril in glomerulonephritic patients since the drug can expose to a superimposed membranous nephropathy. However, we didn't observe the antiproteinuric effect in other renal diseases.

WINEARLS (London): If the hemodynamic hypothesis is to be sustained, presumably the effect on proteinuria would be almost immediate, since looking at the experience in treating patients with renal artery stenosis there is a rapid fall in GFR. Did you measure proteinuria also after the first 24 hrs of treatment?

PONTICELLI: In most patients proteinuria disappeared after eight-ten weeks. Only in two patients there was a more rapid decrease of proteinuria (within two or three weeks).

PETERS: Did you ever measure proteinuria within the first 24–48 hrs from starting the drug?

PONTICELLI: In most patients who were outpatients we didn't make this measurement whereas in a few others we measured proteinuria early and didn't observe any significant reduction of proteinuria.

BERTANI (Bergamo): We have studied the effect of captopril on proteinuria in the experimental model of Adriamycin-induced GN, a model in which there are not very important hemodynamic changes in the kidney, and we have not seen any effect on the proteinuria in a consistent number of rats: it seems to me that, in this experimental model at least, there is no anti-proteinuric effect of the drug.

PONTICELLI: Certainly I do not recommend captopril as an anti-proteinuric agent in general.

CINOTTI (Roma): We all are impressed by these results and I think that the effect of the drug on the renin-angiotensin system may be crucial: how many patients responded with a reduction of proteinuria under treatment with captopril? Did you study in some patients the filtration fraction?

PONTICELLI: Up to now we have just treated 12 patients and all of them had some decrease in proteinuria when compared to the basal values. We didn't study the filtration fraction.

PETERS: As regards the management of these patients in the long-term, my opinion is that measuring the cryocrit, the complement and all the others immunological parameters that we have currently available is not a good guide of treatment. We can only take patients on the basis of the occurrence of their disease and treat them, bearing in mind that this is a disorder which has got a long time to evolve into renal failure and that treatments have serious side effects.

PONTICELLI: In the treatment of cryoglobulinemic renal disease one should keep in mind that this disease is punctuated by flare-ups characterized by nephritic syndrome, severe arthralgias, leg ulcers, abdominal cholic and so on. The clinician has to choose between reserving treatment only to acute flare-ups or trying to prevent them by long-term treatment. I think that most of us in the previous years followed this second approach, but although controlled studies are lacking, we do not have the impression that cytotoxic agents or long-term corticosteroid therapy can really prevent flare-ups. At present my personal feeling is that we should aggressively treat only the severe renal or extrarenal flare-ups of the disease.

MAGGIORE: I agree substantially with dr. Ponticelli. In our limited series we considered ten patients: they received for 9 years very little amounts of cytotoxic drugs and the treatment was limited to the periods in which there was evidence of declining renal function. This is not the praxis today, but there are many people who think that we should do the same also in systemic lupus, that is limit the treatment (cryoapheresis, plasmapheresis, immunosuppressive drugs) to the periods in which there is evidence of disease activity.

PETERS: Is there enthusiasm among those of you who have got a sufficiently high number of patients to mount a controlled trial, examining particularly the question whether drugs or manoeuvres would be likely to reduce the collapse of the cells, as ultimately responsible for ominous prognosis? Is it conceivable the use of long-term large stocks of drugs and/or steroids and/or intermittent plasma exchange, given what is currently known on the natural history of the disease?

CORDONNIER: I was very impressed by the data of dr Ponticelli in which he showed no clinical differences between patients on supportive treatment and those treated with immunosuppressive drugs or corticosteroids. I came to Milan with a protocol, but this protocol bears no very new ideas: it compared plasma exchange on one hand and corticosteroids on the other hand, with immunosuppressive drugs in short term therapy. But it does not take into account new laboratory data about which we discussed in these two days. I am now very impressed by your proposition which is certainly safer, simpler and cheaper. Plasma exchange should be used only in particularly severe cases or for research purposes.

Concluding remarks

J. STEWART CAMERON

It was the XVIIIth Century English writer, Samuel Johnson, who remarked that 'nothing so concentrates a man's mind as the immediate prospect of hanging'. I certainly have had my mind concentrated marvellously over the last two days by the prospect of preparing this summing-up, almost 20 pages of detailed notes. I hope in the next few minutes, if you'll be patient with me, to try and go through the headlines of what I have learned – and I certainly have learned a great deal in this excellent and timely meeting.

Let's begin at the beginnin – the tough end for me, because my appreciation of what was said in the first three talks by Dr. Carson, Dr. Bona and Dr. Agnello, was perhaps at a lower level than in some of the later ones. Table I reminds us that the anti-globulins, both rheumatoid factors and the anti-idiotypic antibodies, – and some of the differences between these two seem to blur a little during the meeting, as we'll hear in a minute – are part of normal living. They are not freaks of nature, they are something that we all have, all the time. They are physiological, concerned with immunoregulation, present almost at birth, and any role they may play in clinical disease is a perturbation of normal immunoregulation, rather than a qualitatively new phenomenon.

It therefore follows that to understand precisely what is going on in this area of medicine, we may very well have to understand precisely what is

Table I. Antiglobulins.

— are coded for in the genome

— are physiological, and concerned with immunoregulation

— the potential for their production is present at birth and generally increases with age

— therefore their role in the induction of clinical disease represents a perturbation of normal immunoregulation

---

going on in the immune response, which is a huge task. Conversely, some of the interest that drives us to search in this area is the fact that it is going to teach us a lot about immunology.

Table II summarizes a tremendous amount of information, which was presented during the first morning, and also in the papers of Sissons and Renversez. Here I'm talking about anti-globulins *in general;* and haven't concentrated, yet, specifically on either rheumatoid factors on or cryoprecitable proteins, which are by no means synonomous. Antiglobulins seem to be products of relatively immature B cells, and Dr. Carson reminded us that stimulators such as EB virus, as opposed to pokeweed mitogen (which activates later mature cells) are particularly strong promoters of immature cells. He also pointed out to us that probably some of these cells producing antiglobulins arise from somatic mutations in proliferating B cell lines. In agreement with this, we heard from Dr. Bona that in the mouse there are many substitutions in the regions of the genome flanking the area concerned with the V_H genes, the genes which code for the variable part of the immunoglobulin G molecule.

One of the most exciting things, I think, that has emerged here is that both in the mouse models that Dr. Lambert and Dr. Bona talked about, and in the human disease which we heard about from Drs. Agnello, Carson and Sissons, there is only a very limited number of epitopes displayed on antiglobulins. The biological significance of this observation in relation to autoimmunity as a whole is obviously important, but in what way we don't know as yet. Another important point for people working in the area of cryoglobulins is that the variations are very limited on the light chain, and very diverse on the heavy chain of the molecule. We are accustomed to talking, in classifications of cryoglobulins (which I want to come back to in

---

Table II. Antiglobulins.

— are produced from immature B stem cells: hence EBV provokes, PWM does not.

— some may arise from somatic mutation in proliferating B cells; many substitutions in regions flanking VR genes

— both mice and men display a very limited number of epitopes on their cryoglobulins

— the variation is small of the K chain, with diverse heavy chains

— there is "cross reactivity" of antiglobulins for other proteins, particularly nucleoprotein

— production is temporaray in health, (but precursors persist in BM) persistent in disease

— how is this proliferation driven?
    — 1° neoplastic proliferation?
    — antigen – driven?
    — is there a difference?

---

a minute) about 'polyclonal' and 'monoclonal' cryoglobulins. It is clear that in the light of the data these terms become relatively meaningless... because, as one of the speakers pointed out, the diversity of the heavy chain will give a spurious polyclonality to the molecule; when in fact the number of epitopes expressed on the light chains may be extremely limited.

Another very exciting area mentioned in Table II – which I am sure will give us much food for thought in the 1990 cryoglobulin meeting in Milan which I hope will be organized, – is this question of so-called 'cross-reactivity' of antiglobulins for other proteins, and in particular nucleoproteins. This 'cross-reactivity' may not truly be a cross-reactivity, since it may reflect the fact that these antibodies, like some monoclonal antibodies synthesized in the laboratory, bind to very small epitopes. During the discussion on epitopes, antigenic sites as small as three serine molecules in a row was discussed as a possible epitope which might account for one or the other of the cross-reactions.*

Production of antiglobulins appears to be temporary in health, and then to be switched off. Again Dr. Carson pointed out that precursors might persist in the bone marrow indefinitely, but it is the persistent production of antiglobulins which characterizes the disease state. The key question, which we have addressed again and again, is how might this persistent proliferation be driven? Is it a primary, pseudo-neoplastic clonal proliferation, or is it antigen-driven? Now, I would just put a point which we didn't raise during the meeting in detail: is there *really* a difference between the two? How would we know that in some of these apparently 'primary' clonal proliferations, there is not indeed a virus or some other DNA driving the proliferation either at T or at B cell level. I think we haven't mentioned hepatitis at all during the last two days, but we must remind ourselves that some of our patients with so-called 'essential' mixed cryoglobulinemia appear to be suffering from hepatitis; if we did not have the test for hepatitis, this we would not detect, and they would remain in the 'essential' group. The word 'essential', as in 'essential hypertension', is a mere cover for our ignorance, and it may be that we will find more and more agents when we have more sophisticated tests. Is it ridiculous to suggest, for example, that there might be a T-cell or B-cell cytotropic virus involved in the induction of some of these phenomena in some patients with what we believe have 'essential' mixed cryoglobulinemia? What role does the environment play in the selection of a clonal proliferation in a 'primary' cryoglobulinemia, with a monoclonal antibody in the circulation?

---

* A moments through suggests that these are only 20^3 (8000) different sequences of three aminoacids at the most, whereas if the epitope is 4 or 5 aminoacids, then the number increaseas to 320,000 and 1.3 million respectively.

Coming down a little more, and coming away from the idiotypic antibodies more specifically to consider the IgM rheumatoid factors, (Table III), it seems from the work presented here that they are often directed against IgG of subclass 3; and this is very exciting. Although IgM antibodies are the predominant class in humans, in the mouse they are usually IgG, as we heard from Dr. Lambert; and are often themselves of IgG3 subclass. This morning also we heard from Dr. Renversez that the IgM antibodies in man do not pick a random selection of molecule from the repertoire of IgG molecules in the circulation with which to bind; and they have a restricted spectrotype, that is a restricted heterogeneity of their isoelectric points. The excuting point was made both by the first three speakers, and by Dr. Renversez, that rheumatoid factors may react preferentially with IgGs which are antiidiotypic for the IgM itself and, – perhaps the most exciting of all – some rheumatoid factors normally react not only with the Fc pieces (which we all know about) but they may react also with the (Fab)$_2$ region. Whether there are homologous regions of small epitopes which occur in both areas, or a true cross-reaction, is not clear yet, but obviously this could provide an extremely small but very stable immune complex, which could be under some circumstances highly pathogenic.

The whole thing of cryoprecipitates is of course that they precipitate (Table IV), and we discussed a great deal what determines that a cryoprecipitate

Table III. IgM rheumatoid factors.

— usually directed against IgG of subclass 3 (in mice, IgG RF are themselves usually IgG3)

— they have a restricted clonotype with cross-idiotypic reactions

— they have a restricted spectrotype, i.e. restricted heterogeneity of pI

— they react preferentially with anti-idiotypic IgG

— Some RF will react with both (fab)$_2$ AND FC regions of IgG

Table IV. What determined cryoprecipitability?

— in mixed cryos, dependent on the structure of the IgM

— cryoprecipitability is also salt and concentration dependent

— associated with a *rise* in binding efficiency of IgM for IgG with cooling

— may depend on crucial amino acid sequences at critical parts of the molecule? Serine substitutions paramount

— there is however no conformational change during cryoprecipitation

— gels or crystals may form
— ? role of carbohydrate moiety
— ? role of fibronectin

develops. It seems to depend, in mixed cryoglobulins, upon the IgM exclusively, and not to depend at all on the IgG antigen, which is a passive participant in the precipitation. However, other physical events, such as salt concentrations and the concentration of cryoglobulins itself, are also important. Dr. Abraham pointed out that some rheumatoid factors have an *increase* in binding efficiency to the IgG against which they react with cooling, which is the opposite from some other immunoglobulins.

Dr. Wang told us about aminoacid sequences in cryoglobulins. He particularly emphasized the role of serine in all the aminoacid substitutions he considered, and the differences in total composition of the protein may seem small. However, if such substitutions are at critical points in the molecule, they can make a very big difference to the structure, electrostatic interactions and to the hydrophobic properties of the molecule. Dr. Abraham also told us that there was no conformational changes detectable by laser Raman spectroscopy during cryoprecipitation. The molecule was not folding and unfolding, it was simply precipitating. We saw also beautiful pictures (which we saw demonstrated *in vivo* this morning from Dr. Mihatsch) of crystals of cryoprecipitate, which can form tubular structures containing a large amount of water, which are probably more visible *in vitro*; as well as the more common gel.

One of the areas which was perhaps neglected in this meeting was the possible role of the carbohydrate moiety. We seem to have forgotten that we are dealing with *glyco*proteins, and not proteins. As most of you will know, there is a considerable literature on the influence of the carbohydrate moiety of immunoglobulins on cryoprecipitability, and this we largely ignored. In the discussion, Dr. Abraham put forward one powerful argument against this being important, on the grounds that light chain Bence-Jones proteins (which are cryoprecipitable) do not have any carbohydrate moiety.

Finally, Dr. Dammaco reminded us that cryoprecipitable proteins are not just IgG/IgM, but that fibrinogen, factor VIII and fibrenectin, can all come down. He denied a role for fibrinogen, but strongly suggested that fibronectin was associated intimately with the cryoprecipitate in mixed cryoglobulinemia, although this was not accepted by all the discussants; this is an area that clearly needs further work and discussion. Incidentally, glomerular fibronectin might well have a role in terms of binding of immune-complexes or the cryoprecipitate within the glomerulus.

What about the role of rheumatoid factor cryoglobulins in disease? (Table V). Well, a lot of data was presented by Drs. Ford, Williams and Naish, and during the discussion, which suggested that antiglobulins are present and persistent in human and animal infections, both parasitic and bacterial. This, of course, may only emphasize their *physiological* role.

That they may play a role in a *pathology* is suggested by the fact that they present in greater quantities in those patients with glomerulonephritis,

Dr. Maggiore and others have shown (at least using aggregated IgG as a probe, which is perhaps open to question after some of our discussion during the last two days) that rheumatoid factors may be present within immune deposits in the kidney, both in primary and secondary glomerulonephritis, and of course in essential mixed cryoglobulinemia.

A very important concept – which I think Curtis Wilson was the first to emphasize ten years ago – is that deposited immune complexes *are not static but dynamic,* and that along with many other interactions with free antigen, free antibody and the complement system (of which we heard from Dr. Gigli this morning) immune complexes within the glomeruli, or in any other vascular bed, are capable of reacting with rheumatoid factors in the circulation in a reversible fashion; this may modulate the disease in a very powerful fashion, both for the better or for the worse, as Dr. Ford pointed out.

Next, we had to ask the question of what determines tissue damage? – but we didn't come up with many precise answers! Dr. Peters, in discussion, reminded us that the *site* of the globulin/antiglobulin reaction may be very important, in terms of its relation to where in the vascular bed it is occurring – at an intravascular or an extra-vascular site. We were reminded also by Dr. Ford that the rheumatoid factors have a particular affinity of IgG on

Table V. RF cryoglobulins and disease.

— are present and persistent in human and animal infections, both parastic and bacterial

— are present in the circulation in greater quantities in those with GN

— are infrequent in 1° GN in circulation, common in 2° GN with vasculitis

— are present within the immune deposits in the kidney in both 1° and 2° GN

— can react with complexes *in situ* and modulate disease

Table VI. What determines damage?

— site of globulin/antiglobulin reaction — IgG on surfaces

— physical properties of complex formed

— failure of RES phagocytosis

— complement activation?

— FC reactions with monocytes?

— growth versus dissolution of complexes

— C receptors in glomerulus?

surfaces, which takes me back to the point made above about the glomerular capillary wall.

The physical properties of the complex formed – which includes a vast number of variables – may also determine what damage may occur; equally, its phagocytosability, and its ability to activate complement. What the role of complement activation, discussed by Dr. Gigli, or reactions of the Fc with the monocytes which may thereby be attracted are yet unknown. We *still* do not know *how* the monocytes get there in such huge quantities, as Dr. Ferrario demonstrated. There is no disease, as he pointed out, in which there are more monocytes in the glomerulus than essential mixed cryoglobulinemia.

The *growth* versus the *dissolution* of complexes is really crucial. What makes 'deposited' immune complexes persist or dissolve in glomerular disease, and what role might rheumatoid factors play in this? Dr. Gigli reminded us this morning that complement receptors of several types are present in the glomerulus, and may play an active role in binding material to the glomerulus; and to these I would add fibronectin, as I have already mentioned. Also laminin, which has recently been shown to bind to $C1q_1$ may play a part. There is a lot to learn about chemical or immunological 'acceptors' in the glomerulus as well as receptors on cells. And finally, there is no doubt that there are mechanisms of which we know nothing at present which determine whether or not damage occurs within a vascular bed.

I am not going to say anything about classifications of cryoglobulinemia (Table VII) beyond what is in the table, except to say that *no* classification is satisfactory, and that while we have the present unsatisfactory ones, we must remember we are trying to co-ordinate different levels of description, of which I have put only three in this table. First we, as clinicians, need descriptions which help us to label patients into slots. Then immunologists want classifications which rest with the fundamental knowledge of immune dysregulation; and finally the protein chemist wants one to describe precisely, in molecular terms, the proteins he is working with. We need all these – and probably several others – but as long as we recognise that we are talking

Table VII. Classifications of cryoglobulinemia.

— No classification is satisfactory

— classification is possible

    — at the level of immune dysregulation

    — at the level of cryoglobulin chemistry

    — at the level of clinical manifestations

several different languages simultaneously, perhaps some of the difficulties in classification will dissolve a little. The main thing is that everybody says *precisely what they are talking about* when they describe patients, or proteins, in the literature and in discussion.

We then went on to the clinical features of Essential MIxed Cryoglobulinemia, (Table VIII) the discussion centering very largely on the incomparable series assembled here in Milan; which raised the immediate question of why this rather rare disease is so common in Italy, and perhaps rare elsewhere. Obviously, both genetic and environmental factors, from what we have already said, could play a part. This obviously needs a dissection in those who have big series (such as here). We learned that the Milanese groups really feel, in their large experience, that the histological changes depend fundamentally on the one hand upon *acute precipitation* of cryoglobulin within the capillary (which is a rapid event), and on the other the *slow aggregation* of immune complexes along the capillary wall rather than within the capillary lumen, which is a much slower process. These two events perhaps determine the histological varieties we see in these patients.

There was good correlation between clinical and histological presentation in their series (although both are variable, and I think this has been everyone's experience). And, again, I think it has been everyone's experience that there is no correlation between clinical events and either serum complement levels, or with the total amount of cryoprecipitable material in the circulation. Clearly, studies need to be done to determine whether one can associate *specific* clinical or histological features with more detailed examination of the cryoprotein. The disease, clinically, is of slow evolution, with a relatively benign course. When we looked at Dr. Tarantino's graph this

Table VIII. Essential mixed cryglobulinemia.

- Rare

- incidence varies country to country
    - genetic factors?
    - environmental provocation?

- histological changes depend on:
    - acute precipitation of cryoglobulin within capillary (rapid)
    - (slow) aggregation of immune complexes in capillary wall

- clinical and histological presentation variable, correlate *well* together

- in contrast, *no* correlation with C levels or cryocrit

- ? Correlation with type of cryo?

- slow evolution (> 65 y)

- hypertension, not GN determines outcome

morning, I think we should have had, above that graph, a graph of the life expectation of 65-year olds living in Milan or around it; because after 10 or 15 years, maybe 30–40 or 50% of them, perfectly well people, might be dead. This raises the whole question of how aggressive treatment should be – and I am not going to discuss treatment, since your've just heard it and it's fresh in your mind.

The very important point that hypertension (of unknown origin) determines the outcome, and the very exciting work that Claudio Ponticelli just presented using captopril, indicates that *hypertension* may be the principal clue to this disease, and that in going for the immunology we are actually looking in the wrong place under the wrong lamp; maybe we should be going for the haemodynamics.

It is getting late. We all have homes to go to. I don't think it would be right to let this session close without a profound and very sincere vote of thanks for our hosts from the three hospitals in Milan, Luigi Minetti, Claudio Ponticelli and Beppe D'Amico – and not the least Dr. Tarantino, who has done a great deal of the work (as many of you will know who have received letters from him). Many meetings are arranged merely to publicize a hospital, for the greater glory of the organizers, or just because some tourist organisation would like to have it. This has *not* been one of these meetings. It is a very timely gathering, it has brought together diverse people, a lot of interests from different areas, and I think that it has produced a genuine fusion of ideas; finally, I hope sincerely that it will actually benefit the future of patients with the diseases we have been talking about. I would like to thank our hosts on your behalf for having us here, and making it such a successful meeting. Thank you.

Index of subjects

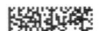